Caregiving 101: A Practical Guide to Caring for a Loved One

by Dave Leffmann PT et al.

Caregiving 101

A Practical Guide to Caring for a Loved One
Dave Leffmann PT et al.

Summertime Publications Inc.

Copyright © 2017 by Dave Leffmann
ISBN: 978-1-940333-14-4 (eBook)
ISBN: 9781940333151 POD (Paperback)
ISBN: 9781549926402 (Amazon Paperback)
Library of Congress Control Number: 2017917841

All rights reserved.
Published in the United States by Summertime Publications Inc
Phoenix, Arizona

1. Health—Popular works 2. Caregiving—Popular works 3. Nursing—Palliative Care
2. Title: Caregiving 101: A Practical Guide to Caring for a Loved One

Cover design by Derek Sparks

Neither the publisher nor the author is engaged in rendering professional advice or services to the individual reader. The ideas, procedures, and suggestions contained in this book are not intended as a substitute for consulting with your physician. As each individual situation is unique, you should use proper discretion, in consultation with a health care practitioner, before undertaking the techniques and actions described in this book. Neither the author nor the publisher shall be liable or responsible for any loss or damage allegedly arising from any information or suggestion in this book. The publisher does not have any control over and does not assume any responsibility for author or third-party websites or their content.

For Karen

This book was written as part of our feeble little attempt to pay forward the wonderful gifts of love and understanding she gave to all who helped care for her in the last year of her life.

It is our hope that wherever your journey leads, your path may be as rich as ours. We hope this work helps.

A portion of the proceeds of this work will benefit
MyLifeline.org

How to Use This Book

If you are picking up this book because you are now in a caregiving situation, you probably don't have time to read a book. You may sit down and read this whole book through, and that's not a bad idea. You can also just search for what you need to read up on right now. Each topic is short and should give you the answers you need without taking much of your scarce time. You may use the Table of Contents in the front, or the Detailed Table of Contents in the back of this book to look up just what you need. You will find good medically sound information in a real, yet succinct way.

This book was initially written to utilize the features of an ebook. In it you will find internal references and links to websites in underlined letters. The chapter subheadings and URLs or website addresses are printed in the link to help book readers find the same sites. We have created a website, https://www.caregiving101book.com/ where you can jump to and specific portions of the book, use the links, see updated sections, and view shared input and stories of other caregivers and professionals. I encourage you to share your story and give us feedback to make this a better resource here as well. You may find our videos at the YouTube channel Caregiving 101Dave Leffmann PT at https://www.youtube.com/channel/UC9EKe42gTxwWLXiHOuJuDrA

If you purchased this book on Amazon you can get the ebook version for a couple dollars. On Kindle or another e-book reader, you can use the "Go To menu" (found by touching the top of the screen) to search the content for a word or phrase. You may also jump to a section through the table of contents on the "Go To menu" or use that to jump to a more detailed table of contents in the back of the book to find just the information you need. The internal links within the book's text will jump you to those sections. On a Kindle Fire, iPad, Tablet, or other internet capable reader the external links should take you to those websites too.

That said, I do encourage you to read Part 1, Being a Caregiver and Taking Care of Yourself, first. It may save your life.

Happy caregiving.

Prologue: Facing Disease

There is no way to do this right or wrong. There is no amount of medical or psychological training for it. There is only the way you will do it.

And you will do it. In your own way.

You have only that choice.

When Karen's cancer was first diagnosed, it was not shattering. It was only a fact. The lump was small, the size of a pea. It was stage zero to one. Treatment was available and the chances were good. It was somewhat more like a broken leg.

Life changed as we headed into treatment, but it turned out not to be an overwhelming change. In fact, during her treatment, my left ACL failed again, and I was also diagnosed with a large cartilage tear behind the kneecap of my right knee. I did have a broken leg—two; I had double surgery. We could convalesce together in this time of medical centers and rental movies. We worked, we lived, we shared, we loved.

But something happened as Karen's treatment concluded. She became increasingly wrapped up in the gravity of *cancer*. She held onto the word so tightly. In the years between her initial diagnosis and the recurrence, it sat pinned on her chest like a badge of survival. She ran triathlon with the cancer survivors group. She began a website and support class for women faced with sudden menopause (she had to take estrogen-blocking drugs following her treatment). She began a project to develop a more attractive compression garment for lymphedema. The cancer did not die with the end of treatment. It clung onto her and changed her life.

Five years later, when we sat in those uncomfortable chairs and absorbed the horrible words "Your cancer has returned—there are lots of treatments, but there is no cure," something else happened. We faced her fear.

It was no longer a specter in the shadows. It was now standing in full view, over us, in every direction. It was our path.

We were suddenly faced with the full realization that life is indeed short. There is no reason to fear the inevitable. We were too busy living it already. Suddenly our priorities changed. Suddenly time became our most precious possession. There was little room for the daily quibbles that might steal from our time together. More than ever we appreciated the ordinary. More than ever we appreciated the very taste and smell of life.

This book has detailed information for lots of different caregiving situations, but it also tells about our way. This is what we did.

There is no wrong way.

You will find your way.

Contents

CAREGIVING 101:
A PRACTICAL GUIDE TO CARING FOR A LOVED ONE I
   CAREGIVING 101 II
   FOR KAREN III
   HOW TO USE THIS BOOK IV
   PROLOGUE: FACING DISEASE V
   INTRODUCTION: ADVANCED BASICS 1
   HOW DO YOU KNOW WHEN YOUR LOVED ONE NEEDS HELP 1
      What You Can Do 1
      Dignity: Practical Considerations 2
      Help Your Loved One with Their Loss 4
      A Caregiver's Loss 6
      New Ways to Do the Things They Love 7

PART I.
BEING A CAREGIVER AND
TAKING CARE OF YOURSELF 9
   CHAPTER 1.
      BUILDING A CAREGIVING TEAM
      (OR, WHAT TO DO WITH ALL THE TUPPERWARE) 11
         Heroes 14
         Training Your Caregiver Team 15
         Creating a Carebook 15
         Managing Conflicts in the Team 21
   CHAPTER 2.
      CALLING IN THE PROS 29
         Finding Good Professional Caregiver Help 29
         Managing Hired Help 32
         Making sure it "Feels Right" 34
   CHAPTER 3.
      AVOIDING BURNOUT 37
         Balancing Caregiving and Work 37
         Getting Paid for Caregiving 38
         Spending Time with Friends or Connecting with Caregiver Support Groups 38
         Planning for Respite Care 39
   CHAPTER 4.
      DANCING IN THE RAIN:
      HEALTHY HABITS FOR CAREGIVERS 43
         Embrace Stress 43
         Stay as Healthy as Can Be 46
         Keep Your Brain Healthy 53
   CHAPTER 5.
      A BRIEF ABOUT GRIEF 57
         Brief Acute Grieving (the Immediate Stuff) 57
         Grief in the Longer Term (the More Subtle and Deep) 59
         Complicated Grief 60
   INTERLUDE—Celebrating the Time You Have 63

PART 2.
LEGAL, FINANCIAL, AND INSURANCE ISSUES 65
   CHAPTER 6.
      THE NOTEBOOK OF IMPORTANT PAPERS 67
         Identity Papers 67
         Medical Information 68
         Financial Information 69
         Records of Your Wishes 69
         Shared Bank Accounts etc. 73

CHAPTER 7.
    THE IMPORTANCE OF EXERCISE 75

CHAPTER 8.
    MEDICARE, MEDICAID, AND PRIVATE INSURANCE 77
        Medicare.. 77
        Medicaid.. 85
        Private Health-Care Insurance 88
        Long-Term Care Insurance 91
        Managing the Bills 92

    INTERLUDE—Backflips... 97

PART 3.
CAREGIVING SKILLS AND ADVICE FROM THE FIELD 99

    CHAPTER 9.
        DOCTORS... 101
        Managing Medical Appointments 101
        Knowing What the Letters Behind Providers'
        Names Mean... 103
        Finding a Good Doctor.. 105

    CHAPTER 10.
        HOSPITALS AND OTHER MEDICAL FACILITIES 109
        Short-Term Medical Facilities (Hospitals) 109
        Helping Your Loved One During a Hospitalization 109
        Rehabilitation Facilities... 110
        Comfort Care, Hospice, and Home Health Care 111
        Longer-Term Medical and Residential Facilities 112
        Choosing a Long-Term or Residential Care Facility............... 116

    CHAPTER 11.
        MEDICATIONS... 123
        Making a Medications List 123
        Giving and Storing Medications 125
        Keeping a Medication Log 127
        Using Basic Charting Techniques...................................... 127
        Paying for the Pills... 129
        Disposing of Unused Medication the Right Way 130

    CHAPTER 12.
        FOOD AND NUTRITION... 131
        Factors that Affect Food Intake 132
        Techniques for Physically Helping Your Loved One Eat......... 137
        How to Use Nutrition to Keep the Gut Balanced and Moving .. 138
        Approaches for Diseases and Conditions........................... 141
        The Brief Summary 149
        Recipes for Shakes, Smoothies, and the Best Comfort Food Ever 150
        The Link Between Exercise, Hunger, Satiety, and Diet......... 152

    CHAPTER 13.
        EXERCISE 153
        Exercise Concepts (More Information Than You Want).......... 154
        Building a Basic Exercise Program 160
        Exercise Throughout the Day 164
        Special Considerations 164

    CHAPTER 14.
        SLEEP... 181
        Sleep Hygiene... 181
        Special Sleep Problems 183
        Disease- and Condition-Specific Approaches...................... 186
        Sleep Medications.. 190

    CHAPTER 15.
        BASIC MOBILITY AND TRANSFERS 195
        Fall Recovery: How to Get Back Up 195
        Fall Prevention 196
        Mobility Aids and Adaptive Equipment............................... 199

    Assistive Devices 208
    Obtaining and Paying for Mobility and
    Assistive Devices 209
    Physically Helping Your Loved One Move 211

CHAPTER 16.
HYGIENE, BATHING, AND TOILETING 221
    Bathing 221
    Oral Care 225
    Toileting 227
    Incontinence and Peri-care 229

CHAPTER 17.
PAIN MANAGEMENT 233
    Measuring Pain 234
    Pain Medications 235
    Nonpharmacological Ways to Help Control Pain 240
    A Sense of Control 240
    Exercise for Pain Relief 241
    Transdermal Electrical Neural Stimulation (TENS) 242
    Acupuncture and Acupressure 242
    Counterirritants: Ben Gay, Icy Hot, and Others 244
    Music 244
    Joy 245
    Meditation 245
    A Sense of Purpose 246
    Gentle Massage 246
    Social Contact 247
    Compassion 247

INTERLUDE—BUDDHA IN PAJAMAS 249

CHAPTER 18.
MANAGING DISCOMFORTS 251
    Anxiety 251
    Fatigue 254
    Shortness of Breath: Dyspnea 255
    Swelling and Edema 258
    Itching 261
    Muscle Spasms and Myoclonus 262
    Hiccups 267
    Dizziness and Wooziness 267
    Constipation 270
    Diarrhea 274
    Wounds or Ulcers 275
    Infections and Compromised Immune Systems 280
    Delirium: The Hard Road 286

CHAPTER 19.
DEMENTIA 293
    Diagnosing Dementia 293
    Treating and Managing Dementia in the Early Stages 296
    Managing Dementia in the Middle and Late Stages 299

CHAPTER 20.
NEAR THE END 305
    Our Vigil 307
    Time with Karen, My Lifeline Post May 29, 2013 307

EPILOGUE 311

CONTRIBUTORS 312

ACKNOWLEDGEMENTS 314

You will find your way.

Introduction: Advanced Basics

How do you know when your loved one needs help

For Karen and me, it was obvious when she needed help: Major disease came with major consequences right away. This isn't true for everyone. Often the lines are fuzzy between someone managing just fine, needing a little help, and needing full-on caregiving. You might spend a little time with your loved one if you're loving and curious. Being around a bit, especially in their home, will tell you lots. What do you notice? Here are some signs, some red flags:

Cognitive Changes

- Uncertainty or confusion with familiar tasks
- Forgetfulness, more than the usual
- Missing important appointments
- Forgetting to take medications or taking more than what's prescribed
- Letting hobbies and interests go by the wayside
- Changes in mood or major mood swings
- A diagnosis of Alzheimer's or other dementia

Mobility Problems and Increased Risk of Falling

- Difficulty walking, not walking straight, walking with feet wide apart
- Trouble getting up from a chair
- Unexplained cuts and bruises

Problems with Activities of Daily Living (ADLs)

- Dirty house, more than their normal, extreme clutter, dirty laundry piling up
- Stacks of unopened mail or an overflowing mailbox
- Late payment notices, bounced checks, calls from collectors
- Poor diet, weight loss
- Cooking "incidents": leaving the stove on, the refrigerator open, the water running
- Spoiled food that doesn't get thrown away
- Not taking baths or showers as they used to, becoming unkempt, body odor
- Smell of urine in the house
- Unexplained dents and scratches in the car

What You Can Do

So let's say you see some of the things listed above, more than one or two. What can you do? Most people don't want to admit they are having trouble. Most people don't want to give up their independence. Most likely they are older than you, they are adults. You need to treat them as such. There are a few ways you may approach this.

You might ask them what's going on. Be prepared to be specific about what signs you're seeing. Decide whether they see those signs too. Find out if they have a plan to address what they are seeing. You might plan on being a bit more generous with your time and just begin helping them with the areas they are having trouble with. This might give you more opportunities to open a discussion. Maybe you can accompany them to some doctor's visits. This also is a good venue for discussion.

Often, concerned family members talk with some of the rest of their family and friends. If you do this, don't just gossip; see who may be available to help. Through this type of discussion, you might begin to build a team (see Part 1, Being a Caregiver and Taking Care of Yourself). You might begin to consider hiring some form of in-home services or reaching for other community assistance such as Meals on Wheels.

Begin to prepare for an emergency. Reading this book is a good start. Most people have an "emergency contact person." If that's you, talk with your loved one about the "what ifs." See if they may agree to begin to assemble the notebook of important papers described in Chapter 6 and some of the pieces of the Carebook described in Chapter 1, Building a Caregiving Team, like the medication list, medical contacts, and other emergency contacts.

Mostly, be thankful that you are there to notice these signs as you try to find the balance between helping your loved one and respecting their independence and dignity.

Dignity: Practical Considerations

I didn't recognize him at first. Julia nodded over my shoulder and said, "Isn't that your old professor over there, Dr. Holmgren?" It didn't take him long to recognize me, and soon we were chatting about old times and how life is now. He and his wife (who is also a physical therapist) were retired now and planning a trip to Tanzania. The topic turned to what I was doing. I was on my way to Phoenix under the auspices of helping sort out the 45 years of things left in our family home. My stepfather, Doug, was moving into a smaller, simpler home close to his son Tim. "Hmm, that's tough." Dr. Holmgren said.

"Any advice?"

He and his wife paused, thinking a long moment. Then in the style of those couples who dance together so seamlessly or finish each other's sentences, they said in unison, "Respect. Maintain respect." Also, "They are still your elders, your parents. We cared for our parents, and we are facing the other side of being cared for now. Even though we may need so much help, with physical things, with memory, with decisions, we are still the elders." And, "You are not there to tell them what to do; you are there to help them." Once again the wisdom of my professor rings true. This time it shines on one of the most basic of human needs.

...Respect

Respect can be found in all those little places where your attitude shines through. It is the extra bit of time you give your loved one. It is paying attention to their concerns. It is supporting them to make as many of their own decisions as is reasonable. This section provides some practical tips.

...Respect Their Choices

If your loved one has advance directives, as described in Chapter 6, The Notebook of Important Papers, by all means respect those choices, even if you don't agree with them. Decisions about end-of-life care is their ultimate choice, and it deserves your respect. If they choose to live in their own home, even if it is difficult, try your best to make this possible. That is one reason you are reading this book.

Respect as many of the small choices as is practical. Let your loved one choose what to wear, what they like to eat, who they want to be with, and whether they want to be left alone at times. Sometimes the smallest of choices, such as how they like their coffee, lets them hold on to their sense of control in a time when control of anything is a struggle.

If they are having trouble with their memory or with their thinking, you can still help them by laying out simple choices for them. If their processing is slow, give them time to think and to choose. There are many ways to support someone in making decisions for themselves. http://www.supporteddecisionmaking.org/choices_brochure can help you help them make their own choices, large and small.

...Give Them Privacy Where You Can
Knock before entering a room, especially if the door is closed, and allow your loved one the time to respond to you before entering. Close the door or a curtain if possible if they are toileting, bathing, or dressing. If at all possible and safe, let them do their private business privately.

Don't discuss their personal issues or information with others without your loved one's permission. Never talk about them as if they are not there, even if you think they are confused, asleep, or not listening. Hearing is one of the last senses to diminish.

...Acknowledge Life's Realities with Dignity, Respect, and Love
How can we possibly discuss the challenge of maintaining dignity without addressing bodily functions? We were initially going to call this section Dignity and the Really Big Fart because, let's face it, bodily functions happen.

Caregiving is one of the most intimate acts of love one can do for another. In this intimate setting, things will happen. In these moments, there is no exact "procedure" to follow. You know the one you are caring for. Let your knowledge and your honest caring guide your reaction.

They may just brush it off, may be a little embarrassed, or may be mortified, and you will have your own feelings. How you both react the first couple of times can chart a course that makes this a nonissue and maintains dignity for you both. If you handle whatever the feelings and reactions are with respect and love, then whatever you both do will be the right thing and will most likely diffuse any negative feelings.

Uncomfortably trying to ignore it might not be the right thing to do if that is not the tendency of both of you. Usually gently acknowledging the obvious, making a little joke, or chuckling a tad less than a giggle might feel right in the moment. Sometimes the best reaction is just an honest acknowledgment of the facts of life. It is, in fact, entirely normal.

...Think About Their Perspective
Talk *with* your loved one, not *at* them. Let them know what you are about to do and how it will help them. Address them from eye level, facing them. Think how it feels to have someone talk to you, towering above you or facing away. Address them by their

name or in your familiar respectful way. Think how impersonal or demeaning it can feel to be called "Sweetie" by some nurse.

Take the time to listen to their concerns. Address them whenever possible. Speak to them as an adult, even if you're not sure they understand. Ask opinions, give choices, and involve them in as many decisions as possible. If their choice seems wrong or silly to you, see if they might have a good reason for their choice.

...Give Them Choices at Mealtimes

Support your loved one to make choices of what they will have to eat. Use adaptive plates and dishes if needed so they can manage more on their own. See Physically Helping Your Loved One Eat in Chapter 12, Food and Nutrition.

If they need food to be cut in small pieces, do that in the kitchen, not in front of them at the table. Allow them the time it takes to finish their meal. If you are eating with them, don't clear your plate until they are finished.

Let them do as much for themselves as they can. Though it might take less time to just do it for them or manhandle their way through a task, giving them the time to do it themselves helps protect their dignity and preserve their function.

...Exercise Your Compassion

As someone faces serious illness, pain, and the loss of control over their lives and that all this entails, they may become excessively angry or agitated over what might seem to you as a little thing. Their anger or anxiety might also be more related to a brain or metabolic issue rather than something you did or didn't do. Try not to take it personally.

Certainly avoid power struggles. You might not be able to control their behavior, but you might be able to control your response. Listening to them and addressing their concern often helps. Focusing on their behavior or their perceived need might diffuse the situation. Blaming them or yourself does not help. It takes more strength to be gentle. You can have that strength.

If you find your patience running out, remember that sometimes it might be the best thing for everyone to take yourself out of the situation for a while; see Chapter 3, Avoiding Burnout. Dealing with difficult behavior is further discussed in Anxiety in Chapter 18, Managing Discomforts, and in Chapter 19, Dementia.

Help Your Loved One with Their Loss

"I can't believe this is happening," she would say as I wrapped my arms gently around her. There was no way I could make her cancer go away. There was no way I could fix this for her. I was just as helpless as she was against it. All I could do was hold her gently.

"I can't believe this is happening," I would echo.

In this way we would hold each other up, leaning on each other for support. In this way we acknowledged that this was truly happening. Actually acknowledging what is happening is the first step in dealing with it. This may be the hardest part for both of you. Simply being *with* your loved one may be the best thing you can do.

Allow them to talk, but try not to pry or push. Sometimes a lot can be said with no words at all. Simply listening, truly listening, in this moment, facing all that is, has tremendous power.

...Anger, Sadness, and the Torrents of Emotions

Many people will talk about how it is not fair, how angry they are at it all. This is normal; see Chapter 5, A Brief About Grief. Let them be angry. Anger may spill over to anyone or anything around them. Try to keep it real, keep it tender, and just understand that this is probably not your fault. You can stand up for yourself where you need to, you are not a punching bag, but understand that sometimes they might just need to hit things.

Eventually the anger may fade into sadness. Each loss, each realization that they might not ever see this or do that again may trigger it. It may come whenever it does, and it may come in waves. It may be at 3:00 a.m. or at the grocery store. Strong emotions don't really try to be convenient. Again, be there. Listen, truly listen. This might take all the strength you have. It is OK to give in and acknowledge your own weakness and powerlessness here. Giving into it is power, and it is how you will avoid breaking. Your own softness and your own vulnerability to it all is your power to listen.

...Things that Can Help

For Karen and me, humor helped. I was careful not to crack jokes about the situation until she could, but laughing in the face of it all brought us perspective. Sometimes it is funny just how pathetic or preposterous a situation can be. It is life, after all. Humor helped us accept things as they were. Morbid jokes were usually avoided, but we didn't try to pretend that everything was normal either.

Journaling helped too; see Keep Your Brain Healthy in Chapter 4, Dancing in the Rain: Healthy Habits for Caregivers. Somehow writing helps organize the thoughts and brings resolution. We didn't try to talk about it when we didn't feel it. We just didn't want to focus on her pain or problems all the time. There was too much other life to focus on. Friends or family who wanted to come over to have Deep Moments in the brief time they were there were gently distracted into another room until they found our rhythm and our normal and could again just be themselves. Karen always had tremendous interest and empathy for others, and this didn't change as she got sick. She still wanted to know what you were up to more than talk about herself, and dragging her through the emotions of it all again was unnecessary pain.

...Sources of Support

Our loved ones do need to talk about it enough to process it all, but they might not be able to talk to you. You might be too close to them, or they might need help to face it or open up. Sometimes it's easiest and feels safest to talk to a stranger, and it's best to have someone who's well trained to help your loved one deal with it.

Social workers are often part of the health-care team and are part of most hospital and hospice staff. They are well trained to help navigate this difficult emotional terrain and can be very helpful. Chaplains and other religious leaders and counselors can help too. If your loved one is part of a church or wants to be, church leaders often have specific counseling training and their own spiritual perspective. Ask if and what kind of training they have. They might be very helpful in ways that no other professional can be.

There are support groups for most major diseases too. You might be surprised at how specific they can be. We found several just for middle-aged women facing breast cancer recurrence. Your social worker or nurse should be able to point you toward one or more. Support groups can offer the empathy of the shared experience of people who are in similar straits. They are often organized and facilitated by mental health professionals. Both the facilitator and the other participants may have insights and experience that can help you both navigate this path. See Spending Time with Friends or Connecting with Caregiver Support Groups in Chapter 3, Avoiding Burnout.

...Rumination

Talking about your loved one's situation is important, but steer clear of rumination. Rumination is what happens when that same pesky thought loop keeps rolling around in the mind. It is not processing or psychological work, as it doesn't resolve or change the emotions associated with the loop. It simply plays the same loop over and over again. This is not walking through the forest to the other side; it is walking in circles.

If your loved one is saying the same things related to their loss, often in the same way with the same expressions and word choices, often several times an hour, this is a clue that they might be ruminating. When they talk about their loss, there won't be an emotional release. There will be no resolution, no decisions, no talk of change or acceptance. You may hear only the same words with the same emotions in the same way. It just feels stuck. Again, look to the professional help of good counseling. If your loved one's ruminating continues, seek a different counselor. Rumination can be more painful and troublesome than just not talking or processing at all.

A Caregiver's Loss

Remember that you are not immune to the losses you both face. Your loved one might even be feeling it less than you are. Allow yourself the time and emotional room to grieve as well. Be gentle with yourself just as you are for them. Allow yourself to process this as well.

Read Chapter 4, Dancing in the Rain: Healthy Habits for Caregivers; you may need to double down your efforts to keep yourself healthy. Look at Chapter 5, A Brief About Grief, for more information on grief and grieving. Allow yourself to talk and process. It is good medicine to talk with friends, family, a counselor, your bartender or barber. Seek professional help if you might be ruminating—you don't want to end up a drunk with bad hair.

Seek help if you are just stuck or are experiencing physical or emotional symptoms. The counselors with your health-care team and your clergy are there to help you too. There are support groups for caregivers as well. Often they are held the same time and right next door to the ones for patients, so you might go at the same time as your loved one.

New Ways to Do the Things They Love

Any illness that brings someone to needing care threatens to take from them their independence, their mobility, and all the physical ways they would play and enjoy their life. It might take their energy, their physical strength, or their desire for many of the foods they love. They may lose their memory, but usually not their memories. The list of loss is long. It includes almost everything in some way. If you think quietly for a moment, you may envision a few of the activities or ways of life that are now slightly out of reach. See how many things that they love you might somehow make still possible or possible again. Karen and I loved to dance. Even when she could barely walk, we would hold each other close and gently sway to the music like we might have done to a slow song at the high school dance. Allow yourself the patience and creativity to find new ways to do the things they love. You might be surprised at how easy and fun this might become.

It is true that if your loved one is dying, they will lose almost everything physical that they knew and loved as a healthy person. There are some things that should never be on this list of losses. Any disease process, no matter how severe or cruel, does not need to take a person's dignity, their ability to love, or their ability to feel joy. Remember this as you reach for new ways to be in this world with them. Help them find new things to love and new ways to be. Focus on what they can do and be creative. If an idea or desire pops up, ask yourself, Why not? or How can we do this? before you just write it off as not possible. You may find that with a little creativity and accommodation, the world is still a very big and interesting place.

There is much to experience, learn, and love. The holes in your loved one's life may be at least partially filled with new joys and new ways to be. You may be surprised that, as they walk down this path, they change and grow in ways you might never expect. As things in their life fall away, there is room for new and more powerful ways to be. This journey is not all about loss. Helping them with their losses may be one of the ways you help them grow. The world is still bigger than we know.

Part I.
Being a Caregiver and Taking Care of Yourself

It's six o'clock in the evening at a high-school lecture room in Seattle, Washington. The seats are filled with mountain enthusiasts who squirm and fidget because their bodies would rather be outside in the hills than crammed into these institutional plastic chairs. We are all here enduring the chairs to learn a bit more about mountain safety and avalanche rescue. The screen behind the instructor pops up an image of a torn mountain, an obvious avalanche with its path of destruction.

"The slide has just happened!" the instructor bellows, waving his arms for extra emphasis. "You stand here above the fracture line. Your friends are now somewhere below you in the debris. What do you do?" Among the first three procedures is "The mountain is obviously unstable, get yourself to safe terrain ..."

This bit, or something like it, is almost always included in the top three priorities in most all type of rescue situations: Keep yourself safe enough, warm enough, fed and hydrated enough, and rested enough so that you, the rescuer, do not become another victim. Even in these most extreme situations, when the dangers are so stark, there is still a strong and conscious effort to keep the rescuer healthy enough to help the victim and not become yet another person needing help.

So now your wife has cancer. Life and death still hang in the balance, only now time is measured in months or years rather than minutes or hours. The terrain you will travel is demanding, unstable, stressful. It's loaded with pitfalls. Instead of hypothermia, you risk the effects of grief and depression. The threat of rockfall is replaced by sleep deprivation or malnutrition. The danger of a second avalanche taking you with it may in your situation be the very real threat of your health failing and your slide from being a caregiver to being another victim requiring care.

When my mom was diagnosed with advanced metastatic melanoma, she and her husband just wanted everything to remain "normal." They didn't want any special fuss. They didn't need any extra care. The rest of the family anxiously stood by as my stepfather took on the load of her care. They fought nobly on, going to appointments, wrestling with complex and difficult decisions, gradually absorbing all the problems as her pain and her health worsened. Trying to keep everything "normal" took its toll.

One day my mom's lone caregiver found himself on the operating table for a quadruple bypass. Chronic stress causes inflammation and constriction of the arteries, and what had been a moderate concern for him quickly became a major life-threatening problem. The family rushed in to help, but now we had two patients instead of one. To make matters worse, we also weren't able to gradually walk into this situation. Neither our parents nor we had any experience with them being patients needing our care.

Mountaineering, like most challenging sports, holds many lessons for living. One of the top three lessons in mountain rescue—to care for yourself—is just as important in your being a caregiver for a loved one. You need to be your best for the one you love in this most difficult time. You also need to take care of yourself so that you remain helpful and do not become another patient requiring care.

Part I, Being a Caregiver and Taking Care of Yourself, provides practical advice to help keep you healthy. It also will help your loved one. Many of the things that keep you healthy will also help your loved one be as healthy and comfortable as can be. I beg you, don't skip Part I, heading straight into financial and legal concerns (Part II) or patient care (Part III). Having been part of treating broken caregivers for more than 20 years, having been through it twice, back to back, myself, and having sought a lot of help in creating this guide, I strongly believe this to be the most important part of this book. That's why it's first.

Chapter 1.
Building a Caregiving Team
(or, What to Do with All the Tupperware)

When Karen got sick, it was a terrible shock to us. It was also a terrible shock to all our friends and neighbors. While we were still reeling from the diagnosis and how sick she got early on, our kitchen was piling high with chicken soup, cookies, and all manner of comforting and really delicious, wonderful treats and foods. A work acquaintance of mine, David, whose wife also was recently diagnosed, was commiserating one day: "What the hell do I do with all the Tupperware?" We had a long, cleansing laugh, as this was truly the least of our problems.

The point is that people really do want to help. A terrible, debilitating, or life-threatening illness or even the realization of your loved one's gradual decline doesn't just shock you and your loved one. It shocks your whole community. To deny these caring people the ability to help is really more selfish than noble. The same grief and horror and desire to make it better that you feel, they feel. Allowing them to help not only helps you and your loved one, it helps them process and be a part of this most difficult and profound time of life. There are so many gifts around us if you only share.

One of the most important things you can do to be a caregiver who takes care of yourself is to not face your caregiving situation alone: to build a team.

Caregiving with a team approach isn't a new idea at all. In fact, this is how tribes of people have been doing this for as long as there have been people. Somehow in our modern culture we've moved away from this approach, so the notion of inviting people in to this most intimate time of life may seem scary. In this chapter I hope to share with you just why and how building a team works.

There is a lovely book and website just on the how-to for building a team called **Share the Care** http://sharethecare.org/. They provide a step-by-step method and tools for two loving people outside the primary caregiver and patient to do this for their loved one. If you feel the notion of building a caregiving team is at all awkward or wonder who might be part of your team, I strongly encourage you to look into Share the Care.

...Friends and Family: Visitors or Caregivers?

Times of illness are stressful, and a strong, active social network helps us process and mitigate this stress. Simple companionship may be the best type of care anyone can have. As illness sets in, your loved one may not be mobile enough to be socially active in the way they are used to. Going to dinners, parties, or outside activities requires more energy and planning or may simply not be possible.

Still, it's very important during a serious illness or injury, or nearing the very end of life, that people maintain social connections to the degree they wish. If you can't go to the party, bring the party to you. Using social media and support websites (see the next section) can help you tell your friends and family when you want visitors and what they can expect.

At the same time, some friends and family members may not be able to emotionally deal with a new illness or disability and may fade away from contact. This becomes part of everyone's grieving and stress process.

Karen and I are blessed with an amazing circle of loving friends and family. Our Framily we called them. Many of them stepped forward to become part of the caregiving team that would carry us through this difficult and profound time. Some, for many reasons of their own, could not participate in this circle and stepped away. You never know how someone will react in this intense situation. How long or how deeply they'd known us, the adventures and adversities we'd shared before, or our link by blood seemed to have little bearing on how closely they could take this walk with us. We could not blame them, only accept that this is what they needed to do at that time. Still, others that were more distant in our community stepped up to help and stepped into the caregiving team.

Perhaps because of our life experiences, we were able to accept the absence of some long-term friends or close family. For many, finding out the hard way who is able to stick with you and who cannot comes as a secondary shock to the diagnosis. If you cannot help but focus on who is not there, it can really add a painful layer to the grief process. It is important to try to let the hurt and abandonment feelings in for a bit, in order to let them go. Talking with a therapist or social worker or, if you have one, your religious clergy can help you work through the absence of previously close friends or family. In the end, you need to focus your energies on the tasks at hand and the wonderful caring people who are able to be there.

Visitors like to be useful. They may enjoy simple tasks such as bringing a glass of juice, or reading a book out loud. For us some went further, doing a load of laundry, or helping with other housekeeping. Early in Karen's illness, the number of times a day I heard "Honey, can I ask you a little favor …" far exceeded the number of times I heard each of my three sisters play "Heart and Soul" as they learned to play the piano in succession. Company in the house of a seriously ill person can help with some of those favors. Wipe away the notion that visitors need to be entertained by you and, instead, leave them to sit, talk, listen to music, or watch TV with your loved one. They know things are hard, and they are there to bring comfort and help make things better. That's why they bring the cookies.

Some of the people who come to be companions may allow you enough confidence to take some "respite" time away from caregiving. Schedule the time and take the time. Respite from day-to-day caregiving is very important to help you run this marathon. It will help you pace yourself to avoid caregiver burnout, compromising your health and the care you can give. Please read Chapter 4, Dancing in the Rain: Healthy Habits for Caregivers for good concrete ways to mitigate stress and keep you and your loved one as healthy as can be.

…Support Websites

Have you ever had a cast on your arm or foot and everyone asks "how'dyadoit?" You might have worn the cast for four to six weeks and over the course of those hundreds of "how'dyadoits," your story morphs out of sheer boredom of repetition: "I fell from a helicopter battling a fire-breathing dragon over the Amazon basin of Africa …" People really do want to know, even if you get sick of telling them. With something like cancer, telling the story over and over also brings on all the emotions of the diagnosis again. This is exhausting and troublesome and, let's face it, you don't have the energy. When Karen got sick the first time, we looked for a better way to tell people and discovered cancer care websites.

Cancer may have more support websites than any other disease, but there are specific sites for most diseases and conditions. Most have been put together by caring people who are giving back after their bout with illness. You may find them by typing the illness your loved one is dealing with into your search engine. I found that adding the words "support website" to the search helps narrow it down a bit.

Websites have many features, including a blog-like function that can easily keep your family and friends informed without having to repeat your story again and again. Your people can share comments, pictures, and their own stories on many of the sites as well. This helps them process. This helps them stay in touch. This also helps you with all the love they pour into their contributions into the blog forum.

Websites also have many tools to help organize people, such as a care calendar function. This feature helps your friends and family know what they can do and when they can help you. The care calendar that we used allowed us to call for help for specific events, such as support for important doctor visits. When the information and the decisions are hard, it's important for many people to have another core person there to help take notes and remember all that was said, and they also lend emotional support by their presence. At one point we were so sick of the bad news in those uncomfortable chairs in the doctor's office that Karen invited a small army of our friends to come for good luck. Sure enough, all the news was good that day and the cheering could be heard down the hall.

Some calendars allow you to create nonspecific or repeating events. Karen created one called "Sparkle Day" in which she asked for help cleaning the house. The care calendar is most effective when care is needed around the clock. With this tool, your caregiving team can organize into shifts and give you and themselves enough time off to remain healthy and helpful.

The site we chose also has a page for specific helpful instructions and information a caregiver needs when care requires more skills. You can relay detailed instructions about your loved one's specific needs. There are places for contacts and a place for what to do in case of an emergency. Sites have other functions such as fundraising vehicles, newsletters, and caregiver mentorship.

Our friend Mary Lou stepped in early on and helped set up our support website. This took a load off Karen and me so we could focus on everything else. Early on, you may want to tap the resources of a technologically savvy relative or friend to help put your site together. While these sites are generally designed to be user-friendly, you may have a bit on your mind. Below are some commonly used general care-calendar sites:

- **Lotsa Helping Hands** http://lotsahelpinghands.com/ was the site we used on our first go-round with cancer. They provide a calendar and blog function that is fairly easy to use. Last time I looked, it did not notify your circle when you made a post, so you might need to create a separate contact list so you may notify your group when you make a post.
- **Caringbridge** http://www.caringbridge.org provides a calendar and blog function for any health journey. Updates can be posted, and members can choose to be notified by e-mail when new posts or events are added.
- **Care Calendar.org** http://www.carecalendar.org/ provides a calendar and blog function that is easy to set up and is password secure. It focuses on meals but can be used for anything you put into the calendar, including links to videos and other information. For this site, you also need to notify your group when you make a post.

- **My Lifeline.org** https://www.mylifeline.org/ was the site we settled on for our second go-round with cancer. We liked the way it notified our "guest list" of when we posted or created an "event." We also found the people there to be, well, truly caring.

Heroes

When word rolled around that Karen was sick, we found great support in heroes all around us. Maureen, a neighbor I had never met, is our friend Mary's friend and a retiring nurse. Maureen gave her time and expertise to help us and became one of our emergency contacts for our caregiving teams. Oh, there were more heroes—Mary herself, for one—people who stepped up way above and beyond anything we might have expected. They did so because it was needed.

You may find that if you lift the veil of privacy from your suffering just a little that the heroes will emerge. Don't be afraid to talk with your loved one's neighbors, the leaders in their church or synagogue, the people in their clubs or social organizations. When you're creating the "my community" list on your care website or opening up your story on social media, be more generous rather than stingy while inviting people in or accepting support. When people do offer to help, consider saying yes. People don't set out to be courageous or noble; they simply are, because they know it's important.

The *Oxford Dictionary* defines "hero" as a person who is admired for their courage, outstanding achievements, or noble qualities. I might define it as someone who sees something important that needs to be done and, without selfish considerations of difficulty or danger, simply goes about the business of doing it.

You may be surprised by the number and depth of heroes in your community. They are among your neighbors, your friend's friends, your distant family, your congregation—or they may just volunteer their help through community volunteer organizations (see the next section). They may very well lend that crucial hand in your hours of greatest need. They do it for many reasons, but mostly because it needs to be done. Your job is simply to open your heart and your home and welcome the blessings of your own heroes.

...Volunteer Organizations

Among the heroes you might find are nonprofit organizations whose local volunteers can offer help.

Meals on Wheels http://www.mowaa.org/ is a national organization with local chapters.

Senior centers and hospice organizations exist in most communities. A simple web search should help you find the ones in your community.

You may find more organizations in your area full of loving people who give and help. Chances are the good people in your state Medicaid office and your local **Area Agency on Aging** http://www.n4a.org/ will know of these and may be able to refer you in the right direction. It is worth browsing their website or calling.

If you have a **social worker** through the hospital or through Medicaid, they can also be a terrific resource for local organizations.

Training Your Caregiver Team

Your friends, family, and good people in your community want to help, but they don't always know how. Effectively harnessing their truly amazing outpouring of love and energy into effective care helps them feel effective and useful ... because with training they *are* effective and useful. I have been truly amazed by the outpouring of generosity and love from our friends and our family. It is one of the great unexpected gifts of this whole adventure. You need only to open your heart ... and do a whole lot more. The main things you need to do are:

1. Ask for help.
2. Let people know how and when they can help you.
3. Keep people informed of your loved one's situation and the specifics needed for their care.
4. Foster communication amongst the team of caregivers.
5. Develop a cohesive well-informed team.

This section provides some tools to help you train your caregiving team.

Creating a Carebook

Set up a notebook to be kept in an obvious place in the house such as the kitchen counter. It serves as a central place for "hard-copy" information for all the caregivers. It should be clearly organized so it's easy to find all the pertinent information caregivers need to help take basic care of your loved one. It should also contain all information needed in case of an emergency. There are many ways a carebook can be organized. I like the following:

Face sheet: This contains your loved one's name, date of birth, address, phone number and other contact information, diagnosis and precautions, and allergies. It also contains contact information for primary caregivers, doctors, and emergency providers and contacts.

Overview of care issues: This is an informal note to the caregivers letting them know the current situation and any specifics regarding care. It should be updated as issues change.

Legal documents: Such things as advance directives, do not resuscitate (DNR) orders, or physician's order for life-sustaining treatment (POLST) can be kept in the carebook or in plain sight, such as taped to the outside of a kitchen cabinet door, so an emergency responder can easily see it. Medical power of attorney and release of medical information, and copies of insurance cards and photo ID, may also be kept in the carebook for easy access in case of an unexpected hospital admission. For more on these documents, see Chapter 6, The Notebook of Important Papers.

Contact list: This may be a more extensive list than that included on the face sheet. It may include all the people on the caregiving team. The backup for each person on the team may be identified here.

Current medications list or "med list": This is especially important if a doctor or emergency medical personnel needs to be called: They will need to know what and how much medication the patient is taking. To help lay caregivers identify medications, create a sheet for each pill, its name, its purpose, and how frequently it should be given. You may include other information here, such as how the medication works, how the body processes it (for instance, eliminated by the kidney in whole form, or broken down by the liver), and possible side effects to watch out for. All this information is available from the pharmacist, the medicine data sheet you get with the medicine from the pharmacist, or online http://www.drugs.com/. We simply kept the data sheet from the pharmacist, highlighting the important bits. We were also careful to cull out those sheets that Karen was no longer using to keep it simple and readable.

Medication log: Anytime medications are being given or tracked by anyone but the patient themselves they should keep a daily chart of meds administered. This should include the amount and time of day and should be initialed by the person administering the med. When you are trying to establish the proper dosages, it is very helpful to note your loved one's reaction or condition at the time. A narrative form works well here; this may look like "3:30 p.m. Ativan, 0.5 mg. Resting heart rate 105; agitated." When dosages are established, the med log may look more like a checklist. Please see Keeping a Medications Log and Using Basic Charting Techniques in Chapter 11, Medications. The med log doesn't need to be beautiful. Remember, it may change frequently, and you've got other things to do.

Other Daily Logs: In more advanced cases or when the patient's mental function is impaired, it is especially important to have a running log of issues from day to day. This information helps with the handoff between caregivers and allows caregivers and medical personnel to look back at events and the patient's condition over time.

If you are trying to sort out different issues, you can use separate tabs for each. You can add a section for anything that is an ongoing or changing issue that you are trying to gain some balance in managing. Do try to keep it simple. If you get much beyond three daily log tabs, it becomes difficult and time consuming to check on or make notes on it all, so things begin to be missed. As an issue stabilizes you can make a final note entry discontinuing that section, but leave the breakout tab and what was written in the book. For more on what to write and how to keep notes that make sense, see Keeping a Medication Log and Using Basic Charting Techniques in Chapter 11, Medications.

Other things: A chemotherapy or treatment log can be kept in the notebook to help everyone know what treatment the patient is getting and when. You can also keep sections on non-medical concerns. Our carebook included a chore list such as watering the plants.

...Training Your Family and Friends in Basic Nursing Skills

Your loved one's condition may require some basic nursing skills. They may be unsteady on their feet or need assistance with getting around. They may need someone to manage their medications or help with positioning to be comfortable or to keep off pressure points so they do not develop sores. The caregiving team may need to watch your loved one's diet closely or monitor their bowel and bladder output for signs of infection or constipation. Your loved one may even need help with changing dressings or managing an IV. Perhaps you've learned these skills from your health-care team, or just by being with your loved one. If you've been doing it a while these things are simple to you but they might be scary for people who are not familiar with them. These tasks are somewhat easy to do incorrectly, but also pretty easy to do right. In other words, you can learn these things, and so can most people who care to.

This section offers one way of training your caregiving team so they can provide these basic nursing skills. In this section we walk you through a training session. If you are comfortable teaching the skills needed, great. If not, consider getting help from your loved one's health-care team. Home Health Care for nursing, physical therapy and occupational therapy can all provide training.

Set Up Teams and Host a Training Session

As Karen's condition worsened, we put out a call for a core team of caregivers. Within a week, more than 20 of our friends volunteered to be there at least once a week. We set up a care calendar so that they worked in pairs. I talked with each person individually, then we held a training session.

The goal of our training session was that everyone involved would be both competent and comfortable in providing care. We wanted them to feel and actually be well supported. We also wanted them to know how much they were appreciated.

There are many ways to do a training. Here is what we did—you may find some value in our format to help you build your own training session:

Gather the Group

We set up our living room comfortably for a large group. We kept everything there as if Karen was there too, though on this night she was tired and not in the mood for a large group. We set out wine and snacks and such, in the same atmosphere as a quiet party. These were our friends, after all. We allowed time for hugs and chatting before tapping on the wine glass to begin.

Introduce the Session

Thank you: We let people know how much we appreciated them and how amazing they were to give of themselves this way.

Confidence: We let them know that the skills they would be learning were to be a very small part of what they were to do. Mostly they would provide love and quality of life.

Communication: We gave them permission to talk with us and with each other about the illness, their concerns, their emotions, and their joys. We encouraged open communication with each other, acknowledging our emotions. We talked about how real and very powerful they can be.

Goals: We set the tone and goals for the group of helping our loved one live deeply, comfortably, and well through the course of this illness.

We set the goals of that training night: to have each of us feel and be competent in communicating with each other in the basic skills we may need, in skills hopefully beyond what we will need (just-in-case skills), and in the knowledge of who and when to call for backup.

Talk About the Nitty-Gritty

We introduced the Carebook, where it was kept, and how to use it. We familiarized the group with each part of the Carebook.

We gave special attention on the topic of whom to call if they needed or wanted help, including when to call 9-1-1.

We discussed the POLST and advance directives (see Chapter 6, The Notebook of Important Papers) and showed them to everyone.

We reviewed the med list, along with where the medicines were kept. We passed the meds around and had people get familiar with them. We introduced the pill caddy and how it was used. We introduced the med checklist and we practiced using it.

Do Some Hands-On Training

The hands-on training was fun and got everyone laughing. The skills were easy for me to teach because I am trained in it as a physical therapist. We also had a nurse there to help with the training.

First we showed positioning. We showed everyone how to accommodate Karen's spine, how to use pillows, and how to help her spend less time on her tailbone and heels.

Next was mobility lab, and we introduced Karen's brace, how and when it should be worn, and how to use it as a gait belt (see Chapter 15, Basic Mobility and Transfers).We trained participants in mobility assistance, beginning with maximum assist transfers, moderate assistance, minimal assistance, and standby assistance. We taught the group how to use a walker and a wheelchair. People paired up and practiced with each other, switching partners frequently.

Then we applied the mobility training to techniques for getting Karen from the bed to the bathroom and using the toilet.

In addition to this training session, I produced some simple videos and provided the group with links to them on our support website. You may use these yourself:

Karen's Brace:
https://www.youtube.com/watch?v=1Fv2RIRVHIQ

Karen's Command Center; Positioning and bed mobility:
https://www.youtube.com/watch?v=pl3EB4TWwLw&t=7s

Karen's Wheelchair:
https://www.youtube.com/watch?v=Q6vpPg98gp8

Karen's Carebook:
https://www.youtube.com/watch?v=uP4WY3F3oRs

Karen's Framily:
https://www.youtube.com/watch?v=L8EfoaOqMYg

Helping Karen Out of Bed:
https://www.youtube.com/watch?v=v1tc1nZf01A

There are also countless other videos with caregiving instruction. Here are some examples:

Walker Use:
http://www.youtube.com/watch?v=uiBHdHZ7w6g

Cane Use:
https://www.youtube.com/watch?v=pTJVaoYTnXw

Stand-Pivot Transfer:
http://www.youtube.com/watch?v=bdgG3mbtvpQ

Quad Cane Use:
http://www.youtube.com/watch?v=VsKJ8-d5Rg8

Bath Bench:
http://www.youtube.com/watch?v=-J9d_8iGYWI

Bathing:
http://www.youtube.com/watch?v=6r5YkjKE7Ao

Alzheimers and Stroke:
http://videocaregiving.org/beyond-video/default.php

It is so easy to post video on YouTube that you may very well want to do your own. It's fun and it allows you to be specific for your needs. See the Producing and Publishing Training Videos section below. MyLifeline.org also allowed us to link the videos on our page in their website. We used the site to notify our team when we had posted anything new as well.

Set Parameters for Calling on Skilled Help

Caregiving is a very intimate act of love. Each caregiver should be comfortable with their role. For some on our caregiving team, it was important for them to know just exactly what they might be expected to know or do. I made sure to give permission for people to speak up and to step back if they felt uncomfortable. I also set parameters for when we would call in certified nursing assistants (CNAs) to take over some of the nursing tasks. For us, this included if wound care was needed, if incontinence, anxiety, or profound loss of cognition occurred, or if Karen required total assist (more than 50 percent help) with transfers getting from bed to chair, etc. Not everyone wanted to talk about these things, but for those who did, I made sure to talk with them.

In the end, we had a wonderful, cohesive team who shared in the caregiving process with Karen. They provided something that few CNAs can: They provided love. That was worth it, for everyone.

I leave you with this quote from Josh, a business executive and part of our caregiving team: "Allowing us to be with her, to share in the precious little time she had, was a gift. It was a gift to everyone who loved her. I was so happy to be able to be with her. There were many people who wanted to be there to share this limited time in her life."

...Producing and Publishing Training Videos

To produce and publish your own custom training videos on YouTube, you will need a smartphone with video capability, a gmail+ account, and the YouTube application. To create a google+ account, simply type "gmail" into your browser and click on "gmail." If you don't have an account already, it will lead you there. Follow the prompts and write down your passwords. If you don't have a YouTube app already, it is free on the internet. For Apple products, you can download it through the App Store or iTunes. You will need your Apple ID for that. For Android and Windows phones, you may download it directly.

The script: Consider what you want to say. Keep each segment short—one to three minutes is a good length. You don't need to rush or pack everything in, as you can do more than one video. Some people like to write out their script. Personally I find it more natural to just know what needs to be said. Talk it through with your cameraperson and other "actors." You may even want to give it a dry run first.

The scene: Have any props handy such as a gait belt or wheelchair. Consider the lighting and background noise. Most modern digital cameras can handle low light well, but the light should be from the front to show your face. The new microphones are pretty good, but you might want to cut the background noise by tuning off loud fans or air conditioners.

The shoot: When you're ready—one, two, three, action, and away you go. Talk to the cameraperson as if they are one of your friends (they probably are). Don't worry about being perfect. It's just for your friends and family, and in this digital age you can always do it again.

Share: After you've reviewed the video, tap the screen and find the "share" button; on Apple it looks like a box with an arrow coming out of it, and on Android it is a small circle with two arrows. If you have the YouTube app, YouTube will be one of your options for sharing the video. You might also have the option to e-mail or message the clip. Video files are usually large, so depending on your setup, these options might not work well.

The title: Give it a title that makes sense; a brief description is optional, as is category. It's usually best with a simple video like this to publish it in standard definition; again, large data files can be more cumbersome.

Viewing options: From here you have the option of making it (1) public—anyone can view it and it will show up on a search; (2) unlisted—anyone with the link can view it; or (3) private—you need to be part of an account to view it. For our purposes, unlisted worked well.

Publish: Now you're ready to hit "publish." After your clip loads and plays, you have the option to share the link. E-mail yourself on this list so you have a record of it too. We used our cancer care website, MyLifeline.com, to post the link on their Learning Links page. We could then easily notify our caregiving team through posting on the site to view the video.

Other options: If you don't like YouTube, there are other sharing platforms, each with a slightly different batch of fairly easy instructions. **Dropbox** is more private, and you might have better control of who gets to view it, but each viewer needs to set up an account. **Vimeo** works much like YouTube but with much less traffic, ads, and clutter. Again, you need an account.

Most likely, if you are a primary caregiver, you may not think you have time for all this. Fortunately, creating training videos is one terrific way people can help support you from their own home on their own time schedule. Luckily, two of our good friends graciously handled most of the training-video production and publishing details. It was usually fun and easy.

Managing Conflicts in the Team

The best way to manage conflicts is to not have any to begin with. Of course, this is impossible in any high-stress situation that goes on for any length of time. This section looks to the work of psychology and businesses' human resources techniques for some tips for communication and conflict resolution:

...Who Is in Charge?

In mountain rescue, we often appoint a leader to coordinate the team and delegate responsibilities. Alternatively, many of the climbing parties I've been on were led by consensus. We know each other well and can make decisions together and switch leads easily. With either style, we rely on our common purpose to pull us together and clear, respectful communication to keep us moving in the same direction while diffusing tensions as they arise.

The advantage of having a leader is that the team has one person to turn to. That one person can be in a good position to see the whole picture, delegate tasks and responsibilities, and ensure that these are carried out. They often take the center position when difficult decisions need to be made.

If there is to be one leader of a caregiving team, that role often falls to the person who is closest to the patient and who is most likely performing the bulk of the caregiving duties. That said, leadership should never be self-proclaimed. It should occur naturally and by consensus of the group. It doesn't need to remain static, either. Leadership can change as the situation changes, by who is present the most or by who is best at something. In caring for my parents, my siblings and I mostly lived far away and came to help in shifts; leadership fell to those who were there at the time. In caring for Karen, it was obvious: I was closest. Still, it was not me who did all the heavy lifting or made all the decisions. I tend to favor group consensus, and everyone played an integral and irreplaceable role, especially Karen.

To be a good leader, try to understand the strengths and weaknesses of each team member, including yourself. Treat each member with respect. Remember, you are only leading because they let you. Without them, you are alone. Respect their ideas and observations. They have eyes, hands, and brains. This is tremendously valuable. Chances are, you are no smarter than anyone else on the team, but together you are brilliant. Respect their emotions and their needs. This caregiving role is hard for your team members too. Watch for signs of fatigue or stress overload. Help them stay healthy.

...Team Member Roles

If you are not the caregiving team's leader, it is your job to speak up if you see a problem or a better way. It is also your job to keep yourself healthy and to ask for help if you need to. Let the leaders on your team know what you can and cannot do. Help everyone look after all the members of the team, especially the leader. Lastly, try not to lead from the back.

I once had a ski mountaineering buddy who, if he didn't like the path the person in the front was making, would fall off the back of the line and go another way. Though he was a fairly competent mountaineer, the team wasted a lot of time looking for him or waiting for him, and it scrambled the direction of travel for everybody. Often we had to scuttle the trip because of him. Being reliable and consistent is important. In the home caregiving situation, nobody has extra time or energy for keeping track of fellow caregivers who just decide to change course.

Caregiving can be addictive, and it is difficult to step away from the person you are caring for. For many people, it is very difficult to read Take Breaks in Chapter 4, Dancing in the Rain: Healthy Habits for Caregivers, which describes the idea of taking breaks from caregiving. Read that section anyway. Consider taking a break and stepping away for a little while. It is probably just as difficult for your brother, sister, or son to consider this. Be gentle in suggesting that a caregiver take a break. Approach the subject tenderly. Let them know that your loved one will be well cared for, and that you know that stepping away is sometimes difficult. Let them know that it is important that they do take some time so they remain healthy and at their best for the ones they love. You may give them this book and let me, the author, take the heat while they take a walk.

If your team is one utilizing group consensus, all the same rules apply as for a group with a single leader. The difference is that in consensus, the whole group works out decisions together, making sure that all is OK with everyone else. Delegation comes in the form of "I can do that" or "Will you do that?" Leadership flows seamlessly from member to member as new roles and challenges arise. Someone is always in the lead, but that changes as the group navigates the changing terrain. The experience can be much more fulfilling this way, but sometimes it is more difficult not to become a herd of cats. Clear, respectful communication is even more important in group consensus.

...Clear and Respectful Communication

Most of the time if you hold the idea of being clear and respectful in your mind, the words you choose and the way you deliver them will convey that sentiment.

Address issues sooner rather than later. Don't let the issue fester. It might even help to have a regular time to talk things out, such as Monday evening after dinner.

Choose a neutral time and place to broach a subject. We liked to talk things out on a quiet walk or in a corner room. The heat of the moment, in front of your relatives or the one you're caring for, or at the grocery store where either of you might be worried about what the neighbors will think, only adds to the tension. Things are tense enough. You both want minimal tension in an environment where you are equals and can share openly.

Consider what you want to say and what you might need to understand from the person. Write down clear examples, and use magazine or online articles to support your point, which can make it less personal. It doesn't usually help to rehearse your speech, as this drags you through it emotionally more than you need, making your brain live through the conflict without resolving anything. It can add to the emotional charge and hurt you more for nothing. Instead, simply visualize the subject clearly, and visualize a quiet, respectful conversation. Think of listening more than speaking.

Consider your role in the conflict. What are your "hot" buttons? What might be your contribution to the problems? Be ready to listen, accept, apologize, and change. When you own your part, it helps the other person own theirs. This will also help you be less defensive and a better listener. Remember, you are seeking solutions and resolutions, not victory, revenge, or beating someone down for their transgressions.

Speak directly to an issue and remain in the present. Don't bring one issue up as a condemnation of the whole person forever. Avoid phrases like "You always …" and "You never …" Avoid past issues. Speak only to this issue, this time, now.

Speak in "I" statements. Avoid damning judgments such as "That is just like you to …" Choose instead the "I" statement. Remember, the problem you are having is yours. If you are frustrated by something, say it like this: "I get frustrated when …" If you're feeling mixed signals, you might try something like "I get confused when …" or "I don't know what to do when …"

Take clear turns talking and listening. If you are talking, try to remain clear and calm. Give them time to acknowledge and paraphrase what you've said. If they try to jump over your time to speak or they step on your words, gently bring them back and remind them to hear you out, then you will listen fully as they speak. Try to gain that trust to communicate.

Be aware of your nonverbal messages. Consider your voice, the tension in your shoulders, your posture, your hands. Are you aggressive, solid and immovable, defensive, defeated, or relaxed and open? Reminding yourself that you love this person, that you are in this together, that they have feelings and needs and opinions too, might help you remain open and relaxed. See this short piece on nonverbal communication http://video.about.com/psychology/8-Types-of-Nonverbal-Communication.htm.

When it's your time to listen, listen. Avoid talking over their words. Avoid defending yourself or spending your emotional attention on crafting your response. Simply try to understand what they are trying to say to you. If there is any question, try paraphrasing it back to them, like this: "What I'm hearing is this … is this right?" For more on listening skills, try http://www.skillsyouneed.com/ips/listening-skills.html.

Respond to criticisms with empathy. Feel the emotions in the speaker. Consider if there might be any truth in their statements before you reach for defense. This is very hard, but you are strong, and you know yourself. To do this will only make you stronger as you open up your soft side in the hardest of times.

Go through listening and talking as many times as you need to understand each other. Try to have an equal word count: you both get to say about the same amount.

When you understand each other, solutions may become apparent. Reach for them. Write them down. This is now brainstorming. Don't throw any solutions out yet. When you have several proposed solutions, review them and together choose what is best, then consider who will do what and when to make the solution real.

Don't be afraid to take some time out. Let things calm down if, during this whole process, tensions begin to rise too high. This clouds reason and makes any clear productive outcome pretty unlikely. Karen and I were very good at this. "Honey, hold that thought, I have to take a walk. We'll talk about this … a little later today." Make sure you do get to talk about it later. Again, don't let it fester.

...Common Purpose

Consider your common purpose. This is the glue that holds you all together. You may want to write it down. For a business, this is called a mission statement. For caregiving, it might be something more like "We gather together our friends, family, and skilled professionals to help our mother live as fully and meaningfully as possible while providing as much comfort and the best, most humane medical care."

Now consider a different statement and how the thoughts in it are different from the previous one: "We gather together our family to help our mother survive as long as possible and help keep her comfortable in her battle with cancer." Consider each element in each statement and how some elements might conflict. Consider each element within each statement and how it might conflict with the other elements in the same statement.

...Concerns that Generate Caregiver Conflicts

Areas that usually generate the most conflicts among caregivers are these:

- comfort vs. fullness of life
- quality of life vs. quantity of life—in other words, how medically aggressive to be
- how much each person can and should contribute to care
- how to do the best job—the particulars of giving good care
- financial needs and division of resources

For all of these concerns, the patient should take the lead and the caregivers should take their cues from the patient. If this is not possible, try to discuss and get a feel for consensus before the concern becomes a terrible issue.

For Karen, these concerns were fairly easy. She could communicate clearly until near the very end. How she led her life let us all know how she felt on the first two issues. On the third and fourth issue, we all gave what we could. On the fourth issue, we all did the best we could. We learned as much as we could and trained each other. Our love kept our words soft, and our common purpose of supporting Karen kept us together. In this and many ways, we are lucky. For many, it is not so clear.

Comfort vs. Fullness of Life

Everyone has his or her own wishes regarding comfort versus fullness of life. Some prefer to have pain gone at any cost; they prefer to be knocked out rather than endure pain. For others, pain is only a moderate issue; they prefer to be as alert as can be with an acceptable amount of pain. If you don't know how your loved one feels about this trade-off, ask. It's best to do this when they can still communicate clearly. If they are unable to communicate their wishes regarding this concern, consider their history and how they have lived their life. If they preferred to be sober, minimized the use of pain medications in past illnesses or injuries, and chose local over general anesthesia for minor surgeries, you may consider they will fall on the less-medicine side of the issue. If, on the other hand, they preferred to avoid discomfort, reached for medicines readily, and were the one to say "Just knock me out, Doc," they probably would rather have medicine and the fogginess it brings than the pain it blocks. Try to avoid placing your own preferences onto the person.

There are several tools to measure the subjective response to pain. Please read Chapter 17, Pain Management, on measuring pain and the complex nature of pain. For Karen, we used a simple number system that goes like this: "How much pain are you having now? 10 is screaming agony, like cutting your legs off slowly; 5 is so bad it makes you stop what you're doing; at 1, you feel it; 0 is no pain right now." For Karen, 4 or above was too much. If we couldn't bring the pain down well with positioning, massage, distraction, or other things, we wouldn't hesitate to use medicine. Everyone on the team knew the number.

This issue encompasses activity as well. The same ideas of comfort versus richness of life can be brought to the person's willingness to travel, go on outings, or even take in visitors. Karen could communicate with us easily if she thought she would like to do something. We did not hold her back, but we did not push her out the door either. We all knew, including Karen, that there might be a price to pay later for her being active. But for her, the price of not being active was far greater.

If you think your loved one would like outings, ask rather than suggest. Be ready to take no for an answer. If you suspect depression, you may consider being a bit more encouraging, but otherwise, no means no. If they cannot tell you directly, watch for signs of discomfort or avoidance. They may have more difficulty than usual in transferring, dressing, or collecting their things. Facial expressions will tell you a lot. If you do get to go out, chances are the experience will be wonderful for everyone.

Quality of Life vs. Quantity of Life

The issue of quality of life versus quantity of life is one of the most emotionally loaded and difficult that any family must face. Remember the Terri Schiavo case in 2005 when it literally became an act of congress? To help sort out this issue in the more immediate sense, we have documents for the patient to ensure their wishes are carried out. Please see Chapter 6, The Notebook of Important Papers, on advance directives, living wills, DNRs, and POLSTs. These documents should be completed as soon as possible, and it is generally a good idea to create them for yourself now, while you're still healthy.

If your loved one has not completed these documents yet, do so now. They will most likely be available at your doctor's' office, at the hospital, or from your social worker. As soon as you can, have your loved one discuss, in as much detail as they can face, what they might want for care and when they might consider withdrawing treatment to favor instead comfort care measures. This is not necessarily giving up. Studies have found that in some cases patients who chose palliative care (care focused on quality of life and relief or management of symptoms) over aggressive treatment not only were more comfortable and higher functioning, but also lived longer. Here is the groundbreaking study http://www.nejm.org/doi/full/10.1056/NEJMoa1000678.

Again, as caregivers, we need to follow the patient's lead. If they cannot tell you directly, try to meet with the family and members of the caregiving team to discuss what your loved one might want. Try to keep your own preferences and beliefs out of this discussion, especially your religious beliefs, as these are the most absolute and might not be that of your loved one. Remember, you are here for them, not the other way around. Remember too that emotions on this issue are intense for everybody. Be as generous with your heart as you can be.

How Much Care Each Person Should Give

A care calendar can help provide a solid graphic presentation of how much time each person on the caregiving team is contributing. Seeing one name all over the dates makes it quite clear who may be contributing too much for their own good, as well as who is not contributing much at all. The calendar function on the support websites mentioned earlier in this chapter will work nicely here. Everyone sees the same calendar.

Not everybody can contribute. Quite a few of our friends and family seemed to fade away with Karen's illness. The reasons for this are as many as there are people, but they are reasons nonetheless. Some people sometimes just cannot be there. It may be important to ask, without blame, without judgment, without expectations, just what a family member or friend can do and what they cannot. The team needs to know so they can act. If someone cannot step into the caregiver shoes, there is no way to force them. You don't want to do that anyway, as a reluctant caregiver is bad for everyone. Simply let them go and be grateful for all who do help.

How to Do the Best Job

Agreeing on how to give the best care is a common problem among medical professionals, so you might imagine how much more difficult it can be for people without all the schooling. Here is where all the skills of communication discussed under Clear and Respectful Communication above will help you. Remember your common purpose. Let best care be your ultimate decision point. Avoid power struggles. Check your ego before the discussion starts and be prepared to be open to the observations, research, and experience of the others on your caregiving team. If the team has a leader, ultimately it's the leader's final say. If it's by consensus and the group isn't with you on this one, you might just need to give in to the group think.

...Check Yourself If You Feel Conflict Arising

OK, so you've read the fluffy team-building stuff and still you find yourself thinking, "That Uncle Bob is a real jerk. Damn if he doesn't always do that. He's gonna make life miserable for everybody." Caregiving for a loved one is a high-stress, emotional situation. Most likely you'll have times when you feel this way about one or more members of the caregiving team. Before any confrontations, give yourself a good self-check.

Have you had enough rest? good food? water? Does your body show signs of excessive stress?

- Is your resting heart rate higher than normal?
- Are your hands cold?
- Are your muscles tight or achy?
- Is your digestion not working well?
- Are you forgetful?
- Are you clumsy?
- Do you feel outbreaks of intense or seemingly inappropriate emotions?
- Are you mad at or negative toward more than just one person?

If the answer to more than two of any of these questions is yes, the problem you're having may very well be yours. These are all signs of excessive, unmitigated stress on the body. If you are feeling these, chances are, it is affecting your emotional judgments as well. Don't let the problem come to a head and then blow up. Put your anger down for a second. Consider instead if you can **give yourself a break from**

caregiving. See Chapter 4, Dancing in the Rain: Healthy Habits for Caregivers. Let yourself get healthy and happy again, then see if the problem still exists.

Check your perceptions with someone else on the team in a nonjudgmental way. Be careful not to sow the seeds of resentment in others on your team. If they see the same things you see, perhaps together you can come up with some good ways to improve the situation. Again, caregiving is a high-stress situation for everyone. If you still have common purpose, and you address the issue with tenderness and understanding, perhaps your relationships will be strengthened along with fixing the issue.

Be extra careful with family; they share your history. They share your genes. No one can push your buttons like a family member. Remember, that goes both ways: they can push yours, but you might be leaning on theirs and not realize it. Take a little extra time for cooling off. You might take that time to reread the tips on clear and respectful communication, above, especially the bits about staying in the present and avoiding damning judgments. Few things are more stressful to a patient than their family fighting about them. Don't let a lifetime of history and the traits you share ruin the rest of your loved one's life.

...Get Help from a Neutral Professional

Say you've done your best to be part of a cohesive team. You all share your common purpose. Everyone is on the best behavior they can manage. You're giving yourself and everyone else involved some extra emotional wiggle room. You've done your best to keep communication clear and respectful. Still, tensions can arise.

Sometimes there is just one person on the team, especially among family, who does not have the same purpose or just cannot get along with the others. The rest of the team is doing well. They all see the same things in this one person and agree that it's a problem. They have tried all the things listed earlier under Clear and Respectful Communication and the problems continue.

As I write this I am remembering a family I know in which three brothers are caring for their mother as she loses her ability to make new memories. One brother is giving everyone difficulty. He seems more concerned with his share of her assets than sharing in her care. He has a long history of being socially awkward. He has difficulty in relationships, no girlfriend or partner, and few if any friends. He has difficulty holding a job. Still, he is family. Arguing doesn't work. Anger doesn't help. The mother is tortured by the strife in her family.

To resolve it all, they chose an impartial third party whom they all could trust: their mother's lawyer. They began with small issues on which they might all find common ground. Any agreements they worked out together were recorded by the lawyer and signed by all, and each brother received a copy. The two caregiving brothers focused on being fair. They did not play games or try to bargain. This was not haggling with a used-car salesman, this was their mother near the end of life. They remained respectful and honest, and at the same time they did not run away or give in to their brother's tantrums. They did their best to keep communication open and as clear as possible.

In the end, the difficult brother chose to step away from all his exorbitant claims. He chose instead to take some time away and then to focus on helping his mother, as well as he could, to make the most out of what remained of her life.

What did they do here? Look again at the list in Clear and Respectful Communication. Consider each item, especially the part about getting help. In most cases, help is available to help keep communication positive and productive.

If your caregiving situation has a **social worker** already, they can be a terrific referee and help with resolutions. Check with your **local nonprofit** related to the disease, disorder, or condition. A **family lawyer** also might help if they are neutral and the matters are more in their realm. Don't use *your* lawyer, they are not neutral. You might also seek out a **family therapist**.

For more on conflict resolution consider these sites:

http://adulted.about.com/od/training/tp/conflictresolution.htm

http://video.about.com/stress/5-Effective-Tactics-for-Conflict-Resolution.htm

http://www.edcc.edu/counseling/documents/conflict.pdf

Chapter 2.
Calling in the Pros

Despite all the best efforts of you and your team of caregiver heroes, there may be a time to call professional caregivers into your home. There is no shame in this. You and your team are not giving up. These folks have walked this road before. They are usually quite experienced, skilled, and knowledgeable. They can be a tremendously helpful part of the team. Professional help can fill gaps in difficult times so other caregivers can rest and rejuvenate. They can perform tasks that may be beyond the comfort level of your team. They can help lead, teach, and often defuse potential growing conflicts that are common. Asking for experienced paid help means you care more for your loved one than for your own pride, so don't be afraid to reach out for help.

We had set parameters for when we would call on paid caregivers. This helped put everyone, even Karen, at ease. It allowed us to step back from our caregiver roles for a time and be just friends, family, lovers again.

Finding Good Professional Caregiver Help

So how does one find these elusive nightingales of mercy? The first and maybe the best resource are the people in your caregiving team: your friends, neighbors, and the people all around you. Chances are, they know someone who knows someone who has been very effective in a caregiving situation.

Many professional caregivers are well connected. If they can't take the case, they may know someone who can. This is how we found the best caregivers for my mom.

If you are connected with hospice, a comfort care nurse, a social worker, or a caseworker, they may be able to help you find the right professional caregivers. They may know individuals for hire as independent contractors, or they may work with an agency that places paid caregivers.

Also, if you live near a school with a nursing program, the admissions people there may know of aspiring students who need work experience. Students are usually bright and enthusiastic, but they do often lack experience.

A **home-care agency** is a company that employs and often trains and oversees caregivers in various aspects of health care, including professional home caregivers. They usually have set hours and shifts, though this may be negotiable. They charge you a fee and may work with third-party payers like your state's Medicaid program or your private disability insurance. You can find an agency yourself online using keywords such as "home care."

Self-directed care falls somewhere between hiring a caregiver yourself and using an agency. In this model, the agency can help introduce you to the caregiver, help train them, and help you with managing the financial resources available for paid caregiving. One agency I talked to, **Consumer Direct Care** http://consumerdirectcare.com/, actually helps you with payroll and taxes and sometimes acts as a bridge between your Medicaid coverage and the paid caregiver. Even with all this assistance, this model is less expensive than going through a traditional agency, and the savings can result in higher pay for the paid caregiver. Higher pay usually attracts better caregivers.

Some states have allowances written into their Medicaid program for the self-directed care model as well as many other wonderful services. To find out about programs and resources in your state, search for your **state Medicaid office** www.Medicaid.gov or just type "Medicaid" and the name of your state into your search engine. You may also be able to search out such agencies yourself with the keywords "self-directed care," "self-determined care," or "person-centered care."

...Selecting the Right Professional

So many questions revolve around bringing someone into your home:

- Will they be able to be there at the right times?
- Do they have the skills and abilities your loved one needs?
- Do they possess the temperament and personality that work with your loved one and your team?
- Most importantly, do they connect and care well for your loved one and just "feel right" to you and your loved one?

Trust your gut and the feedback from your care network, and invite your loved one to participate in the selection if they are able.

If your loved one needs more medically related skills from a paid caregiver, such as wound dressing, care for lines like IVs or catheters, more advanced bowel or bladder care, or more advanced help with mobility, look a bit more closely at the letters behind the caregivers' names. Below is a short list of what some common abbreviations mean in relation to training and expertise. Requirements and specific skills-and-practices acts—laws that say what each type of caregiver can and cannot do—vary somewhat state by state.

Companion. This is more of a job title than a professional designation. This person may or may not have any formal training yet they can be critically important in helping someone who cannot be left alone safely. They might help with meals, light housekeeping, laundry and transportation. They cannot help with medication and probably cannot help with any more advanced nursing care. You also may see the general home care designations of direct support professional (DSP), and caregiver. People working under these designations may or may not have experience or training.

Certified nursing assistant (CNA). This is probably the most common professional designation in caregivers both for in the home and in facilities such as hospitals and nursing homes. In most states, they can perform basic medical-related tasks such as changing a dressing and caring for lines (like catheters or IVs) under the supervision of a nurse or doctor. In some states, this designation is written NAC or NA-C. To earn the certificate, they must complete 75 hours of coursework and hands-on skills work, as well as take a written and skills test. NA-R means they have taken the coursework and registered but have not yet received their certificate.

Certified medication aid (CMA). This person works under the supervision of a nurse or doctor and can administer most medications but not by central lines or chemotherapy depending on the state.

Personal care attendant (PCA). This means the person has completed 16 hours of coursework (about three days) plus specific orientation to that case.

Attendant care worker (ACW). This designation began in Arizona as a base level of training required for that state's Medicaid reimbursement. It is now gaining favor as a benchmark for other states. It requires that people sit for an examination that includes a written test and a practical skills test. Generally the coursework to be ready for the test takes about 40 to 60 hours of focused learning.

Home health aide (HHA). These people are usually capable to do many of the same basic tasks as CNA's but their focus is more on care in the home. The formal education requirements vary state by state. However, all states do require training for someone to be *certified* as an HHA, with the minimum at the time of this writing being 75 training hours.

...Going Through the Selection Process

Once you know the kind of professional help you want, make a list of candidates. I like to create a folder for each one or at least a page of paper with their name, contact information, their work experience, and any notes. On this paper you can write reminders for the questions you might want to ask during the interview. Here is a link to a fairly generic but nicely comprehensive list of possible interview questions from Care.com http://www.care.com/senior-care-senior-caregiver-interview-tips-p1145-q7744646.html When you are interviewing, write down the answers in a way that makes sense to you. Also record your overall impression of the person. I like one to five stars and a quick note as to why. Then you're ready to contact them.

Phone call. Chances are, when you call you will leave a message and ask them to call back. If they don't call back, cross them off your list. Don't give out your address until you are ready to set up an in-person interview. Try for at least five candidates to interview.

Telephone interview. You can ask many basic questions quickly in a phone interview. Describe the days and hours you will need and the level of specific needs your loved one has, such as minimal assist with bathing, dressing, toileting, help with mobility, etc. You may ask about the person's availability, transportation (do they have a reliable car?), allergies, whether they smoke, etc. You can ask about their work history, especially their last few jobs and why they left. You can ask what types of clients they like most and least. If they still seem like a good fit, you are ready for an in-person, in-home interview.

In-home interview. For the best chance to see the person interact with your loved one and gain a good sense of your loved one's reaction, do an in-person interview in your home. Your loved one is really the person making the choice. It's their care. Introduce the candidate to your loved one. Does the interaction feel right? Is the person respectful, interacting well, fitting in with your family? Take your time, don't rush. Be open. Listen. Be prepared with your care plan, the Carebook, and your interview sheet. Explain fully your needs and expectations. You may review their availability, training, prior work history, how their last job ended, and anything else that wasn't answered well on the phone.

Because I know what I'm looking for, I like to give the person an opportunity to work a little in the interview process. Can they help with whatever is needed at the time? Is there a skill you know is needed, like a maximum assist transfer? Can the candidate do it with you? Ask what their questions are. Listen, and be honest in your answers. Ask for at least three references, two of which should be professional references from people they have worked with. You may also consider a background check. Each state has its own and you may find the form by typing "background check form" and the name of your state into your search engine. Lastly, talk about salary and any benefits. You will need their social security number if you are going to hire them legally.

Cultural considerations. You may notice that many agency caregivers are immigrants. This is not necessarily a problem. In some of the Muslim cultures of Africa, the Philippines, and Southeast Asia, caring for people in need is more honored than in our culture. If you are considering hiring an immigrant, can you and your loved one put aside any prejudices that may exist? Questions that are most important are more about the ability to understand each other's communication and whether your loved one is able to connect with them comfortably.

References. Yes, actually call the people the candidate says will give a good review. If it's a professional reference, ask about the specifics of what the person did there. If the candidate stated what they were paid, you may confirm it. Confirm why they left the position. Watch for words like "difficult," "challenged," or other negative words. Don't be afraid to ask whether you should hire the person. Many human resource policies will not allow a reference to tell you more than the dates of employment, but ask any questions you want, to get what you need. I like to ask things like "Would you hire them again?" or "Hypothetically, is a person like her great with nonverbal patients?" to try to get at the information you need.

For a good video about hiring an in-home caregiver, check this YouTube from Washington State's **Department of Social and Health Services**
https://www.youtube.com/watch?v=L3skIWEmpas&feature=youtu.be.

Managing Hired Help

Once you have hired your new helper, be there to help familiarize them with care and routines. This will make everyone more comfortable and give you a chance to watch them work with your loved one. Again, are they respectful? Do the two interact well together? You can also get a better view of their skills. Once they are up and running, you will want to stop by unannounced. It's just another way to check up on their good work.

Don't be afraid to let a paid caregiver go if the fit isn't good. You're paying them, you're the boss; think of it as moving the employee on to a better-fitting job. Everyone benefits from a good match, and nobody benefits from a poor match.

...Salary and Benefits

Wage information varies region by region and over time, so I won't give specifics here. You can look up expected salaries for your area by searching "salary" and the professional designation, for example, "salary CNA Seattle" or "salary home caregiver." Salaries are considered for 2000 hours per year, so you may calculate an hourly rate by dividing the salary by 2000.

...Payroll and Taxes

If you are hiring from an agency, the caregiver is an employee of the agency so you do not need to worry about the payroll. If you hire a caregiver directly, they are your employee or a contractor. The simplest way to handle this is to file and provide them with an IRS form 1099 for independent contractors at the end of the year (or the end of their work for you, if that happens first). Keep track of your payments by tracking the checks in your bank account and/or get a receipt book.

...Paying for In-home Caregivers

When my mom was sick, her neighbor told us to get a pocketful of $100 bills and just go out and find good caregivers. This is in fact what many people do for shorter-term in-home care.

Under Finding Good Professional Caregiver Help earlier in this chapter, we discussed **Medicaid.** Maybe that agency can help; they can be tremendously helpful with many resources for those who qualify. Many states have opted in to a waiver system that allows Medicaid to provide in-home support for people. To learn if your loved one qualifies and find out more about how Medicaid can help, see Chapter 8, Medicare, Medicaid, and Private Insurance. You also can look up your state's website with the keywords "Medicaid" and the name of your state. One of the most clearly written and informative sites I've seen is **LongTermCare.gov** http://longtermcare.gov/medicare-medicaid-more/Medicaid/.

Medicare and most private health insurance policies do not provide for home health aides or caregivers. They will provide for "skilled" in-home care. This means skilled medical services such as physical therapy, occupational therapy, speech therapy, and skills that require a nurse or nurse's aid under the supervision of a nurse if the person is homebound. They will do this for a limited time following a recent hospital stay for the illness or injury being treated and require medical necessity and physician's orders.

Medicare supplements do not pay for in-home caregivers. They also tend to follow the Medicare guidelines listed above and are mostly focused on helping pay the amounts Medicare does not cover.

The **Department of Veterans Affairs (VA)** provides caregiver help to veterans registered at a VA for health care. They can provide support to caregivers as well as other professional home health services. Programs include home-based primary care, home health aides, respite for family caregivers and a variety of other caregiver services. The website www.caregiver.va.gov/ is an excellent website for family caregivers to find support and services. There is also an established VA's Caregiver Support Line 1-855-260-3274 toll-free to ask about caregiver support services. Each VA has a Caregiver Coordinator who can help caregivers find out about how to qualify for additional benefits.

The Aid and Attendant program may give increased allowances to qualifying veterans to help with long term care and respite care (see below). If you don't already have a VA caseworker, contact your VA health care team for your specific case. If your loved one is not already registered at a VA, find your local VA office by typing "Veterans Affairs" and your city into your search engine or go to www.va.gov.

Various Veterans Service Organizations can you navigate the VA system and help with getting VA benefits. The Veterans of Foreign Wars (VFW), Paralyzed Veterans of America (PVA), Disabled American Veterans (DAV), and other Veteran Service Organizations may also help you navigate the system.

Private **disability insurance** does not directly pay for in-home caregivers, but **Social Security Disability** (SSDI) might through Medicaid. If your loved one is already enrolled in SSI, check with their caseworker or your local Social Security office.

Private **long-term care insurance** or combination life insurance and long-term care insurance usually does pay for home health aides and companion services.

This is private insurance you buy when you're healthy. There are many rules to follow. Read your policy carefully and ask a trusted advisor to help you decide when to start using the insurance, because most policies limit the total time you can use them. Be aware that once your insurance company gives the OK for a service, you may need to pay out of pocket for an "elimination period," and once you start using the insurance for anything, it may start the clock ticking on a payment window that closes according to the time stated for your policy.

Some **life insurance** policies may allow for your loved one to tap into their life insurance benefit in the form of an accelerated death benefit (ADB). Your loved one may be able to use this if they are terminally ill or have a life-threatening diagnosis, needs long-term care services for an extended amount of time, and/or is confined to a nursing home and incapable of performing activities of daily living (ADLs) independently. Typically this amount is capped at 1 percent of the death benefit per month for home care, 2 percent for nursing home care, and 50 percent total. You may want to consider that taking a lump sum of money in a person's name may create a situation where their assets exceed the amount allowed by Medicaid or Supplemental Social Security and may jeopardize those benefits.

Chapter 8, Medicaid, Medicare, and Private Insurance, has more about all this, including links to help you find a good lawyer.

Making sure it "Feels Right"

I leave you with this story about hiring Karin, a most wonderful caregiver who helped us when my mom was sick.

Karin is a registered nurse (RN) and has a company called 24/7 staffing.

She identifies herself as a terrible businesswoman.

24/7 is a tax ID and a loose network of caregivers of different backgrounds and educational and credential levels, from RNs, respiratory therapists (RTs), and CNAs to folks with no credentials who are low-cost and there to be companions.

Karin doesn't take a fee or percentage from the other people in her 24/7 network.

She gets her work entirely by word of mouth; the work comes to her. Usually friends of friends, family, or other people who have gone through caregiving situations say "I know someone …" If she cannot or will not take the case, she often can turn to one of her contacts in 24/7 who she feels will be a good fit. Likewise they may turn to her.

The most important thing to Karin when deciding to take a case is the "fit." It's a feeling that she should be there with this person, with this family, in this home, helping them through this journey. The moment she met my mom, Karin knew she should help us. They reached out to each other, shook hands, and Mom smiled and then took Karin's hand in both her hands. Their hands were warm together. She was meant to be there.

* * * * *

Often our most complex and important decisions are not made on what we think of as a rational basis. They are far too complex for the little wedge of neurons on the front of our brains for that. We make decisions about who to let into our homes, lives, and caring hearts because it feels right. There is so much more to it than all these forms and questions can outline. Of course we did the interview, checked the references, did all the steps listed above, and they all checked out ok. Those are important to avoid a nasty situation and help provide structure, but this is how Karin decides to take a case: if it is a good fit. This is also how we decided too. It felt right.

Chapter 3.
Avoiding Burnout

If you've read chapters 1 and 2 you've learned that you need to create a team and how to reach for professional help. In this next section we'll teach you more about keeping your life in balance as part of keeping yourself healthy for your loved one.

Balancing Caregiving and Work

When my mother was diagnosed with metastatic cancer, I was the owner, manager, and one of the physical therapists in a busy outpatient physical therapy clinic. I was the boss, which really meant that I bore the responsibilities toward all the employees, our patients, and the people who referred them. I hadn't taken any significant time off in years, working rain or shine. But this was different and everyone knew it.

I sat down with the rest of the staff and we figured out how to make time for me to help Mom and my family without letting everyone else at the clinic down. We talked to our patients and their physicians. We got help. My siblings and I all made the time, and our employers and the rest of our families understood and did their best to make it possible for us to care for Mom.

When the need to take care of a loved one arises, you will figure out how to make some room in your busy life, and most people will help you too if you are open, communicative, and asking for support. It is part of life.

Most managers and employers are people who understand and honor the responsibility you're faced with when your loved one needs you. It is important to talk with your employers and managers to help them to understand. See if you can plan creative ways together to allow you to have the time you need without letting them down on your work responsibilities. You may be able to telecommute, have a compressed work schedule, or use flex time. You may job-share, cut hours, or take family leave to gain more time to be home.

Learn your company's policies. Your human resources department or employee handbook will probably have it outlined pretty clearly. In the United States we have provisions in the **Family Medical Leave Act** http://www.dol.gov/whd/fmla/ that give basic requirements to all large employers. You may be eligible for up to 12 weeks per year without risking your job or benefits.

Work provides grounding through its challenges, teamwork, and social contact. It is a link to "normal life." Be creative in finding solutions to balance your work with your caregiving needs. Most employers and managers appreciate an effort to do what you can to keep your end up there.

But remember that you are not superhuman. Your employer, manager, and the HR department may be able to help you with emotional and physical support. Many companies have employee assistance programs that can help with resources, counseling, and effective strategies to help manage the stress and extra workload. It is in everyone's interest that you keep yourself healthy, effective, and as happy as can be.

Getting Paid for Caregiving

Decreasing your role in your job often comes with less pay and more financial burdens. In some ways, we as a society have tried to compensate for this a little. There are several ways a caregiver, even if it's a family member, can get reimbursed for some of their time and effort.

Some **insurance policies**, especially long-term care policies, permit family members to be paid as part of the insurance benefit. Unfortunately, they often exclude family members who live in the same household. Still, it might be well worth it to review all your health-care, long-term care, and disability insurance policies. Life insurance may have clauses that pertain to disability as well. You may find it easiest to call your agent rather than wading through the policy yourself.

The Veterans Administration has provisions under the Aid and Attendance Pension Benefit for veterans. For veterans injured in the conflicts after 9-11, a special law was passed in 2010 providing additional benefits with relief for caregivers. If your loved one is a veteran, call the **Department of Veterans Affairs** (1-877-222-8387) to learn more.

Some states have programs to help people pay for caregiving. Most often these are offered through your state's **Medicaid** program. The names of these programs vary state by state, but many have common buzzwords like "Participant Directed Care," "Consumer Directed Care," "Caregiver Supports," or "Community-based Services," which can help you find them. To look into these programs, contact your local state Medicaid center or go to the **National Resource Center for Participant Directed Services** http://www.bc.edu/schools/gssw/nrcpds//.

In some states, **Medicare** supports a consumer-directed care model. If your loved one qualifies for Medicare, the agency may be able to help train and provide people in your caregiving team with some reimbursement. You can find out more about this by searching with the keywords "self-directed care," "self-determined care," or "person-centered care." We also discuss consumer directed care in Chapter 2, Calling in the Pros.

If your loved one has savings or other assets, you may be able to work out a **caregiver contract** so they can reimburse you for your time and expenses. Keep in mind that any contract you work out needs to have the blessing of the rest of the family and anyone else who may have interest in their estate. This might be one option to discuss at a family meeting. There are huge emotional pitfalls here. I strongly recommend you consult your loved one's or your family attorney (not your own attorney) when creating any type of caregiver contract.

Spending Time with Friends or Connecting with Caregiver Support Groups

We are social creatures. Connection is one of the ways our bodies mitigate stress. Oxytocin (the love hormone) is a stress hormone, secreted from the pituitary gland in response to, among other things, **stress** http://en.wikipedia.org/wiki/Oxytocin. One of its many effects is to help us create an internal environment that is more ready for connection. Oxytocin is protective of the heart. It helps the heart rebuild stronger after a high-stress event. In many ways, opening your heart to others heals the heart.

Even the most introverted of people need connections with others to keep themselves healthy. We don't necessarily need to be with people who are going through the same things we are. In fact, I'm not sure this is always good. We tend to mirror the emotions of those around us. We tend to be happier if our neighbors are happier whether we are close to them or not. Allowing yourself time with vibrant, healthy, happy people is remarkably restorative and will keep you able to bring that happiness to the one you're caring for.

You don't necessarily need a party, though I rather like parties; just one healthy, caring friend will help you rebuild your spirits. They might give you an ear, but sometimes it's more important to share a laugh or just some time than it is to share your troubles. They don't necessarily need to be very close to you. Sometimes, random connection with strangers is the best. They do need to be emotionally healthy and not too needy themselves. We probably all know someone we might call an "energy vampire." This is not the connection you need now.

That said, it might be difficult to connect with people who do not share your experience or cannot relate to what you are going through. Support groups are fantastic for this, as the room is full of people who share this common thread of life. There you may find someone who reaches their hand out and says, "I feel your pain" and actually means it. A moment when eyes and hearts meet may be more powerful than an hour with a good bartender. I believe we need both: time to connect and time to laugh. Either way, we need to be with others.

Planning for Respite Care

One weekend early and deep into Karen's illness, our friend Mary Lou came to the house while her husband, Chris, took me by the ears and dragged me off to the mountains, giving me, and Karen, respite from the intensity of our situation. This is no small thing. It became a pattern for how we would care for Karen, a cornerstone of what made the whole experience work.

Respite means a short period of rest. And it can come in many forms. Professional or volunteer caregivers in your home—and, in fact, the whole team approach to caregiving—could be considered a form of respite care as you and your teammates relieve each other. You may see and hear the term *respite* as you navigate the journey of caregiving. It may be applied to seeking help from family and friends, community organizations that help, and adult day care programs. It might be overnight and short-stay programs offered at nursing homes and some assisted living facilities, adult family homes, and other care facilities. Emergency services can also stand in for a caregiver if they have problems.

You need to know the term *respite*, both to be encouraged to take a rest regularly and well, and to help you search out resources. Chances are that if you type "respite care" and the name of your city into your search engine, you will find a plethora of services and resources to help. The most useful site I have found is for **Access to Respite Care and Health (ARCH)** http://archrespite.org/consumer-information; it has good descriptions of the various models of care, how to choose a program or provider, and how to pay for it. Because ARCH has done such a terrific job, here we need only stress a few points about it:

- **Plan for respite times** before you begin to see or feel signs of stress or burnout. Take some time now to locate, choose, and secure services so it is there for you.
- **Use respite care regularly.** Have set times off on your calendar so you know when they are coming. It's like knowing where the top of the hill is when you're cycling up a steep grade. You can push harder if you know rest is coming.
- **Use respite care wisely.** Take that time to get fully away from your caregiving situation. Do things that are important or joyous to you. You may also consider attending a caregivers support group in this time. Some respite care models include separate support groups for you and your loved one.
- **Have your carebook ready for the respite caregivers.** Your carebook, or a copy of it, will help them to have a basic history, your recent notes, your team's contact information, and your medical team's contact information. It will also help them to know the routines and your loved one's likes and dislikes. If you don't have the carebook yet, **Aging Care** https://www.agingcare.com/siteimages/RespiteCaregiverChecklist.pdf provides a respite caregiver checklist form you could use instead.
- **Check in with your respite caregivers** and your loved one when you return. "How did it go?" will tell you a lot. Notice any changes in your loved one's condition. Are they rested or more stressed?

...Consider Your Loved One's Needs

When deciding what type of respite-care model would work best, consider the needs of your loved one first:

Is travel difficult? Are they at high risk of hospital shock (see Delirium in Chapter 18, Managing Discomforts)? If so, in-home care assistance may be your best option. Finding and hiring an in-home caregiver for respite care is pretty much the same as hiring for regular in-home care (see Chapter 2, Calling in the Pros). Even though you may be hiring them for only a short period, respite for you and your caregiving team should be a regular event, so that short period should be repeated. This will also give you and your loved one a chance to try the caregiver out, as they may become a more frequent part of your team should you need it.

Would a change in scenery help? Could your loved one use some social interaction besides you, perhaps some activities? Adult day care or many of the other out-of-home models could be a better option. Hospitals and nursing home respite-care programs can offer more medical care, whereas family care homes can offer a homier environment. Group homes, hospitals, nursing homes, and other specialized facilities provide emergency and planned overnight services, allowing caretakers 24-hour relief. Many hospice programs also offer both in-home and facility-based respite programs that are included in the hospice care program. Caregiver retreats and respite camps, available in some areas, are often specific to diseases or conditions such as Alzheimer's or Lou Gehrig's Disease (ALS). These often combine respite with education and support.

The different models (and resources to help pay for them) are all nicely discussed by the ARCH team. The different care models and facilities and how to choose one that is best for your loved one are also further discussed in Chapter 10, Hospitals and Other Medical Facilities.

...Paying for Respite Care

When considering what options are available to you financially, resources vary greatly state by state. Again, the ARCH team is the clearest and best-connected website I have seen. It has a very straightforward and comprehensive description of different types of programs, including the Lifespan Respite Program, hospice, Medicaid, the National Family Caregiver Support Program, and Veterans Affairs programs. They include links that will steer you to resources in your state. Generally, here is an overview:

Private insurance does not cover respite care. Some long-term care plans do, but as with in-home caregivers, be careful with your policy's exact rules.

Medicare does not cover respite care at this time.

Social Security Disability Insurance (SSDI) may cover in-home care. Check with your local office to verify your loved one's eligibility.

The **Veterans Affairs** provides 30 days per year of inpatient respite for veterans who qualify. If your loved one has VA benefits, speak with your caseworker.

Medicaid does cover respite care in some states through a waiver program if the state governor chose to accept it. This is available to people who qualify for Medicaid benefits.

Individual state programs http://archrespite.org/respitelocator/respite-locator-service-state-information-map for respite care (and many other ways to help caregivers) are available in states that are enlightened enough to realize that you are doing them a huge favor, caring for a loved one at home in the least restrictive (and least expensive for them) environment.

Many **foundation grants and nonprofit organizations** are out there to help. These are usually local, funded and run by good people who understand the importance of the help they are giving you. Again, ARCH has a good link base.

* * * *

The main thing is that you and the other members of your caregiving team do take measures to avoid burnout: balance caregiving and work, spend time with friends or support groups, and take respite regularly. Remember the lessons of mountain rescue: keep yourself warm enough, hydrated enough, and on safe terrain ... take care of yourself, take the rest you need, so you can continue to do your best for the one you are caring for.

Chapter 4.
Dancing in the Rain:
Healthy Habits for Caregivers

This chapter is about how to stay happy during the most difficult of times. No one expects, and you shouldn't either, that you will not find yourself uncontrollably weeping at an intersection or dumbfounded by stress at the grocery store. No one expects these most difficult times to have no effect.

I was recently at a seminar on the effects of stress on the brain, and the instructor used "being a primary caregiver" as the most stressful situation, one giving the most deleterious long-term effects on the brain. You don't need to read the details here of the nasty bits; it will only add to your stress.

You do need to know and use techniques and habits to help mitigate the effects of stress and keep yourself (and your loved one) as happy as possible. You need to turn this distress into **eustress** http://en.wikipedia.org/wiki/Eustress.

Embrace Stress

Stress is not always a bad thing. Our bodies are loaded with protective and regenerative responses that not only make us more resilient to the negative effects of stress, they help us stay strong, fight disease, and keep sharp minds and close relationships. So much of our response depends on our attitudes and habits. In one very elegant study, people who did not have the attitude that stress was bad for them did not have the mortality usually associated with high-stress life events. In fact, they actually fared better than those people who did not perceive themselves as being under stress.

Think of the last time you were about to rise to the challenge before you. Perhaps you were up to bat or at the starting line of a race. Perhaps it was your turn to speak at a meeting and you had something important to say. Can you remember your racing heart and quickening breath? This was your body getting ready to perform. This was the physiology of courage. In this physiology, our blood vessels dilate and our bodies produce stress hormones such as cortisol, adrenaline, and oxytocin. Our minds and our bodies become ready to perform. Afterwards, we are ready to rest, relax, and connect deeply with the people around us. Health physiologist Kelly McGonigal gave an excellent **TED talk** on this http://www.ted.com/talks/kelly_mcgonigal_how_to_make_stress_your_friend.html.

...Be Prepared

Though this might seem impossible, try to read ahead in this book and practice the basic skills in Part III, Caregiving Skills and Advice from the Field, before you need them. If you feel a little more prepared and a little more like you can handle the situations as they arise, you are less likely to have the deer-in-the-headlights feeling of panic or helplessness. Take a little of the down time you have. You can read this book, consult with nurses or other health professionals, look at the videos, and practice your skills and prepare your team. A little sense of competency makes a huge difference not just in how well things go, but also in your stress response.

...Take Breaks

Taking a break is the rest part of the stress-rest cycle. One of the most important reasons to build a caregiving team is so that you, the primary caregiver, can take breaks. Get yourself out of the house, out of the situation, and away, doing something not related to caregiving. Even the most dedicated nurses and doctors do not work 24-hour shifts end-to-end, over and over again. Calculate your hours: see how much time you are really "on duty." If you are like most caregivers, it is probably well over 100 hours each week. No one can work this many hours, week after week, month after month, and be expected to be able to perform. Even if their work is not stressful, they simply break down from the load of it.

Your caregiving work is stressful. Even when you are sleeping, if you are still in caregiver mode, you are probably not fully resting. To be at your best, try to be off at least 30 hours per week. That means being "off duty" as a caregiver an average of about 4.5 hours per day. If that sounds like a lot, consider that you will still be on 11.5 hours plus another 8 hours of "sleep time" seven days per week. For more on this, including in-home and out-of-home services so you can take breaks, read Planning for Respite Care in Chapter 3, Avoiding Burnout.

...Recognize Times of Crisis

"Let's climb the North Face of Mount Robson," Johnny Johnson said to me, grinning with excitement and confidence. I met him learning to climb glaciers with his father. I had one season of this under my belt now and was young and overly confident. We had done a few climbs together and had just run a one-day ascent on Mount Rainier, hitting the summit in just over five hours. The funny thing about when you feel cocky is, nature always finds a way to show you yourself.

So there we were, most of the way up the rock portion of Mount Robson, when Johnny fell apart. The route was steep with sharp, somewhat loose stone, which was unprotectable. This meant we couldn't use a rope. If we fell, we would quite possibly fall all the way to the bottom. We were about 2000 feet off the deck when his nerves just gave out. Stress hormones and neurotransmitters built up too high and something just snapped. In an instant he became a mass of blubbering goo.

Falling apart like that can happen to anyone. I've seen it happen to strong people, more than twice. It's like a broken leg or bonking (when your metabolism goes awry and you run out of energy), only it's your central nervous system. Like so many people faced with a crisis, on Mount Robson I became hyperfocused, hypervigilant, and very matter-of-fact. I also seemed to possess nearly unlimited patience and energy. Johnny and I unloaded all unnecessary provisions for this section and secured our packs to the rock, then climbed in baby steps up to relatively flat ground. There we tried to calm him and hit his reset button.

We then proceeded with the 2000-foot vertical crawl down the mountain, sometimes roped on a body belay, with him tied to me without tying to the mountain. Sometimes I physically placed his hands and feet on holds as we descended. We spent a long time with nothing under our heels but air and the icy river below. About 11:00 p.m. we forded that river and made our way back to camp. Now, safe on flat ground, it was my turn to fall apart. By the time we hit camp, I could hardly move. Johnny made me dinner while I lay in the tent with my reserves spent and my nerves shattered.

There are two lessons here for the caregiver. The first is that everyone's nervous system can snap under prolonged stress. Watch for the signs:

- Are your thoughts racing and hard to control?
- Do you feel anxious, overtired, numb, or overly emotional?
- Are you having trouble concentrating or solving more involved problems?
- Does it take you longer than usual to do simple or routine tasks?
- Do you get distracted?
- Do you make mistakes?
- What is your resting heart rate?

If your resting heart rate is more than five beats per minute higher than normal and/or you feel or observe symptoms or signs, take special precautions:

- Get help.
- Get rest.
- Eat, but avoid junk food.
- Get exercise (I like hitting a punching bag).
- Talk with people if that helps you.
- Double-check all vital work.

Count the medications before you give them. Double-check that all things are secure before you move the one you care for. Double-check your setups. Check your calendar for appointments and responsibilities. Be careful to leave everything in its place.

Mostly understand that what you are experiencing is normal, but dangerous. Schedule a time when you can be "*off*" as soon as reasonably possible. R&R is important.

The other takeaway is that you may experience any or all of these things *after* the crisis has subsided. This is especially confusing because, externally, things are calming down. Now is the time to allow for rest. Allow yourself to slow down for a little while. You may need only a few hours. You may need up to a few days. As soon as energy returns, though, pick up all those healthy habits that helped you before the crisis began. Journal about positive things, exercise, spend time with friends and loved ones. Blow off some steam. You'll be OK … as long as you give yourself room to fall apart a little.

...Step Outside Yourself

"I'll have the trout special, please." Four hours later, I was intensely aware of the folly of my request. We were on our way into the Huayhuash mountain range in Peru, the same mountains where Simon cut the rope to let Joe Simpson fall in *Touching the Void*. We weren't even in the mountains yet, only in this remote town at the end of the last dirt road traveling eastward toward the mountains. Now I was lying in a cot, shaking uncontrollably or jumping up to sprint across the courtyard to the toilet. Sit, kneel, or both.

Sometime that night I was reminded that we Americans are quite a bit taller than the locals. I saw a flash of light and felt my head snap back as I hit the bathroom doorframe. I noticed in a curious way as my feet sort of passed by me in midair. "What are those doing there?" I wondered. Then I landed hard on my back.

Lying on the concrete floor with a lump on my forehead, my strongest sensation was a kind of queer amusement about just how pathetic this all was. It was hilarious. Then I remembered why I was running.

In times of extreme stress, many people report a sensation of being outside themselves, just calmly noticing the events and sensations. This sense of detachment and looking back on yourself, or meta-analysis, allows you in hard times to take an honest, non-panic-ridden assessment. Sometimes it is key to making clear decisions when otherwise you might crumble or panic.

Several meditation practices strengthen this phenomenon. See Mindfulness Meditation later in this chapter. You don't need extreme stress or full meditative practice to use and strengthen this effective tool. Try the following:

Calming Exercise: Four Count Breathing

1. First calm yourself a little. You can do this.
2. Then gently inhale smoothly while counting off four seconds in your mind.
3. Without pausing, exhale smoothly, also counting four seconds silently in your mind.
4. Continue this for three more breaths, in and out.

This exercise is often calming and centering. It allows you a moment to step out of the scene and helps activate your parasympathetic (calming) nervous system. It's quite pleasant and much easier on your head than the bathroom door header.

Now you can take another moment to see this scene simply as an observer. You may notice your body's reactions or the environment. Feel your heartbeat. Notice your temperature. Are your hands cold? Are they clenched? Notice the scene around you. You may find it amusing or ridiculous. You may sense the scene more fully. Take notes of your own signs of stress.

Simply taking a moment to notice activates your prefrontal cortex, your rational mind. Now it can help you return to the situation and help you make more rational decisions and take more calm actions.

Stay as Healthy as Can Be

It may seem obvious, but in order to continue functioning well as a caregiver, you must take care of your own health, not just your loved one's. This section focuses on strategies for maintaining your physical health while you are caregiving.

...Sleep in Sleepless Times

This section is just as important for the patient as it is for the caregiver. The body of scientific evidence elucidating the importance of the full spectrum of sleep to both mental function and physical recovery is overwhelming. Don't just pretend you can go without good sleep. You can't for long.

Try to keep the same regular sleeping hours you normally did before all this happened. Well, good luck with that. If you're like most primary caregivers on the night shift, your sleep is interrupted and there are many nights with little or no sleep. If you can't sleep your regular hours, here are some other options to help replace the sleep you need:

Take micronaps: Sometimes a 15-minute nap will refresh and rejuvenate you. If you are sleep-deprived or, more importantly, REM-deprived, your body may drop right into the rapid-eye-movement (REM) stage. Set a timer so you don't have to worry about sleeping too long. Lie down, but you don't need to be in bed. Take your shoes off, but you don't need to undress. You may do this up to three times each day.

Take a siesta: A one- to three-hour nap after lunch is common in many cultures. You know the after-lunch sleepies? You may use that to your advantage. Instead of reaching for tea, reach for a pillow. Just a few brief cautions about napping, however: Don't sleep past 4:00 p.m., as you may throw off your regular diurnal cycle and have more trouble getting to sleep at your regular time. Be sure to wake up fully after the nap; a bit of exercise or physical activity helps with that. Be sure to go into your regular presleep routine and go to bed at your regular time, even if you did take that siesta.

Meditate: Body-focused meditation works well to rest the body, and 15 minutes may be considered by some to be equivalent to a full three-hour sleep cycle. Here is a simple instructional manual on meditation techniques http://www.learning-modern-meditation.com/sleep-meditation-1.html. The techniques will be easier to master at first with an external guide such as a recorded voice. There are many sources for guided body-focused meditation—here are a few samples:

http://www.youtube.com/watch?v=obYJRmgrqOU&list=PL5602F9BEFDB2CFE7&index=26

http://www.youtube.com/watch?v=dbLzoOIuhhs

http://www.youtube.com/watch?v=DsmuKeOtXV0&list=PL5602F9BEFDB2CFE7

If you have trouble falling asleep even when your situation allows you to go to bed, you may try some of the following suggestions to help ease you into sleep:

- **Try performing a body-focused meditation** lying down and self-guided. It will relax you and you may fall asleep doing it.
- **Enjoy a glass of warm milk or chamomile tea** before bed. Both are mild sedatives. Careful not to drink so much volume that it has you getting up to pee often.
- **Have a turkey sandwich** (or any turkey) 30 minutes to an hour before bed. The tryptophan in turkey is a mild sedative. Consider how you feel after Thanksgiving dinner.
- **Take a hot bath** about an hour before bed. You can add any leftover chamomile tea to your bath for a little aromatherapy. Afterward, your body's cooling is a signal to go to sleep.
- **Have a "pre-sleep routine".** These are the things you do every night just before going to bed, such as brushing your teeth, stretching out, or journaling. Your routine just before sleep time signals your brain that it is time to go to sleep.
- **Avoid exercising with intensity** more than a relaxing walk or an easy stretch within an hour of bedtime. That tends to be excitatory.

- **Turn away night lights** so they do not shine in your face as you're trying to sleep. Though they may be important for your loved one to get around safely, they can keep you from falling asleep.
- **Put the cat out,** or any other noise-making, blanket-stealing creatures that disturb your sleep.
- **Avoid any reading that tells a story** or gives you images in your mind's eye. Choose something nice and boring, like this book or a technical journal like *Grey's Anatomy*—or even the phone book.
- **Avoid computer work, movies, or television.** If you must look at a screen before bed, use amber glasses. The blue light (same color as a sunny day) triggers your brain to be awake. For more on amber glasses, see https://www.lowbluelights.com
- **Avoid caffeine past noon.** This includes many soft drinks and teas, which may be robbing you of deep restorative sleep.
- **Avoid sweets before bed.** Sweets may help some people sleep, the sweet (even imitation sugar) does kick in their insulin system and they end up having low blood sugar and feeling low energy or sleepy. The drawback is obvious: Any sugar scoured from the bloodstream due to insulin goes straight into the fat cells.
- **Create a worry journal** if you lie awake perseverating on your worries (we call that monkey mind). Write down the issue, what you are going to do about it, and when you will do it. Assign a time to worry about it, to figure it through, and to address it. Then put the book away on the shelf. Address the issue in its time, not during your sleep time. If you can't do anything about it, why worry? If you can do something about it, why worry?

...Eat Right

If your house is like my house or most caregiving homes, all that Tupperware was initially full of comfort foods. When people feel bad, they typically reach for the ice cream, cookies, or mac 'n' cheese. So when they think you might feel bad, they reach for the same foods to help make you feel better. This might be great if you are sad for a day or two. But caregiving is a marathon, not a sprint; most caregiving situations for life-threatening diseases last months or years. Those "comfort" foods make people feel good for minutes, but in the long run will make them feel worse.

In this section we'll try to give you what you need to know about what to eat and how to create an environment where good food is the norm.

Ask for Good Food

The first thing to do is send out the message of what types of foods will be most appreciated by you and your loved one. Again, people want to be helpful. Don't worry—no matter how strongly you say "Bring veggie soup, not cookies," there will still be plenty of cookies.

Try to keep all the sweets and comfort snacks in one place rather than scattered about the home. This will make a reach toward them a more purposeful act and help decrease your impulse junk-snacking. If you do have trouble with impulse junk-snacking, make that one place somewhere that takes a little effort to get to, like a cupboard in the garage or basement. It's there if you really want it, or there for guests, but not in your face all the time. Oh yes, and avoid the fake sugars as well. It turns out that your body triggers many of the same unwanted responses to fake sugar as it does to excessive real sugar.

Plan Meals

Plan meals and create a menu for the next three days to a week. Include healthy foods and target foods. Go shopping, and fill your home with the good food that will be ready for you when you want it. It's OK to cook enough to make leftovers for later. It's also a good idea to have some nutritious, easily prepared meals ready for when you can't cook. You may try cooking with a crockpot or other slow cooker; you can prepare a meal in advance when you have time, and it will be hot and ready for you later.

It is also a good idea to have plenty of foods on hand that are specific for the needs of your loved one (see Chapter 12, Food and Nutrition) but you may need to keep separate food for yourself. If their diet is becoming restricted or their appetite fickle, avoid eating what they eat just because it's there. Chances are, you really don't want cream of rice or boxed mac 'n' cheese every day, though these foods sound great if you're on chemotherapy.

Keep Regular Mealtimes

Eat every three to five hours. Avoid skipping meals, especially breakfast. Have protein as part of your breakfast. This helps avoid large swings in your blood sugar, keeping your energy up and giving your body the building blocks it needs to repair itself.

If you are less physically active as a caregiver than you were before you were thrust into this role, reduce your caloric intake accordingly. Monitor your weight. It could go up or down in this time. Eat accordingly.

Eat a Balanced Diet

Protein is a must. You should get about half a gram of protein for each pound you weigh. For example, if you weigh 180 pounds, you should eat 70 to 90 grams of protein per day. If you are exercising hard (burning off stress), you may increase this amount up to 50 percent. This is not as much as you think. A 6-ounce can of tuna contains 40 grams of protein; 6 ounces of lean meat (chicken, pork, or beef) contains 52 grams; one egg has 6 grams; a cup of milk has 8 grams. A cookie, however, has almost none.

Choose quality **fats**. Omega-3 fatty acids help reduce the risk of depression, dementia, and age- or stress-related disruptions in brain function. This short TED talk discusses depression and includes omega-3 http://www.youtube.com/watch?v=drv3BP0Fdi8. For more information and research around these benefits, see http://en.wikipedia.org/wiki/Omega-3_fatty_acid for some basics. For more scholarly articles, check out these:

http://www.ncbi.nlm.nih.gov/pubmed/19523795

http://www.ncbi.nlm.nih.gov/pubmed/21382308

http://www.psychosomaticmedicine.org/content/72/4/365.short

Cold-water fish such as salmon, mackerel, halibut, sardines, tuna, and herring contain substantial amounts of omega-3 fats in the form of EPA and DHA. Flax seeds, walnuts, soybeans, and pumpkins seeds contain another form, ALA. For a list of foods see http://circ.ahajournals.org/content/106/21/2747.full.pdf.

Select foods with an anti-inflammatory effect: Omega-3 fatty acids, **fruits and vegetables** (especially brightly colored or dark-green vegetables), and fiber-rich grains. Have vegetables raw or only lightly cooked. Avoid the overcooked, mushy broccoli. This is not a nursing home.

If pitting edema (the swelling caused by excess fluid, usually in the legs) is a problem for your loved one or you, **avoid adding salt** and avoid processed foods and salty snacks.

High-tryptophan foods such as turkey may be helpful to counteract serotonin loss due to chronic pain and/or stress. **Tryptophan** http://en.wikipedia.org/wiki/Tryptophan is a precursor to serotonin. It is also helpful to encourage sleep. You may be familiar with the after-Thanksgiving sleepies.

Consider a **Mediterranean diet**: lots of fresh vegetables and fruits, fish, mild amounts of poultry, a little red meat, and long social mealtimes and physical activities. For more information look at www.oldwayspt.org.

Bring **healthy snacks** with you on long doctor or treatment visits. Avoid the vending machines and be on the lookout for good food in the cafeteria. Ask the cashier if they have fruit, and if they don't, ask if they will get some. Check out online food delivery services or salad bars, etc.

Use **smoothies or shakes** to augment your and your loved one's diets. You may augment them with protein supplements. Be sure to read the label to check the amount of protein in a serving against the total amount of a serving: There should be more than half protein. Whey protein is very complete and is most easily absorbed by most people, though not tolerated by some. There are several other sources for protein powder. There is even hemp protein. Bananas and frozen berries work well and are almost always good in a smoothie. If you or your loved one isn't eating vegetables, try mint, parsley, watercress, or spinach in the smoothie. You may find the taste surprisingly refreshing. You may add more nutrient rich ingredients like cooked nettles, wheat grass or dandelion leaves that help fill the gaps in your nutrition (and let's face it, it sounds cool) See Recipes for Shakes, Smoothies, and the Best Comfort Food Ever at the end of Chapter 12, Food and Nutrition.

The services of a **nutritionist** should be available to you and they should be able to help you with some good advice.

Bon appetite.

...Exercise for the Caregiver

When I consider this section, I am reminded of an earlier time in my life, one in which I used exercise to handle my stress:

Damn, that ex-girlfriend pissed me off. I mean, the whole thing started out bad, then just got worse. And now I am burning up the highway between Ellensburg and Seattle with my foot down and steam squeaking from my ears. How did I become the red-faced guy screaming at the windshield?

As I passed the last of the Cascades, instead of continuing to sit in the car, I pulled off at Mount Si. Instead of driving mad and taking that anger home, I began walking uphill, then I was running uphill. By the time I was most of the way to the top, I was sweat soaked but more excited than angry. I scrambled to the summit and looked down. My anger and frustration were somewhere far below. All those problems that had been so big and overwhelming were now tiny, as if they could fit in the palm of my hand. My body and soul relaxed and took in the view.

Most of us who have any history of being physically active know a story like this one. Most of us have felt the grip of powerful negative emotions slip away as we work up a good sweat. This effect is an important tool in your arsenal for keeping healthy during this most stressful time of caregiving. Volumes have been written about the details regarding the effects of exercise on the stress response. Here is one example of one detail: Exercise helps your body process excess cortisol http://en.wikipedia.org/wiki/Cortisol.

Cortisol is one of the chief stress hormones. In normal conditions, cortisol suppresses inflammation as well as a number of other fight-or-flight-related effects. The drug cortisone is a synthetic analog of cortisol. If that fight-or-flight response never happens, and if cortisol levels remain elevated over an extended period of time, it actually causes increased inflammation in multiple sites in the body. Long periods of elevated cortisol have been linked to a wide range of inflammatory health problems, including heart and vascular disease, memory processing problems, emotional problems, and body composition (that is, where you store your fat, body weight regulation, etc.) problems. Exercise, especially intense exercise, seems to simulate the fight-or-flight response your body needs to process the excess cortisol and helps you reset it to normal levels.

What is the best form of exercise? Anything you'll do. Most importantly, anything you enjoy. It's even better if done with other people. A punching bag, a chin-up bar, and a bicycle have helped me through a lot of difficult times. For others it may be tennis, weight lifting, running, or hiking. It doesn't matter that much exactly what you do. It matters more that you do it.

A workout group gives you time with friends and exercise. Research shows that being accountable to someone outside yourself is the greatest factor in being regular and effective with any exercise program. If you are currently involved in any exercise activities with friends or a group, now is the time to keep that up, not quit.

It is also important to have some exercise you may do alone. Your schedule may be tricky now and a bit haphazard. You may find yourself at an odd hour or two with the energy and availability, but no tennis partner. Can you still hit against the backstop, or maybe hit the gym?

Exercise strongly at least twice per week and moderately five days per week. Work up a good sweat. Let your body say "Ahhhhh" after. Enjoy the relaxation response that comes naturally after a good exercise session. This increases blood flow to your brain during and after, helps your muscles relax and reset their normal resting tension, and also helps you develop a real (not just emotional) hunger, which helps you regulate your appetite. Furthermore, the relaxation response you experience after exercise helps improve your rest and allows you more deep, restorative sleep.

You should be aware of one possible side effect. For someone under a lot of stress, exercise can trigger intense but short-lived emotions. This can also happen with massage or other forms of therapeutic touch techniques. We usually just tell patients that it can happen so they are not shocked if it does. Still, I sometimes find it amazing to have all those emotions just coming out of me as I pedal up a strong hill. I reach the top and feel empty yet full, like you're supposed to feel after a good cry. By the time I'm home, I'm right as rain, like my old self again. That right-as-rain feeling after a workout is stronger and better after a group workout.

While writing this section, I thought I should include a basic exercise program here. I write exercise programs every day. I'm a sports and orthopedic physical therapist after all. But what is exercise for one person is torture for another and hardly moving for yet another person. I have, however, emphasized the importance of exercise in all three parts of this book even if it's just for a grin. Here I've included some resources you can explore to help you find a simple program that is at your level, toward your goals, and fun for you:

Conditioning for Outdoor Fitness, by David Musnick and Mark Pierce http://www.mountaineersbooks.org/Conditioning-for-Outdoor-Fitness-P373.aspx, includes basics on dos and don'ts, nutrition, and rest and has many good pictures and descriptions of functional exercises for strength, skill, and cardiovascular fitness.

Core Performance and *Core Performance Endurance,* by Mark Verstegen http://www.coreperformance.com/about/team/corporate-management/mark-verstegen.html and http://www.barnesandnoble.com/s/core-performance-endurance-mark-verstegen?dref=1, were originally given to me by one of the most experienced and accomplished track and field coaches I've ever had the good fortune of meeting. The programs are effective and easy to follow.

The **National Institute for Health** (NIH) Web page for exercise for seniors http://www.nlm.nih.gov/medlineplus/exerciseforseniors.html links to exercise videos of multiple types and provides a generous amount of information regarding exercise and health, including exercise for specific conditions. Here is one workout within the site for a gentle, simple home-based program http://www.nia.nih.gov/sites/default/files/workout_to_go.pdf.

...Spend Time with Friends

Chapter 3, Avoiding Burnout, discusses the importance of spending time with friends or connecting with a caregiver support group. It's important to double down on that notion here, as it's one of the most important healthy habits. I will always remember stepping off the plane after returning from the intense caregiving for my mom and right into a group birthday party. The warmth, the hugs, and just being there with and for happy people who had nothing to do with caregiving was like dipping into a cool lake after battling through the hot jungle. I could literally feel the stress leaving my body.

For many caregivers, this presents a difficult paradox: How can I leave my loved one when their need is so great? How can I spend any time being happy when they are suffering? If you are trapped by this paradox, remember that you need to take care of yourself so you may be your best for them. If this time with friends is how you spend some of your limited time away from caregiving, then laughing and connecting with those friends may be one of the best things you can do and a healthy habit you should keep.

Keep Your Brain Healthy

Both pain (and fear of pain) and chronic stress cause changes in the brain, including up-regulation (hypersensitivity) of the stress response of the *amygdala* (regulates emotions) and degradation of the *hippocampus* (processes memories). Changes in these structures are recognizable on MRI images in as soon as six weeks: Your *prefrontal cortex* downwardly regulates the stress response in the amygdala to help spare the hippocampus. All this is to say, as a caregiver you are stressing your body and your brain, so it is important to help your brain stay healthy too.

...Mindfulness Meditation

After breakfast we drive to the water's edge to watch a coming storm. Karen is tired from the efforts of morning, the doctor visit, the meal out, the little bit of walking she was able to do, everything. Without talking we clasp hands, settle back, and enjoy each other's company. I focus on our touch. I can feel her breathe. I feel my own breathing. The sensations of the moment fill my consciousness: the familiar position of the driver's seat, sounds of rain, smells of newly wet concrete mixed with saltwater spray. I feel my relaxed breathing, her relaxed breathing, us together. I am fully with her as if our souls dance and embrace all around us as our bodies rest. Rain intensifies. We are transformed together. Time rushes both backward and forward through our joined experience. She squeezes my hand just a little, then she lets go a twitch that reminds me that she is really very sick and her time is short here. I gently squeeze her back. We open our eyes. The rain is slowing. We look into each other's eyes and smile. It is the same smile she gave me the very first time I asked her when I would see her again.

Mindfulness meditation can happen almost anywhere. It is the art of being completely in the moment, experiencing it fully. It is the discipline of gently bringing your awareness back to the present moment when it inevitably wanders. It is a simple gift you give yourself. It is, for your brain, an exercise, like lifting weights with your prefrontal cortex. It is also rest and relaxation for the rest of your body.

The exercise of mindfulness meditation helps to strengthen the prefrontal cortex and also helps greatly with mood stabilization or sadness and depression. People who use the practice routinely improve their scores on almost all tools we use to measure happiness. Mindfulness is a very useful tool for anyone experiencing chronic excessive stress—that means both you and your loved one.

Jon Kabat-Zinn did not invent mindfulness meditation. It has been practiced for thousands of years. He did, however, bring it to the forefront of western medical practice. He is a doctor, a scientist, an author, and a teacher. As such he deserves mention here. His work is highly recommended for pain control, mood stabilization, and helping mitigate the effects of chronic stress. For more information, see his books http://www.soundstrue.com/shop/authors/Jon_Kabat-Zinn?gclid=CKKrs4_7qLYCFYdxQgodryMAjg. In this lecture he did for Google, he guides a meditation for the group http://www.youtube.com/watch?v=3nwwKbM_vJc.

Most likely, by the time you are reading this you and your loved one have probably been experiencing high levels of stress, anxiety, and/or pain for some time. You might find that your ability to maintain focus (being mindful) is already strained. Try beginning with something easy and short:

Visual Counting Exercise

1. Picture clearly in your mind the number "10." Hold it in your mind long enough to explore the visual image. See its edges, its depth, the color, its size.
2. Now turn to the number "9" and do the same.
3. Continue this visualization through to the number "0." If your concentration wanders, simply notice that and gently return to the number.

Perform this practice once or more each day until it is easy to focus through the whole exercise. Now you are ready for the more traditional practice of focusing on your breath. Try setting a 15-minute timer and practice once or twice each day.

Many people find the practice easier to start with guidance from a teacher or recording of a teacher. Many such recordings are available. For example, here is a brief "how-to" http://altmedicine.about.com/cs/mindbody/a/Meditation.htm. Again, I refer to the work of Jon Kabat-Zinn mentioned above.

...Positive Journaling

This practice is exactly what it sounds like. Pick a time in the day, such as before bed or after dinner, to write about three or more good moments or things that happened that day. This may take only a couple minutes and may be as simple as a bullet-list format, but it helps your brain experience the best of life several times over.

For your brain, living an experience in your mind's eye is almost as the same as living it in real time. When you journal about a positive moment or event, you gain the benefits from that experience all over again. Read back through your journal and again reap the benefits. As you make positive journaling a habit, your mind begins to look for positive experiences to write about. You spend more mental energy experiencing the positive moments and pause in them long enough to record them into long-term memory.

To record long-term memories, your brain echoes the same circuits over and over again for several minutes up to several days. Each time it echoes the circuits associated with a positive experience, you gain the benefit from all those helpful neurotransmitters and make the connections between those cells stronger. You are "exercising" those parts of your brain associated with happiness. (If you find there is some overlap between "positive" journaling and "gratefulness" journaling—see below—don't worry: a little cross-over is OK.) Here is a simple example:

> ***Positive Journal, February 6***
>
> *A most excellent day.*
>
> *After morning chemo, I turned to Karen and announced "We are now free for the day." We enjoyed a fisherman's diner for lunch. We danced gently at Gas Works Park. We talked deeply and held hands. We kissed in the car and looked at rainbows.*
>
> *Also, I looked into the current medical bills and found that insurance was actually covering things. Thank you, ACA.*
>
> *Karen had dinner with her girlfriends.*

I wish you happiness in your positive journaling.

...Gratefulness Journaling

The practice of gratefulness is deeply imbedded in most of our religions. There is good reason for this; it appears to be one of the key factors affecting our level of satisfaction and happiness. The massive volume of writing on this subject spans spiritual, philosophical, and scientific literature. It is probably much more volume than you want right now. Brother David Stendi-Rast provides one elegant and contemporary voice on the subject in his books http://www.gratefulness.org/books/dsr; he also gave a presentation on TED http://www.ted.com/talks/david_steindl_rast_want_to_be_happy_be_grateful; and here's a beautiful piece featuring his words, also on TED http://www.ted.com/talks/louie_schwartzberg_nature_beauty_gratitude.

Gratefulness journaling works the same way on the brain as positive journaling. In this case, the practice tunes the mind's awareness of stimulation that invoke feelings of gratefulness and strengthens the ability of the brain to generate those feelings. These positive effects reverberate on many centers in the brain. To put it simply, it can tune the brain to be more grateful. Karen began this practice in December 2012. The effect on her and all those around her was profound.

The practice is simple and very similar to positive journaling. Pick a time of day to write down three or more things you are grateful for. If it is a person, take a moment to hold them in your heart and mind. Feel the warmth for them that your gratefulness gives. Wish them well in your heart and mind. You may tell the story of the day in journal form or simply write a bullet list as you reflect on the day.

As with positive journaling, your mind will begin to look for reasons for gratitude and people to feel warm toward. And as with positive journaling, your brain will experience the positive emotions of warmth and gratitude several times over. Again, each time the experience echoes, the circuits associated with it get stronger. Here is an example:

> *Gratefulness Journal, December 21, 2012*
>
> *Morning: Well, what an appropriate day to write and be and be thankful. The Mayan calendar ends today, and I'll be fine!!! Speculation abounds about this day in our history, but what a rich, rich day it will be, and I have thanks abounding.*
>
> *Hannah: OMG! She loaned me three of the greatest wigs last night. They are so fun and transform me into such different looks. If I have to go bald, this will make it super fun. I will try to make it not so scratchy on my bald head. This scratchy fact may limit use, but boy oh boy was it fun. I totally see the appeal.*
>
> *Laura, Lori's friend, is visiting from Chicago and has offered to assist my office. Assist she did. What a glowing wonderful soul she is. It was such a treat to be with her yesterday. Headway was made and I thank Lori from the bottom of my heart.*
>
> *Snowshoe; OMG! I went snowshoeing. I cannot believe it. It was some of the most beautiful snow I ever seen. Dave took his time and spent the day with me, having to let a perfectly good powder day go by so that I could feel more comfortable tonight for Solstice. What an amazing man he is ...*

> *Solstice; yeah! I can do it! We will bring the party much, much, much closer in so that I can play in the snow. This will be sooooo gorgeous and wonderful. What a way to end the world, to hike into an open meadow with some of your best friends, build a huge fire, eat, drink, and be merry.*
>
> *It is so amazing—my life, that is. I have gathered some of the most amazing people around me. They have been steadfast in their love and friendship. They give their time and energy, love, concern, money, and ... well, you name it. I love my life. I love my life. I will live now.*
>
> <u>*Evening*</u>: *What a day! I am flooded with happiness and relief, and love, and happiness, and happiness, and happiness.*

You also may notice the positive effect that this practice has on those you interact with. As people feel your positive, grateful intent, they may mirror it back to you or forward toward their next interaction. I believe this was one of the strongest factors in creating the "bubble of love" that surrounded and sustained us.

...Random Acts of Kindness: Gifting

Giving a simple gift gives many positive emotions and, thus, physiological effects on our minds. The act of intentionally setting out in your day to see what you can give and then taking a moment to reflect allows those positive effects to reverberate and amplify. The practice is powerful.

In the popular book *29 Gifts in 29 Days* http://www.amazon.com/29-Gifts-Month-Giving-Change/dp/B003NHR6T0, Cami Walker describes the intention and act of giving at least one gift a day and then reflecting on that gift. In the TED lecture "How to Buy Happiness" http://www.ted.com/playlists/4/what_makes_us_happy, Dan Gilbert describes some of the findings regarding happiness, creativity, productivity, and gifting. I believe these may work in a fashion similar to positive journaling and gratefulness journaling.

Karen and I did not intentionally choose this practice, as we did many of the other things described in this section. Somehow, though, without intentionally meaning to, I found myself gifting in the months following Karen's passing.

I believe some care must be taken if you choose giving as a way to generate some happiness. Many of us know people who give so much of themselves that it begins to have negative effects on themselves and sometimes those they give to. Anything that generates dopamine and endorphin release (reward and good feeling) can be addictive. Still, it is a very good practice.

For more information, see this short video of Cami Walker talking about her gifting experience http://www.youtube.com/watch?v=Vj2YhqXYEiE.

Chapter 5.
A Brief About Grief

So all of a sudden there I was, behind the wheel in the left-turn lane of a large intersection, sobbing uncontrollably. It just came over me suddenly, like it does sometimes, only this was a bad place for it. Something had to give. My right hand knew what to do and took action. It jumped up and across my right cheek so hard it snapped my neck like that of a boxer just before going down. It was quite a bit harder than I expected, but it worked. I was present again. I was turning left.

I pulled over and began to laugh at myself. The thought of what somebody might have seen if they had been looking through my windshield at that moment rolled over me. I could hear the "Honey, you'll never believe what I saw …"

A few minutes later I was calm, normal, almost myself again. I was feeling a bit raw, but it was almost as if it had never happened. I drove on to continue the search for the wheelchair that we had just begun to need that morning.

* * * * *

A lot has been written about grief. There are theories and books. There are steps and lists and stages of the grieving process. Elizabeth Kubler-Ross and David Kessler wrote one of last century's early contributions with the five stages of grief: denial, anger, bargaining, depression, and, finally, acceptance. Roberta Temes describes three behaviors: numbness, disorganization, and reorganization. I also found a description of seven stages of grief.

The authors of these lists describe that grieving does not come in any particular order, has no particular time frames, and does not necessarily touch each item in their list—or any items, for that matter. Still, we describe it in terms of lists. Making a list about the wide range of emotions that one can experience makes us feel as if we have a little more control of this profound and difficult time. It gives us structure, even if that structure is scant. I believe we have these descriptions of grieving because we are trying to get a handle on something that has no handles. We make lists because we, as human beings, like lists.

Brief Acute Grieving (the Immediate Stuff)

We may not know about time frames or what exactly the griever will experience, but we do know that profound loss can create profound emotions. The parts of the brain associated with sadness can become much more active. They can inhibit the centers that control motivation, memory creation, attachment to others, and executive function. They can hijack the emotional centers altogether. In other words, a wide array of brain regions are affected and the results of that will squeak out in a wide variety of ways. Very strong emotions can be triggered by something outside yourself, like the scent of your loved one's perfume or a color that she wore, or from within, such as a thought or memory. It may even be a thought that never reached your conscious mind, so the emotion really just seems to come out of the blue.

Sometimes powerful, even overwhelming emotions can come on suddenly and leave just as suddenly. They might not always be sadness. Frustration, anger, anxiety, giggling fits, or almost any type of emotion or impulse can roll on slowly or can occur suddenly and then leave a few minutes later. For these types of events, it may be best to recall the third rule of hallucinogenic tripping (from our pals in the '70s): "If anything really weird starts happening, relax, enjoy it, it probably won't last that long."

In other words, don't freak out about the fact that you're freaking out, because that doesn't help. It only adds another layer of trouble. Simply understand that it is part of the experience, it isn't dangerous, it isn't abnormal for someone going through this, and it too will pass. As a physical therapist working on patients' scarred traumatic injuries, I find that patients sometimes will experience a short, intense emotional response. I simply inform them before we begin the procedure that this could happen. If it does happen, the patient, having been warned, simply understands that it is normal and lets it pass.

You also may feel different effects over a longer term. The centers associated with intense sadness can **suppress our motivational centers**. If that is happening, you won't feel motivated to do anything. It will be very difficult to have purpose. It may be difficult to get out of bed, get dressed, interact with people, go to work. If this is coupled with decreased connection with others, it can be tremendously isolating. Accepting that this is normal and not blaming yourself for these feelings is a good first step in dealing with it. Again, you're not freaking out about the fact that you're freaking out. You can allow yourself some time in pajamas; three days is a good rule.

But here is where I differ from some of the list makers. I believe it is important to get these centers of your brain started up again. Ask for help. Have your family members or friends come get you out of bed and take you out to do things that you enjoy and are important to you. Understand that you probably won't enjoy the activity or your family initially, but do go, even if just to go through the motions and have contact with people who love you. Hopefully they will forgive you later for your nasty behavior.

Executive function suppression may also occur with grief. You may find your decision making is impaired. Test it with simple inconsequential things like choosing a new brand of ketchup or cereal at the grocery store. If these decisions are slow or difficult, chances are, it's probably a bad time to talk to the real estate agent. Concentration, memory recall, and memory creation may also be impaired. I like the simple self-test of mental arithmetic, such as number doubling. This is taking a number in your head and continuing to double it until it gets too difficult and you lose concentration. Can you do a three-digit, four-digit, five-digit number, and so on? If you think you are having too much difficulty, try spending a few minutes thinking happy, loving thoughts toward someone and then play this game again.

You may notice other things too. You may notice you are more clumsy, have more aches and pains, get hurt doing simple or repetitive things, have trouble getting to sleep, or have trouble staying asleep. Again, a wide array of brain functions and, thus, body functions are affected when your sadness meter is on high. Step outside yourself a little to take an inventory of these signs and symptoms. You may not be able to fix these things right away, but you can make accommodations for them in your daily life. You may need to be more careful about where you put the car keys or, if your symptoms are severe, avoid driving.

You may need to be better about self-monitoring your feelings toward others. If you are mad at someone, then someone else, then a third person that morning, the anger is probably from you, not from something they did. If you are tripping on the stairs, you can expect yourself not to play such a strong game of tennis. By all means, play tennis, but you can laugh at how bad you are that day. Give yourself allowances and take double precautions for anything you see as being affected. Remember, these things also are temporary. They too will pass. Go back to some of the same practices that kept you healthy as a caregiver (and are useful for the patient too) in Chapter 4, Dancing in the Rain: Healthy Habits for Caregivers, such as exercise for the caregiver, positive journaling, and mindfulness meditation. This will help to restore your brain and body to their full glory and help you continue on in a healthy life.

Lastly, don't be shocked or feel guilty if you are not terribly sad. You may have "processed" it all along the way as it occurred, grieving in the moment. It's possible you feel it deeply, but your brain did not reach the tipping point to make any of the issues discussed in this chapter happen to you. Mostly, do not force emotions on yourself or reach for emotions you think should be there. Simply experience what is. That is enough. You may even consider yourself lucky if you don't spend three days in pajamas or end up slapping yourself in the left-turn lane. Simply make the left turn and get on with the business of living.

Grief in the Longer Term (the More Subtle and Deep)

I wrote the words above while Karen was still sick. Now, eight months after she passed, I am reading them again for probably the 15th time. They are still true and still very helpful, even to me, who wrote them. But these words do not give enough weight to the terrible depth of the experience. So much is written in our world under the horrible pressure of sadness. I could certainly write more. My journals are peppered with pages of words trying to make sense of times that sometimes have no sense at all. What wasn't in the initial draft above is that sometimes the effects of grief are subtle and insidious. They are much more difficult to recognize as grief. You might not be able to hear what's playing in the background inside your head, but the dark noise still affects your mood, your interactions, and your choices.

Again, be gentle with yourself. Allow yourself time. Even if the larger waves of grief are waning, it is important to continue the practices to make you healthy. Again, consider regular intense exercise, positive or gratefulness journaling, and meditation. You should probably add *fun* to the list. I believe that helps a lot. Have you ever tried to be sad on a swing set or frown while skipping?

Be gentle with the ones you love, too. Your mood will affect how you feel about them. How you feel will affect how you react to them, and that will affect how they treat you. It may be subtle enough that you and the people you love don't recognize your behavior as grief. Apply the mad-at-three-people-in-one-morning rule more broadly than just that morning. How many of the people close to you are you mad at or are mad at you? Is it more than three? Reconsider your emotions. Consider apologies. Consider how much you appreciate them. Consider ways to bring them joy. This is part of the practice of gratefulness and gifting. It may help with rebuilding your feelings of appreciation and love and your relationships.

I believe you still may need to make a conscious effort to get out of the house and be with people. Though you certainly should take some time alone, excessive isolation can allow grief to become depression. Contact and connection help guard against the dark ruminations that drive depression. We are social beings, and our minds are stimulated by contact. Stimulation helps. For extroverts, this is much easier. For introverts, it may feel awkward and take what feels like an overwhelming amount of energy. I feel it's critical to muster yourself and spend that energy. You can rebuild it soon enough in your alone time.

With longer-term, more subtle grief, our decision making may be subtly impaired but not enough to show on the changing-ketchup-brands test. Double-check your larger decisions with people you trust. Write out the logic. Read it back to make sure it makes sense. Reconsider your decision on days when you feel good. You probably will need to make some major decisions as you begin to rebuild your life. If you have doubts, ask for help.

In the longer term, it is important to find purpose again. For so long your purpose and focus were about the person you love who was sick. When that person is gone, they leave a hole not only from when they were healthy, but also from when they were sick. We all need a reason to get up in the morning, and now, more than ever, you need to return to your prior passions and find new ones as well. The world is different now and you have much left to give.

Complicated Grief

When grief continues and slips into depression, it becomes what we call "complicated grief." If you feel like this is happening to you or to a loved one, get help. Bouts of major depression can have long-term effects on the brain and on people's lives. We need to treat this like the physiological illness it is.

One in four people who lose their partner will face complicated grief. We don't know exactly what chooses those people, but we do know some of the contributing factors.

Thyroid disease: The thyroid regulates metabolism and energy. We think thyroid disease affects up to 10 percent of sufferers of complicated grief. Tests for thyroid function are simple. Go to your doctor and ask about a thyroid test.

Substance use and abuse: Most of the time when people self-medicate, they choose the wrong drug. Alcohol is a depressant. Despite what the country songs tell you, it only makes depression worse. Any drug that impairs brain function is not healthy to do to a brain that is already having trouble functioning. It's hard to heal and reorganize when you're all doped up. If you suspect that this is a problem, understand that this too is a disease. Seek help. Seek treatment.

Sleep disturbance: Sleep insufficiency, especially of stage three and four restorative sleep, underlies many slow, difficult disease processes. Probably the simplest test lies in the answer to these two questions: Do you feel rested in the morning? When was the last time you got a good night's sleep? Treating sleep disturbance may be simple, or it may be complicated. To get started, see Sleep in Sleepless Times in Chapter 4, Dancing in the Rain: Healthy Habits for Caregivers, and Chapter 14, Sleep.

Avoiding or not being allowed to grieve: The theory on this contributing factor is that, in the grieving process, memories (internal triggers) and associations (external triggers) are gradually processed without the emotional weight that delivers strong blows of sadness or anxiety. Thus, avoiding or not being allowed to grieve prevents the brain from reprocessing these emotional triggers of grieving in combination with less-powerful or destructive emotions. Even if the person doesn't think about what caused their sadness, these circuits of triggers and emotions can run in the background below their conscious level of awareness. Every time these triggers and emotions fire together, the circuits get stronger.

One of the key brain regions associated with sadness is called area CG25, which lives between the *hypothalamus* and the *prefrontal cortex*. This area is very active with incidents of sadness. In grief or depression, the area can become hypermetabolic: its cells become too active and too interconnected and don't seem to shut down. This area's overactivity can alter or shut down function of most other parts of the brain at any given time, leading to a wide range of symptoms or experiences. Stimulating the area causes sadness, negative thinking, social disengagement, lack of motivation, increased cortisol, and decreases in the neuropeptide BDNF, which is crucial to healing neurons and developing new neuron connections.

I suspect that the neural circuits associated with grief, if not disassociated from their strong emotional load, continue to stimulate area CG25. When life spins out of control, the problem only gets worse.

Treating complicated grief is like treating depression—which is, of course, beyond the scope of this book. What I can say here is that if you are reading these words and thinking "That's Aunt Mary" or "Yeah, that's me," please do get professional help. You wouldn't ignore a heart condition; why would you ignore a brain condition? Good medical treatment can help in many ways:

- **Medications and other treatments** can increase levels of certain neurotransmitters to support and improve the function of certain brain cells.
- **Tests** can address and help thyroid function, sleep disorders, and substance abuse and addiction diseases.
- **Cognitive tools** can help with the negative mental cycling and rumination so frequent in this disorder and help people process sadness.
- **Emotional and cognitive assignments** can help stimulate the brain, counteract some of the effects of the disease, and get you back into life.

Many tools and techniques for dealing with depression are discussed in Chapter 4, Dancing in the Rain: Healthy Habits for Caregivers; Eating and Depression in Chapter 12, Food and Nutrition; and Sleep and Depression and/or Anxiety in Chapter 14, Sleep. You can also find a good discussion on physical exercise and a basic exercise program in Chapter 13, Exercise.

All the things said earlier in this chapter about grief still apply with complicated grief, such as don't freak out about the fact that you're freaking out. And if you're not making decisions well, remember that now is not the time to talk with your real estate agent. Addressing rumination and negative or self-destructive thought patterns is a must. Returning to social and enjoyable activities is crucial. Mostly, see if you can do something every day that makes you feel alive.

I leave you with this thought from Winston Churchill:

"If you must walk through the valley of the shadow of death ... just don't stop."

Interlude

Celebrating the Time You Have

When you're falling off a great cliff, you could scream and kick helplessly at the air, or perhaps you could celebrate the flight, doing as many back flips as you might possibly be able to. The ground is coming either way.

No one can tell you how get the most out of life. Living fully means whatever it means to you. I don't believe it means to live without fear or hardship, for they are certainly part of life. I think that to accept the fear and embrace the hardships, to dive in knowing that it might be difficult and do it anyway, helps us grab hold of the very essence of life.

Loving deeply, be it people, creatures, or just this wonderful world and all the experiences and adventures it offers us, breathes life into each moment. In this way we live passionately, thoughtfully, in this present moment.

Consider those who might spend their whole lives wrapped up in what was or worried about what will be, never actually being here now. Faced with the imminent sense that life is indeed finite, that the ground is coming, we are *here now*.

Being in the present moment is another of the great unexpected gifts of this whole experience. I don't remember when Karen and I made the decision to live deeply, to celebrate each breath even if it hurt, to do what we can as we can. Even so, it turns out that this became the most important decision we ever made. Somewhere between a bucket list and the joys of the normal, mundane moments seen anew, we found love again. We found meaning. We faced death. Life stared back at us. What else could we do? Kicking at the air never works anyhow.

* * * * *

Part 2. Legal, Financial, and Insurance Issues

"Other lawyers wonder how I manage to choose such nice families."

I'm speaking with my mom's estate attorney. Her affairs are in order, wonderfully in order. Everything is clear.

"They wonder why so few of my families end up in litigation," he says. "It's not about being nice. My families are no nicer or any less litigious than anyone else. It's because we set everything up clearly so that everyone knows what their role is and what to expect. If everything is clear, there is very little room for arguments."

One of the best ways the care *receiver* can help their loved ones is to make everything as clear as possible. Unlike Part 1 and Part 3, written for the caregiver, Part 2 is written for the care receiver. Much of the information in this part of the book is here to help you help the ones you love as they care for you. Your most trusted caregivers and family can help you set your affairs in order, along with your lawyer.

Chapter 6.
The Notebook of Important Papers

Many people likely have done much of the work of putting their legal and financial houses in order already. For those who haven't or aren't sure whether they've covered everything, let's start with creating a **notebook or folder for copies of your important documents and instructions**.

This chapter describes the basic list of what goes in your notebook of important papers. The list here is a bit long, but that's because not everything here will apply to every person. As we further discuss some items, the list of what applies to you will shorten. You don't need to fret about how long the list is just yet.

To begin with, **your address book** will help your caregivers contact and inform your friends and relatives about your situation. This collection of names and contact information may be just as helpful for your caregivers as it is for you. Make sure you provide them with access to your address book or a copy of it, or a list of the people in it they should know about and contact for you. If you don't keep a written address book, it's time to create one. This can be a separate book from the Notebook of Important Papers, but it needs to be there in some findable, readable form that your loved ones can access and understand.

Identity Papers

Typically if you are a citizen and you aren't planning on leaving the country, a copy of your drivers license or personal identity card is enough to satisfy most requests for identification.

Divorce records and death certificates of spouse or parents may be necessary for someone trying to manage your bank or financial matters, as the banks may question if your spouse, ex-spouse, or parents might have claim on or control of your accounts. If you've never divorced or are remarried, or if your parents would be too old to be reasonably living, divorce records and death certificates may not be an issue. If you share your spouse's last name, marriage certificates are not usually necessary either.

Military service records are required if you will be dealing with the Department of Veterans Affairs. Below is a list of identity papers that you might potentially need to include in your notebook:

- Copy of drivers license
- Copy of passport
- Citizenship papers
- Social Security number
- Birth certificate
- Marriage certificate
- Death certificates of spouse or parents
- Divorce records
- Military record or, more exactly, record of military service

Medical Information

You will definitely need the first two items on the list below: your doctor's contact information and your insurance information. Health records, current medication list, and family history will help your caregivers. If you don't have this information, next time you are at your primary-care doctor's office, you can request it. Some medical records have a face sheet with a current medication list, current issues list, and allergies. This is what you and your caregivers want.

- **Doctors' contact information.** List your health-care providers by specialty. Indicate where your medical records are kept—this is usually with your primary-care physician's office. Many doctor's offices now have on line systems which allow their patients to do things like refill prescriptions, see test results or make appointments. Check with your doctor's office to find out what their system requires if you want to grant someone access in this way.
- **Insurance policies**. List your policies, including health, life, long-term care, disability, etc. Include policy number, contact information for your agent or the company, and instructions as to where to find your files with the complete policies. Some insurance companies have internet access to account and billing information. Collect and record the information you need to access the site. Contact your insurance company customer service to ask about granting access for someone you would designate to represent you to also access the site.
- **Health records.** Include a brief overview of your health records, such as any allergies—especially to medicines; history of ongoing health problems such as high blood pressure, osteoporosis, cancer or history of cancer, joint replacements, major bone breaks or other orthopedic problems that you still notice, and anything else that affects your health or may affect your treatment.
- **Current medications.** List what meds you are currently taking, including how often you take them, dosage, and what these medications are supposed to treat. If you've had poor reactions to certain medications in the past, you may write that here too.
- **Family medical history.** Include cancers, heart disease, brain disease or dementia, and anything else you think is important.

...Authorization to Disclose Personal Health Information

Health-care facilities and doctors' offices normally have an ethical code of protecting peoples' medical information. Now there are strict rules codifying this within the law we call HIPAA (Health Insurance Portability and Accountability Act). If you want to give someone other than yourself and your next of kin access to your personal medical information, you may need to sign an authorization to disclose personal health information. This will be kept on file at that office where you sign it.

Medicare has its own form, of course, called the Medicare authorization to disclose personal health information. You can fill it out online at https://www.medicare.gov/MedicareOnlineForms or call to request a copy (1-800-633-4227).

Financial Information

Anyone trying to help you manage your accounts and your financial matters will pretty much need everything on this list that you have. Sorry. Hopefully your records are clear and you can easily pull this together.

- **Any bank and financial institution accounts you have.** List them all, and include account numbers and your contact at the institution(s) if you have one. Include instructions as to where to find your financial files. You may include the approximate value of your accounts and the date of this valuation.
- **Information regarding your home.** Include instructions on where to find your files for deed and mortgage information, title, house insurance policy, etc.
- **Information on any other assets you have.** This might include a business you own, rental property, shares or interest in financial ventures, etc.
- **Information regarding your car.** Include the location of the title to your car, the car insurance policy, and the car keys.
- **Any debt accounts you have.** Include credit cards, car loans, home equity loans, etc.
- **Your attorney.** If you have one, list your attorney's name and their contact information.
- **Your tax files.** Instructions as to where to find your information for your federal, state, and local filings.
- **Any safe deposit boxes.** Include their location, a brief list of their contents, and where to find keys. You might wish to make arrangements for a trusted caregiver to have access to your safe deposit box(es).
- **Any safes or lockboxes.** If you have any, include their location, their contents, and where to find the combination and/or keys.
- **Any other security information.** Include a list of your computer and internet accounts and passwords, any other kinds of lock locations and combinations, and any other keys that the person you choose to represent you might need.

Records of Your Wishes

Each item in this list is described in greater detail in this section. Different states may have different requirements, but this list should give you a very good general idea.

- Advance directives
- Physician's orders for life-sustaining treatment (POLST)
- Letter of instruction
- Ethical will
- Last will and testament
- Durable power of attorney
- Living trust documents

...Advance Directives

These are your "what if" documents. Basically, these documents come into play anytime you cannot make decisions for yourself.

Medical Power of Attorney

The first part of an advanced directive appoints your medical power of attorney (which also may be called your **health care proxy**). This is a person designated to make medical decisions for you should you be unable to do so. They can help guide medical professionals with your wishes about what they should or shouldn't do.

This document doesn't grant any power over financial decisions or duties. That is what the durable power of attorney is for (discussed later in this section).

Usually people designate a first person and a second person in case the first for some reason cannot fulfill the responsibilities. If you don't have a medical power of attorney, there is a usual "order of surrogacy" that the state where you reside may apply in an attempt to designate one for you:

1. Guardian
2. Spouse
3. Adult children
4. Parents
5. Adult siblings
6. Grandchildren

You can see that this list may create problems, as the surrogate the state designates may not be the person you think should speak for you. Also, there may be more than one person in a group, such as more than one adult child. Consider the words of my mother's wise attorney: Eliminate the ambiguity, and you may eliminate potentially painful arguments.

Living Will

The second part of the advance directives is the **living will**. This document is where you may be as specific as you can be about what you might want done when, and when you might not want that done anymore. It covers such scenarios as, if you are in a permanently unconscious state, would you want treatments such as CPR, defibrillation, ventilators, and artificial feeding?

These are difficult scenarios to contemplate and difficult decisions to make. If your mind is not clear on these questions, or if you are having difficulty thinking of them at all, you might want to open the discussion with your most trusted doctor, mentor, or clergy. If it is difficult for you, think of how difficult it could be for your family if they don't know your wishes. You don't want your loved ones trying to guess about these things. Any arguments about these decisions can be catastrophic.

There is a very good little book to help you that many hospital and hospice organizations have for their patients called *Hard Choices for Loving People* by Hank Dunn http://hankdunn.com/purchase/hard-choices-for-loving-people. The Conversation Project http://theconversationproject.org/ is also there to help you talk about end of life care. Take time to think through your choices well. These are *your choices*.

The living-will form is very simple, but it varies state by state. It is available at most doctors' offices, hospitals, hospice organizations, and nursing homes. You may find your state's form online by searching "advance directives" and the name of your state. The form needs to be signed by two "disinterested witnesses." This means a friend who is not related, not a spouse, and not in your will. In most states, this form does not need to be notarized unless there is no other witness. Give copies of this form to your primary-care physician for your medical records and to your medical power of attorneys, keep one in your records, and put one in your notebook of important information.

Make sure your medical power of attorneys understand your choices. Your preferences may change over time, and you are free to redo the advance directives anytime. You can also just destroy the documents, write a revocation, or just tell your doctor and your medical power of attorneys. Also, this document is in effect only while you are unable to voice your own decisions. If you become clear and able to communicate again, all is back to normal—you will make your own decisions.

...POLST

The physician's order for life-sustaining treatment (POLST) is a simple one-page form your physician or most any care facility should have. It may vary somewhat state by state. The POLST gives instructions to caregivers and first responders regarding your wishes about CPR, medical interventions such as ventilation, and intravenous (IV) fluids. It's an important document for anyone to have who is facing serious illness or frailty, because using these more heroic measures to prolong life might only cause more pain and suffering.

It is a physician's order, so it needs to be signed by your doctor, their physician's assistant, or their nurse practitioner. It can go in your medical chart if you are in a care facility. If you are at home, it should go in your Carebook or in an obvious place where a first responder might look for it, such as on the outside of the refrigerator or the front of a kitchen cabinet. You can also keep a copy in your notebook of important papers. Like any physician's order, you can change it at any time; the most recent one overrides any previous order.

...Letter of Instruction and Ethical Will

A **letter of instruction** is not a legal document and you don't have to write one ... but you may want to. A simple letter to your loved ones can help you convey your deeper wishes for your life, their lives, and the many things you have learned and may want to share. It begins as a blank page. You are free to write what you want. You can discuss how your more personal effects should be carried forward.

I remember Karen's things were to be given to people who would love them as she did. This inspired our creation of gift boxes. You can discuss how you would like your life celebrated, particulars of your wake or funeral, even your obituary. These things can be described in a will, but in a letter of instruction, they can be more personal, without the constraints of the legal document.

In an **ethical will** you can share stories, give blessings, and discuss hopes for the future. If, like this e-book, you use a digital format, you can share music, poetry, and pictures. You can do anything you want. You can even tell little Johnny one more time to quit hitting his sister. There are books written to help you; *Ethical Wills: Putting Your Values on Paper* by Barry K. Baines, MD. You can find many amazing examples of ethical wills by simply searching "ethical wills" online.

...Will

Your last will and testament is the legal document regarding your wishes and instructions for your executor as to what should happen with all the material possessions of your estate. Even if you have only a few personal items and tangible assets such as a house or car, you should create this with the assistance of a qualified estate attorney. With an attorney you may discuss probate and vehicles that may make probate simpler or avoidable altogether, such as trusts and joint tenancy.

The notebook of your important personal documents should not necessarily contain your will. It should, however, have the contact information of the attorney who is holding your will or specific instructions on where your will is kept. If you keep a copy of your will, your notebook of important papers should also state where that copy of your will is kept, who the executor is, and the date of the last revision.

Think again of my mother's wise attorney's words. I do not recommend plug-and-play will formats you may get off the internet for exactly that reason. Doing it right is doing a favor for your loved ones.

...Durable Power of Attorney

There may come a time when you want to designate one of your loved ones to be able to manage your financial and legal affairs. The durable power of attorney is a legal document that allows you to designate a person or people to act in your behalf for legal and financial concerns. You are then the principal, and they become your *attorney in fact*. Most people designate a second person as well in case the first can't perform the duties for some reason.

What you designate your attorney in fact can do for you can be as general or specific and limited as you want it to be. Normally the document takes effect on signing, but you can make it provisional on something like your doctor's certification that you can't at that point make decisions or speak for yourself (springing power of attorney). You may use a general form or may draft one with your lawyer. Chances are, a lawyer will also provide good legal advice regarding uses and options. The form must be signed and witnessed and, in some states, notarized. A copy should be kept by your attorney, one should be kept in your records, one should be given to your designated attorneys in fact, and one should be included in your notebook of important papers. You will want more copies for your financial institutions—they will usually make a copy of the one your attorney in fact brings in.

For an example of a general durable power of attorney form, try http://www.free-legal-document.com/free-durable-power-of-attorney.html and for a springing power of attorney try https://www.justice.gov.nt.ca/en/files/power-of-attorney/Springing%20Power%20of%20Attorney.pdf.

To use the power of attorney document, have the attorney in fact present it (along with adequate identification) to your financial institutions. If you can go with them, all the better. The institution may have them sign an affidavit and may have a short waiting period for consulting their legal staff before accepting it. Once that institution has established the person as your attorney in fact, they may act in your behalf to do all the things that you would do.

They are bound by the document and by law to be prudent and exercise reasonably good care in what they do for you. They are legally bound to act in your interest. When a person is signing something as your attorney in fact, have them designate that they are signing for you, something like "Karen Morgan, by Dave Leffmann as her attorney in fact."

Shared Bank Accounts etc.

Wouldn't it just be easier to add your loved one to your bank account rather than designating a power of attorney? This would allow them to make your deposits and pay your bills without the formalities and legal cost associated with a durable power of attorney or a living trust. In some cases, this is a good idea. If you fully trust the person, if your account is relatively small, and if you do not anticipate needing or qualifying for Medicaid, then yes, having a shared bank account is simpler.

There are a number of things to consider before choosing this route, however. If the account is shared in such a way that any of the people on the account (tenants) can conduct business, like writing and signing checks or paying bills (rather than all the tenants needing to sign), then any of the people on the account can withdraw funds, even all the funds, and do whatever they want with it. Also, they have access to bank statements, so they can see exactly what you have in your account. If a tenant has a debt, their creditor can seek funds from that account to satisfy the debt.

In the eyes of the IRS, adding someone to your bank account is like giving them a share in your funds. It may be subject to gift tax. The annual exempt amount at the time of this writing is $13,000. If you add one person, they will need to pay federal income tax on half of any amount over $26,000 in your account. If you gave them anything else that year, it will add to the amount subject to gift tax. Also, it will count against the IRS's allowable lifetime maximum per recipient per benefactor. The IRS tries to be fair, they won't count any contributions the person you added makes to your account. They will need to be able to show the IRS proof of their contributions (with deposit slips for instance).

Medicaid's eligibility requirements stipulate that the applicant not give large sums of money or assets away or sell things at far below market value for five years before applying. This is to keep people from hiding their assets in order to qualify for Medicaid. If a shared bank account is titled so that either can sign (Sally *or* John), Medicaid looks at the full amount in the accounts, even joint accounts. If the account is titled so that both must sign (Sally *and* John), then Medicaid will see it as a gift and may apply a five-year waiting period to be eligible.

Money in a joint account will automatically transfer to the surviving tenant. This means it is not subject to probate. It also means that it is not subject to your will, so it may bypass some of your other loved ones when you consider how you want your estate disbursed. This situation can be contested in court and can become a huge source of family problems. Again, consider the wisdom of my mother's attorney.

Some states allow the creation of a convenience account. This allows someone you designate to access the account for your benefit only. It is kind of like having a power of attorney for that account only. The signer (not a tenant) does not own the money in the account—they only have access to it and are answerable to you.

This very good article on pros and cons of joint accounts also has links to other great legal articles http://www.elderlawanswers.com/be-aware-of-the-dangers-of-joint-accounts-7575.

...Living Trusts

A living (or revocable) trust sets aside certain assets you designate into a separate account. This is like a separate ownership. It then allows you to name someone to manage the trust: the trustee. In this document, you can name yourself as trustee and then name a successor trustee in case you are incapacitated or pass on. Unlike the durable power of attorney, the living trust extends beyond your life. It is another way assets avoid probate. It may save your loved ones enough money and heartache to easily make up for the attorney's fee in setting it up. The terms of the trust can act as terms of a will.

The down sides are that all your assets will need to be renamed or retitled to be in the name of the trust. The trust must file its own taxes as well. If you are the grantor creator of the trust, as well as the trustee, the IRS sees through this and you can simply account for the income on your personal income tax filing. Naming someone else as a trustee gives them the ability only to manage items in the trust. They will still need a power of attorney to act in any other affairs such as signing contracts for you and so on.

...Estate Planning (Here's Where I Punt)

There are many other aspects to estate planning. This is a book about caregiving, so any information in this chapter does not constitute legal advice, and any discussion beyond the basic tools described in this chapter should be with your estate attorney.

Chapter 7.
The Importance of Exercise

If you're reading this, you are probably swimming forehead-deep in the thick of all the legal, financial, and insurance paperwork. You might just take a few minutes to go out, work up a good sweat doing whatever you love to do, feel better, clear your head, get some good ideas that solve some of these problems you are facing, and come back to finish reading Part 2 of this book. Exercise is so important to our general health and well-being that the subject just sneaks into every part of this book, even this one. Yes, this book was written by a physical therapist.

    Enjoy.

Chapter 8.
Medicare, Medicaid, and Private Insurance

Private insurance companies are not there to help you. They are there to sell you a policy; then, when you make a claim against that policy, they are there to fulfill their legal obligations. Some of the more enlightened companies believe that it is actually good business to help you, and some of the kinder and more caring claims managers take this as their mission. If this is your experience, consider yourself lucky. Otherwise, be very wary of the details of the policy.

Medicare, Medicaid, and the Department of Veterans Affairs are federal programs or agencies that are actually there to help you. That is their mission. That is why we created them. However, they have fallen prey to people who have abused their help to the tune of, by some estimates, billions of dollars. So, like any great bureaucracy administered by lawmakers and bureaucrats, they have imposed cumbersome and sometimes ridiculous rules. These rules, which may have initially been intended to protect them from abuse, now stand in the way of them helping those who need it. Just to make matters a little more difficult, these government organizations don't employ salespeople like the insurance industry does. Your interaction may be with someone more intent on the rules than you might like.

Still, in these seemingly blank gray monoliths of government institutions, the people are in fact people. They have ears and eyes and hearts. Just like you. And they do want to help. It is their mission. It is why they go to work every day.

My mom used to say, "They really want to take care of this, they just don't know that yet." She was a tax accountant who routinely dealt with an even bigger governmental monolith: the Internal Revenue Service. This was kind of her soft-spoken battle cry as she would then go about the patient, somewhat meticulous task of calmly showing them that they really did want to take care of things and decide in her favor. I hope you may hold on to her bit of wisdom in all your dealings with our third-party-payer system of health insurance, Medicare, and Medicaid.

Medicare

Medicare is a federal health insurance program for people 65 and older, as well as people of any age with certain disabilities or diseases. It was originally created during the Johnson presidency in response to the plight of older Americans struggling with being unable to afford medical care. This was a time when we were building hospitals and other health-care institutions all over the country. It began with parts A and B and, over the years, has been modified and expanded to include parts C and D.

Over the years the rules and exceptions have evolved with amazing complexity. In this chapter, we hope to give you an overview but there's much more to it than can be explained here. 1800 MEDICARE (1-800-633-4227) and your Statewide Health Insurance Benefit Advisors (SHIBA) may be your best two resources to help guide you through the details that are important to you.

> If you are 65 years old or older and are not enrolled in Medicare, enroll now, at the next enrollment period. If you don't currently have health insurance, there is no good reason for not enrolling, and sometimes there are waiting periods and penalties if you don't sign up as soon as you are eligible. Jump straight to Enrollment and Premiums below, or go Medicare https://www.medicare.gov/ to enroll.

...Parts Overview

Medicare part A: This is federal hospital insurance that began in 1966. It covers hospitalizations, home health care, hospice, and the first 20 out of 100 days of skilled nursing care (see What the Plans Cover later in this section) and you will pay a deductible.

It doesn't cover doctors' charges in the hospital. That is covered under Medicare part B (see below) and only at 80 percent. It doesn't cover a private room unless medically necessary, phone and TV if the hospital charges extra for these, or personal-care items like razors or socks. To be considered an inpatient, you have to be "admitted" to the hospital. Just staying the night, such as if you spend the night in the emergency room, doesn't necessarily mean that you were admitted.

Medicare part B: This is federal outpatient insurance that began in 1966. It covers outpatient care, doctors' charges, home health care, durable medical equipment (DME), and some preventive services. With these plans, you have nearly full choice of doctors, hospitals, and everything else, but you may have to pay deductibles and co-insurance payments (copays). Because there is a low premium to pay, most people are not enrolled automatically when they turn 65. If you go without some form of coverage after you are eligible, there is a penalty when you do sign up.

Medicare part C: These are the managed care plans for Medicare which began in the 1990s. Another name for these is Medicare Advantage plans. These subsidized plans are run by private insurance companies, and they follow similar managed-care models (health maintenance organizations, preferred provider organizations, etc.) offered by private health-care insurance discussed later in this chapter. There are different levels of coverage you can buy, but the plans must meet at least a base minimum of coverage set by Medicare. Because Med C is run by different companies that differ in different regions of the United States, the plans vary by company and by region. In many plans, you are restricted to using the company's providers or risk paying partial or full costs yourself (private pay). All plans include all benefits and services covered under Medicare parts A and B. They usually include drug coverage and may include other benefits too.

Medicare part D: This is federal drug coverage plan began in 2003. This plan was pushed through under George W. Bush, so ... well, the way it works is quite convoluted and leaves many people scratching their heads. You may see what I mean later in this chapter when I get more into the specifics of how Medicare works. In short, these plans are administered by private insurance companies and they vary by company and by region—similar to Med C. To get Med D coverage, you need to sign up and will pay a premium. There is also a penalty for going without drug coverage and then signing up later.

Medigap policies: Also called Medicare Supplemental Insurance, these are private insurance plans that promise to cover part or all of the copays that Medicare A and B do not cover. Most of these plans do not expand coverage; they only cover the copay, coinsurance, and deductible amounts. Medicare pays first, then the Medigap plan fills in.

...Who Is Eligible for Medicare

Generally, you are eligible for Medicare if you:

- are nearly 65 (eligible on your 65th birthday but can sign up three months before that)
- paid into the system with Social Security taxes for 10 years
- are a US citizen or meet the "Lawful Presence and Residency requirements"

You also may be eligible if you have a disability, have ALS (Lou Gehrig's Disease), or have end-stage renal disease. To find out if you are eligible, go to https://www.medicare.gov/people-like-me/new-to-medicare/getting-started-with-medicare.html.

...Enrollment and Premiums

Enrollment in **Med A** begins three months before your 65th birthday and extends three months after. After that, you have to wait for the next annual enrollment period: January 1 to March 31. Coverage starts in July. If you have COBRA (employer-based insurance that can be extended after you leave that employer, if you pay all premiums), private insurance not with an employer group, Tricare (military), or Medicaid, you still need to apply. If you are over 65 and coming off of your employer's insurance, you have eight months to apply. If you are switching coverage, the period is October 15 through December 7, with change implementation on January 1.

Some people will be signed up automatically and for free. If you are already getting benefits from Social Security or the Railroad Retirement board, you may receive your red, white, and blue Medicare card in the mail three months before your 65th birthday. If so, you are signed up. If you expect a card and it didn't arrive, call to make sure they have your correct address (1-800-772-1213).

Because there is a cost to **Med B and D**, or **Med C**, the federal government does not sign you up automatically for those. Most people will need to sign up. The costs to you are low, subsidized by the Medicare system, so even at the highest rates the costs are much lower than purchasing private health insurance.

For **Med A and B,** enrollment forms are available through the office of **Social Security**. It's probably easiest online at https://www.ssa.gov/medicare/apply.html for Med A only or https://search.ssa.gov/search?affiliate=ssa&query=medicare+application for a more general link that directly allows access to Med A and B application and other helpful applications and information.

For **Med C, Med D,** and **Medicare Supplemental Insurance (Medigap)** plans, perhaps the best tool is the handy **Medicare Plan Finder** tool https://www.medicare.gov/find-a-plan/questions/home.aspx. Because these plans are all offered by private insurance companies, Medicare offers this tool that works from your zip code. This tool also helps you compare plans, considers your current medication list and pharmacy, and gives you Medicare's star rating system, which actually does seem to be helpful. It gives you a nice spreadsheet format with plan basics, including estimated annual costs, copays and deductibles, and a link directly to the enrollment process.

What if you don't want Med D? You don't have to get Med D, but if you have no insurance and do qualify for it, the premium costs are so low that it would be silly not to sign up. Remember that if you wait, that cost will go up due to a penalty for not signing up right away and that will stay with you forever. If you have prescription drug coverage based on your current or previous employment, your employer or union will notify you each year to let you know if your prescription drug coverage is creditable. Keep the information papers they give you. Call your benefits administrator for more information before making any changes to your coverage. **Note:** If you join a Medicare drug plan, you, your spouse, or your dependents may lose your employer or union health coverage.

There are exceptions and more specifics to the enrollment period rules for people who have other insurance or are currently receiving assistance from state or other disability programs. Also make sure you let Medicare know if you have any kind of other health-care coverage. There is a place for this on the application, and you can also do this by calling **Medicare's Benefits Coordination and Recovery Center** (BCRC; 1-855-798-2627). You will find more details in section 2 of the "Medicare and You" booklet you get from Medicare. If you need one, type "Medicare and You" and the year into your search engine.

Getting Help

Your state may have programs that may help people with low income, but not low enough to qualify for Medicaid, to pay the Medicare premiums and costs. **Medicare Savings Programs** can help with Med A and B premiums, copays, and deductibles. **Extra Help** or other Med D assistance programs can help with prescription drug costs. Contact your state's insurance commissioner or health insurance benefit advisor to see what your state offers and whether you may qualify. You can find a more complete discussion on this in Paying for the Pills in Chapter 11, Medications.

Penalty for Not Signing Up Right Away

To try to add incentive for people who would choose to not have insurance, then just sign up when they get sick, the rule makers have added a late enrollment penalty to **Medicare B and D.**

If you have insurance—say, through your spouse's employer plan—there is no penalty. There are some funny exceptions to this: If your coverage is through the Department of Veterans Affairs, a retiree plan, a COBRA plan, or an individual plan not related to your employer, someone in the rules department decided that they *do* want you to sign up for Medicare as soon as you're eligible. If you have doubts about how this rule will apply to your insurance, call -800-MEDICARE for assistance.

If you currently have drug coverage benefits—say, through your employer group policy—contact that insurance company before you sign on to **Med D.** If your drug coverage is dropped because you joined Med D, you might not be able to get it back.

For **Med B** (and if you have to pay for **Med A**), the late-enrollment penalty adds 10 percent per 12-month period that you are late. For example, if you are late by 28 months, that's two-plus years, so add 20 percent of the $121.80 per month (in 2016) for Med B, which would be $24.36 per month (in 2016), to the base rate.

Med D gives you a two-month (63-day) grace period, so that 28 months you were late in enrolling in Med B would be 26 months late in enrolling in Med D. Add 1 percent per month, times the base rate of $34.00 per month (in 2016), which would be

$8.84 per month (in 2016), which gets rounded down to $8.80. This penalty stays with you for the rest of the time you have Medicare—essentially the rest of your life.

Choosing a Plan or Switching to a Different Plan

The **Medicare Plan Finder** https://www.medicare.gov/find-a-plan/questions/home.aspx/ allows you to look through the Med C and D plans offered in your zip code area and compare by costs and benefits, and it gives a rating system based on customer experience and oversight agencies' experience with the companies. The site actually is easy to use and works well. Open enrollment is October 15 to December 7. Med C and Med D plans change each year, so it's a good idea to review the plan and medication **formulary** (list of the drugs they cover) before these dates.

Whether you're looking into Medicare for the first time or wanting to change plans, it's important to think about what you need in health-care benefits:

- Does the plan you have, or the ones you're looking at, include your primary-care doctor?
- Does it include the specialists you want?
- Is your new medication covered?

If you're already in a Medicare Advantage plan and want to **switch to a new Medicare Advantage plan,** simply join the plan you choose during one of the enrollment periods. You'll be disenrolled automatically from your old plan when your new plan's coverage begins.

To **switch to Original Medicare,** contact your current plan or call Medicare (1-800-MEDICARE or 1-800-633-4227; TTY users should call 1-877-486-2048). If you don't have drug coverage, consider joining a Medicare Prescription Drug Plan (Med D). You may also want to consider Medicare Supplement Insurance (Medigap).

If for some reason you want to **disenroll from Medicare**, call Medicare (1-800-MEDICARE or 1-800-633-4227; TTY users should call 1-877-486-2048). You can also send a letter to the plan to tell them you want to disenroll. Like enrollment, disenrollment takes place at certain times. Don't just stop paying the premium—that's breach of contract. For Med C or Med D, contact the company that runs the plan. If you drop your plan and want to re-enroll later, you will have to wait for the next enrollment period and may have to face the penalty. This is to keep people from enrolling only when they want to go to the doctor.

...Getting Help Navigating the System

Medicare programs are complex, multilayered, and frequently changing. They have evolved over time as successive political administrations have added programs and tweaked the rules, all the while wrestling with a contingent in our national politics trying to make Medicare fail because they believe it shouldn't exist. Medicare has struggled with fraud and abuse by its users as well as with all the internal problems of any large organization. To try to convey all the complexity of this system in this book and to try to read and absorb all of that as a caregiver would be silly.

Fortunately, there are good people to help you figure out Medicare. Each state has a **State Health Insurance Program** (SHIP). Within each state SHIP office, a staff of helpful volunteers work to help solve health-insurance and Medicare/Medicaid problems for good people like you. The names vary by state but you can link to your state's **SHIP** https://www.shiptacenter.org/.

Medicare itself is quite helpful, though there is usually some hold time to reach them by telephone (1-800-MEDICARE or 1-800-633-4227; TTY users should call 1-877-486-2048).

Your local **Area Agency on Aging** has resources and helpful people who may be able to help you navigate the system or at least point you in the right direction. Find your local agency by typing "Area Agency on Aging" into your search engine or enter your zip code in the national site http://www.n4a.org/.

Elder law attorneys and assistance can help. The **National Academy of Elder Law Attorneys** https://www.naela.org/ can help you find one in your area. The **National Legal Resource Center** http://nlrc.acl.gov/Services_Providers/Index.aspx can help connect you with legal assistance and other resources in your state.

There is more information in this book regarding Medicare and paying for specific needs in the chapters that deal with those issues: See Longer-Term Medical and Residential Facilities in Chapter 10, Hospitals and Other Medical Facilities; Paying for the Pills in Chapter 11, Medications; and Obtaining and Paying for Mobility and Assistive Devices in Chapter 15, Basic Mobility and Transfers.

...What the Plans Cover

Med A

Hospitals: Medicare A pays for the first 60 days of hospitalization with a deductible only. Then you pay a copay and deductible for days 61 through 90. This can be quite a lot of money. You have 60 days of "lifetime reserve days" in a hospital for above 90 days. Inpatient psychiatric care is limited to 190 days in a lifetime.

Skilled-nursing facilities: Medicare A can pay for 100 days in nursing homes following a medically related three-night hospitalization. It will pay the first 20 days in full, then require a copay for the next 80 days. The copay can be quite high, adding up to thousands of dollars. Still, it is a fraction of the total bill, and they have negotiated (if you can call "take what Med A pays or not be able to serve most of your clients" a negotiation) a lower rate than you could get on your own.

Hospice: Medicare A pays fully for hospice care, except you will pay a $5 per-prescription copay for outpatient drugs. You pay 5 percent of the Medicare-approved amount for inpatient respite care.

Med B

The list of what is covered and how much you will be responsible for under Medicare part B is far too long for this book to tackle item by item. The "Medicare and You" booklet's section 3 has this in an alphabetized easy-to-read format. There are specific notes about coverage in the different chapters of this book. What I can say here is that long-term care is not covered under Med B (or Med A or anything else in Medicare). Neither are dentistry, dentures, hearing aids, eye exams and glasses, cosmetic surgery, or acupuncture. An excellent site on costs and benefits is https://www.medicare.gov/your-medicare-costs/costs-at-a-glance/costs-at-glance.html#collapse-4808. Find out more about long-term care regarding Medicare, Medicaid, and the VA from this good site http://longtermcare.gov/medicare-medicaid-more/. If you need a Medicare and You booklet type "Medicare and You" and the year into your browser for a pdf download.

Med C (Medicare Advantage Plans)

These plans are offered by private insurance companies and their contracted providers. Medicare pays them a fixed amount each month for your care. They must cover all the services covered in the Med A and Med B plans except hospice and clinical research (which may be very important for cancer patients), and they may offer you more services at less out-of-pocket cost to you. Most offer a drug benefit program that serves as their Med D portion, and they may offer vision and dental. There are several different models, which reflect the models of insurance currently offered by private insurance companies:

- preferred provider organization (PPO)
- health maintenance organization (HMO)
- fee-for-service model
- medical savings accounts
- HMO fee-for-service plan

These plans have all the benefits and difficulties of private insurance. This is discussed in Private Health-care Insurance later in this chapter. Many of the models of these plans limit your choice of providers, and you may pay more for Med C plans than for a combination of Med B and Med D plans. Rules of the Med C plans may change from year to year. You need to read the contract sections called "Evidence of Coverage" and "Annual Notice of Change."

Other Medicare Plans Beyond Med C

Medicare also has a few plans that private insurance does not have that could be tremendously helpful. These aren't necessarily Med C.

Special needs plans (SNPs) cater to a special group (such as people who live in an institution like a nursing home or who have HIV/AIDS) defined by each plan. These plans generally have a network of providers, require a primary-care physician and their referral for specialty care, and offer drug benefits. These plans do try to encourage coordination of services in an attempt to keep people as healthy as possible.

To qualify to be enrolled in an SNP, you would need to have Medicare A and B or Medicare C. If you live in a nursing home or other institution, or need nursing care at home, you may qualify. You may also qualify if you have a severe or disabling chronic condition or have both Medicare and Medicaid. The plans vary by region. Check with your social worker to see if you might qualify and if this could help.

Many states have programs for All-inclusive Care for the Elderly (**PACE) plans** from Medicare and Medicaid that help people who would otherwise need nursing-home-level care to remain in the community (their home). PACE provides many services, including prescription drugs, doctor and other practitioner visits, transportation, home care, hospital visits, and nursing-home care when necessary. To qualify you must be 55 or older, be certified in your state as needing nursing-home level of care, and be able to safely live in the community with the help of PACE.

There is a premium cost for the long-term care, but if you have Medicaid, you won't have to pay the premium. If you think this could help you, find out more at https://www.medicare.gov/your-medicare-costs/help-paying-costs/pace/pace.html.

Medicare Cost plans are offered by some private insurance companies in some parts of the country. These plans offer many of the benefits of a PPO plan but allow you to see an "out-of-network" provider too.

Med D

Med D is also contracted out to private insurance companies. Like Med C, plans differ by different regions and are not necessarily standardized. You need to pay close attention to the policy details. All plans have a specific formulary of the drugs they cover. Drugs that are not on the formulary are not covered, and you will need to file an exception if you hope to get those drugs covered. Check to see if the medications you need are on the formulary of the plan you are considering. Keep in mind that some medications can be ridiculously expensive, more than $20,000 per year.

Plans may contain some interesting language that makes getting coverage for your prescriptions more difficult. You can ask for an exception for the rules below, but that's yet another hoop to jump through and no guarantees:

Prior authorization: This means that you and/or your prescribing doctor must gain authorization from the insurance company before they will cover the drug. This may make things difficult if it's something you need right away.

Quantity limits: This limits how much of a medication you can get at one time. You should be able to get a month's worth.

Step therapy: This means you must try one or more similar, lower-cost drugs before the plan will cover the drug your doctor actually recommends.

Now, your doctor must be a Medicare provider for Medicare D to cover the medication. They do give a three-month provisional period for your doctor to enroll. Chances are, the doctor has strong reasons of their own not to be enrolled, so they won't enroll just so you can get Med D coverage.

Most Med D plans have a deductible. This means that you will pay the full cost of medications until the deductible is met. Then there is a copay amount and/or a coinsurance amount—you pay a percentage of the cost.

Then there is the **doughnut hole:** After you meet your deductible, there is a gap in coverage that begins after you and your plan have spent a certain amount for covered drugs (noncovered drugs aren't included in figuring the amount). Once you are in the gap, you pay 45 percent of the cost of brand-name drugs and 58 percent of the cost of generic drugs (they cost a lot less). After a certain amount adds up in copays, co-insurance, deductible, and shared cost, you enter catastrophic coverage, in which you pay only the copay amount. This is an annual phenomenon, so it resets each year.

There are some bright spots in the Med D plan. You can still get medications by mail, but you will need to confirm that you need them each month. Ask your provider or pharmacy about this.

If you take medication for more than one condition, you may be eligible for a free review of your medication program. Ask your provider about the **medication therapy management** (MTM) program.

Medigap

Medigap plans, or Medicare Supplemental Insurance plans, are standardized and labeled A through N and Medicare Select. Plans E, H, I, and J are no longer available to buy. You can compare benefit packages in the "Medicare and You" booklet at about page 100. Medigap plans do not work with Med C, only with Med A and Med B. Some plans have a drug benefit that can take the place of Med D, but you cannot have both Med D and a drug provision in your Medigap policy.

As with all private insurance, read the contract carefully. Costs can vary widely, and some plans have escalating premiums as you get older. By the way, there aren't group plans; a spouse must get their own policy. Because Medigap policies cover only what Medicare covers and only help with copays, co-insurance, and deductibles, they do not provide long-term care like nursing homes or in-home assistance. They also do not cover glasses, hearing aids, or dental care.

...Do All Doctors and Providers Accept Medicare?

Most do, and most medical facilities (hospitals, rehab units, etc.) are Medicare certified. This means that they meet certain Medicare criteria that should help them be better providers, and they agree to accept Medicare assignment. Assignment means that they accept the allowed payment amount from Medicare (and your copay, deductible, and co-insurance) as payment in full and won't bill you for any charges above this amount. Charges are almost always above this assigned amount. Assignment also means that providers will file the Medicare claim for you free of charge. https://www.medicare.gov/physiciancompare/search.html allows you to search their rolls for providers, or you can ask the provider if they accept assignment. If they aren't Medicare certified and don't take assignment, or are beyond the number of Medicare cases they accept, you may be responsible for the entire bill. They could accept assignment for individual services. If they don't, they may still submit a claim for you. It's better to get agreement in advance for this.

Some doctors have a **"private contract,"** which means that they contract with you not to accept Medicare. You don't have to sign; you can choose a different provider. If you do sign, you are bound by whatever the contract says. Medicare and any Medigap plans won't pay. There are some rules. Your provider must tell you if they have been excluded from Medicare—which means they lost their Medicare contract, usually due to problems with the provider. Also, they cannot make you sign a contract for urgent or emergency services.

Medicaid

Medicaid is a federal program that provides a medical safety net. It was set up to help with medical care for people with low income and few assets. The programs are a partnership between federal and state governments, so there are federal guidelines and minimums, but each state runs its own program. Medicaid may have a different name in each state and may have different provisions. To find the name of the program in your state, type Medicaid and the name of your state into your internet search engine. Chances are, you will find links to the current eligibility levels and to the application process.

Prior to the Affordable Care Act (ACA, known as ObamaCare), Medicaid set the minimum level of support at the federal poverty line (FPL). In 2014 the ACA increased that level to 133 percent of the federal poverty line (meaning you can be Medicaid-eligible with a higher income level). Your state may have opted to expand this further by raising the amount of income and assets you can have and still qualify.

...What's Covered

The assistance Medicaid provides may differ in each state, but there are minimums that all states must provide. All states cover inpatient and outpatient hospital bills, nursing homes (not covered by Medicare and most private insurance), doctors, laboratory work and X-rays, and transportation to medical care. This is a terrific benefit to the people who need it.

Some states cover hospice, personal care, prescription drugs, and self-directed care services (the last is described in Chapter 2, Calling in the Pros). The Medicaid program has offered states a "waiver" program to help fund home care and community-based settings (home caregivers and other services), but not all states have accepted this funding or made these provisions in their programs. Copays, deductibles, and percentage payments and premiums within Medicaid are also set state-by-state, and some states are more generous than others. To see the federal site for Medicaid benefits and link to eligibility and other pages, try https://www.medicaid.gov/medicaid/index.html . What your state covers is probably listed on your state's Medicaid website.

...Applying and Qualifying

If you think you eventually will need and qualify for Medicaid, start the application process now. It's easier than it used to be, but it's still complex. You won't get it done in an afternoon. Again, you can most likely find the application porthole through your state's **Medicaid** website. You can also find it nationally through https://www.healthcare.gov/medicaid-chip/getting-medicaid-chip/. You can also apply through your state's **Health Insurance Marketplace** (HIM) https://www.healthcare.gov/get-coverage/. Your states Medicaid office, SHIBA, your local Area Agency on Aging, and your Aging and Disability Resource Center can all help you with the application.

The information on your application should trigger the HIM algorithm to forward it to Medicaid or Children's Health Insurance Program (CHIP). Even if your application doesn't qualify you for Medicaid, it very well may qualify you for other subsidized programs. Filling out the application is a good first step. As soon as you can see that you will eventually become eligible, gain a relationship with your caseworker. They will be one of your most helpful contacts. Remember that they really do want to help.

Important: If you have limited Medicaid coverage, when you fill out a HIM application and are asked if you have coverage now, don't check the box saying you have Medicaid. Check "none of the above" instead.

The Spend-Down

Some people may qualify for Medicaid on income level alone or if they currently are on Social Security Disability (SSI). Many older people, though they have little income, may have too many assets and will have to go through a somewhat painful process called the "spend-down." We as taxpayers through our federal government decided that we want to help people, but not if they can afford to help themselves. In other words, Medicaid assistance will start only when the person's assets are nearly exhausted; as of 2016, the maximum allowable assets are $2,000.00 not including some basic assets we need to live like a home, a car etc. There are fairly strict provisions against cheating, such as hiding money in trusts or transferring assets at below-asset value.

Keep good documentation of all the expenses that you had during the spend-down. If you are not superorganized, at least don't throw anything away. Put it all in a bankers box and date it by year, or even by month. Plan on keeping it tucked away in your attic for seven years.

Some parts of Medicaid have an **"Asset Recovery Provision"**. This means that Medicaid will take back some of the money it spent on someone's care after they died if they have a substantial amount in their estate. You don't necessarily need to weed through all this during times of high stress; just don't throw any records away.

Don't intermingle funds: If a caregiver spends anything out of their own account or they intermingle their account with yours at all, they should keep all documentation, keep it clear when and what they paid for and out of which account, and when and how they were paid back, if they were reimbursed.

Give yourself and everyone involved plenty of emotional room as you go through the spend-down process. It's not easy to spend all of your assets—your life savings, essentially.

As far as giving a caregiver access to your accounts, set it up early and through power of attorney rather than through sharing accounts (that will be considered by Medicaid as your giving them half the account—in other words, hiding your money). By the way, even a power of attorney authorization does not provide online banking access. This is not allowed by law, to help keep some unscrupulous relative from carting off all your money. For more on these topics, see Chapter 6, The Notebook of Important Papers.

Is Your House an Asset?

With real estate, Medicaid's eligibility rule is a bit different: When a parent adds a child's name to a real-estate deed, it may be treated as if the parent is making a gift of 50 percent of the value of the house to that child. Adding the names of two children would be deemed a gift of two-thirds of the value of the house, etc. Under Medicaid rules, such a gift can cause a period of disqualification from receiving Medicaid. This can cause trouble if the parent applies for Medicaid within five years of signing the new deed. For more information on real estate and joint ownership pertaining to **Medicaid**, try https://www.agingcare.com/Articles/joint-bank-accounts-affect-medicaid-168094.htm.

This may also be a concern to speak with an estate or elder law attorney about before making any changes; see Getting Help Navigating the System earlier in this chapter.

There is a Medicaid provision to protect a spouse from ending up destitute due to someone's care called the **"Spousal Impoverishment Provision."** For more on this, search "Medicaid Spousal Impoverishment Provisions" online.

...Once Accepted
Once you are accepted by Medicaid, in most states most bills will be covered with little or no copay or other costs to you. This only makes sense, because it is generally for people who have little money. Still, there are quite a few things that aren't covered. Most states don't cover dental, vision, or hearing, for example. Also, as for every other third-party payer, the provider must be accepted by, and accept, Medicaid coverage for payment. See Managing the Bills later in this chapter.

Medicaid will often send new forms to **verify eligibility**. Fill them all out and send them in promptly. Follow up with your caseworker to make sure they were processed. Some caseworkers advise faxing the forms in rather than relying on the mail. Sometimes you will get the same form with a more threatening cover letter. This may be because what you sent in has not been processed to the point of stopping the next letter, kind of like crossing in the mail. But it may just be a similar-looking but different form, or perhaps the first one failed to get processed. Follow up on every letter. Speakerphone works great for being on hold. I hope you like the on-hold music.

Private Health-Care Insurance
The biggest change for Karen and me under the Affordable Care Act (Obamacare) was that we didn't go broke, declare bankruptcy, and go on the public dole due to Karen's illness. Before the ACA, insurance policies were written in terms of a policy's maximum benefit. This was often done in both an annual benefit and a lifetime benefit. This clause protected the insurance company from the sometimes-catastrophic costs associated with a major illness like cancer.

It protected the insurance company, but it left the sick person and all who love them hanging in the wind of misfortune. Generally, once they ran out of coverage, the insurance company wouldn't help them and no other insurance company would touch them. Medical bankruptcy was the most common form of bankruptcy in the United States.

The maximum-benefit provision also left the medical providers hanging. They often ended up eating the costs and passing those costs on to everyone else. This is when we began to see $4 aspirin and other ridiculous medical costs. Eventually the public, through Medicaid or other government programs, had to pick up the cost as the family lost all their assets.

Under the ACA, however, insurance companies had to write their policies in terms of the policy's maximum out-of-pocket cost. This protects the sick person and their family. The family has to pay up to the out-of-pocket amount in a year, and after that the insurance company actually has to act like, well ... insurance.

Medical bankruptcy rates have dropped dramatically. Despite this, medical costs remain high. No one complains when they receive too much money, so we won't hear hospitals say much about this. Insurance companies aren't complaining much either, since premiums are regulated in relation to their expenditures. The net result is that insurance companies are charging their best customers (people who are at very low risk of getting sick) more.

The creation of the **Insurance Exchange** allows individuals to buy insurance with a buying power similar to that of large companies. You don't have to buy insurance through the exchange, but if you do, it should automatically consider your income level for tax credits, assistance, or even Medicaid. If you do qualify for assistance, you may be best off opting for a silver-level plan. Healthcare.gov https://www.healthcare.gov/choose-a-plan/plans-categories/ describes it all in easy-to-understand language and has links about tax credits and assistance If you are buying or changing policies, consider the whole costs, not just the premium. Most plans provide a cost summary so you may see what your projected deductible, copays, and percentage pays might add up to be.

...Types of Plans

There are still different types of private insurance plans. There are lots of letters depicting different models. Here are the main ones:

Fee for service: This is similar to the traditional medical model that most of us had before the 1990s. You are pretty much free to see any medical provider you want as long as they accept the insurance plan. The provider bills the insurance company (third party), and the plan determines how much the insurance company will pay the provider. There is usually a deductible (what you must pay each year before the plan begins to help), copays (a fixed amount you pay for an office visit, medication, or service), and/or a percent pay (a percentage of the bill that you're responsible for). Most plans cover most medical care, but not everything. In some plans, an insurance company will have an allowed amount that they will pay for a procedure. In some plans, you will be left to pay for anything above their allowed amount.

Preferred provider organization (PPO): PPOs have a network of doctors and other providers that they contract with to accept their rates and play by their rules in order to have access to the PPO's patients. You pay more if you go "out of network." These plans may have particular trouble if you want to travel out of state or even to a different region within your state. Check with your doctors to be sure they are in the PPO's network.

Health maintenance organization (HMO): In some cases, the doctors and other providers are employees of an HMO and work in HMO-run facilities. Many HMOs contract with outside facilities to provide services too. The organization may have its own rules about referrals and what tests and procedures it will do or pay for. Most HMOs require you have a primary-care physician (PCP) who acts as gatekeeper and case manager for all your care. HMOs may even have philosophies of care that permeate through the organization. These organizations can be quite restrictive about access to care outside their organization.

HMO point of service: This is an HMO network that allows you to go outside their network with a higher copay or co-insurance.

Exclusive provider organization (EPO): These plans usually only cover the bills when you use their specific contracted providers (except in an emergency). An EPO plan can cost less in premiums, but it is the most restrictive regarding which providers you have access to.

Medical savings account (MSA): These plans allow you to put your premiums in a "savings account." If you are enrolled in Medicare, they deposit money in your account too. There is usually a pretty high deductible, then you access the money in the savings account to pay for care. Medicare MSA plans don't offer a drug benefit: you still need Med D or other drug coverage.

...Knowing the Plan

Plans come in different levels of cost sharing—what you pay and what they pay. There is now some standardization in the language of the levels, using the names of precious metals (platinum, gold, silver, bronze), and catastrophic care. Generally, the more the plan pays, the bigger the premium.

It may be helpful for caregivers jumping in to help you with your medical care to know the basics of your plan. The type of plan and the metal level is usually contained in the name of the plan; for example, "Wise Essentials Bronze EPO." The basic literature of the plan should provide a summary of costs that lists your deductible and maximum out-of-pocket amounts. It should also include (often in table form) what's covered and at what level of reimbursement. Now you know the basics of what the plans pay for.

...Reading the Contract and Watching for Pitfalls

In the Contract or Benefit Booklet, the list of what's covered is detailed out. Perhaps the more important list is the Exclusions, or what's not covered. *Anything not covered is also not included in the maximum out-of-pocket amount.* Here are some other important pitfalls in some contracts:

Most HMOs, PPOs, and EPOs—and now even some point-of-service plans—require a referral, prescription, or even preauthorization for medical care to be considered covered. Most of us are familiar with a **prescription**, the little piece of paper the doctor hands the patient. A **referral** is a level above that: an arrangement made by the doctor's office (the referral coordinator) with another provider, such as a physical therapy office. **Preauthorization** is the highest level: the insurer must be contacted and agree to any services before they are performed; this is usually handled by the provider's referral coordinator. **Medical necessity** is the lowest level of requirement: a reviewer reading the medical notes would find that the treatment is within the usual standard of care and accepted practice for the nation and region.

Plans with a prescription drug benefit usually have a **formulary** of the drugs they cover. If it's not on the formulary, you might have to pay for it on your own. Like Med D, these plans might have "step-up" language requiring you to "fail off" (respond poorly) to less-expensive medications before they will cover the actual drug your doctor prescribes.

The maximum out-of-pocket expense does not apply to provider network–based plans—HMO and PPO plans—if care is received from **out-of-network providers.** The doctors and other providers that work in a hospital do not necessarily work for that hospital. Most don't. While the hospital may be in the network, the anesthesiologist on duty that day, or sometimes whole care units, in the hospital may not be. Their bills aren't subject to your policy's "in-network" rules, and your out-of-pocket maximum doesn't apply. Bills unfiltered by insurance can be huge. Before having any hospital admission or medical procedure done, speak with the admissions office or business office to gain some assurance that all your providers will be covered by your insurance.

Fortunately, since the ACA, health insurance Benefit Booklets are written in plain English, so they are readable. You can also look at the company's website and call their customer service.

...Having Someone Else Help You with Your Health Care

If you are having someone be your caregiver, call your insurance company's customer service. Give verbal **authorization** for the insurance company to talk with your caregiver. If you are unable to talk, most companies provide an authorization form from the customer service department or from the company's website. If your caregiver is your power of attorney, send in a copy of that paperwork with the form. These are people. They will appreciate a letter explaining the circumstances.

Also, with each of your usual providers, before any procedures or hospital or facility admissions, talk to the business office or billing office or even the admission or front-desk people. Ask if *all* the providers on your case are contracted with or are preferred providers with the insurance company.

Make friends with the claims managers. When you do find someone helpful or have a good and meaningful conversation with someone in one of these offices, see if you can get their contact information. Develop a relationship with these good people. They may become your first point of contact for any further dealings as the bills roll in. See Managing the Bills later in this chapter.

Long-Term Care Insurance

Most forms of private health insurance follow the same general rules as Medicare: If they do cover long-term care services, it is typically only for skilled, short-term, medically necessary care. Like Medicare, the stay in a skilled-nursing facility must follow a recent hospitalization for the same or related condition and is limited to 100 days. Coverage of home care is also limited to medically necessary skilled-care physical therapy, occupational therapy, speech therapy, nursing, etc. Most forms of private insurance do not cover custodial or personal-care services at all.

...What Is Long-term Care Insurance?

Unlike traditional health insurance, **long-term care insurance** http://longtermcare.gov/costs-how-to-pay/what-is-long-term-care-insurance/ is designed to cover long-term services, including personal and custodial care. This can be in a variety of settings such as your home, a community organization, or other facility.

Long-term care insurance policies reimburse policyholders a daily amount (up to a preselected limit) for services to assist them with activities of daily living (ADLs) such as bathing, dressing, or eating. You can select a range of care options and benefits that allow you to get the services you need, where you need them. The cost of your long-term care policy is based on:

- How old you are when you buy the policy
- The maximum amount that a policy will pay per day
- The maximum number of days (and/or years) that a policy will pay
- The maximum amount per day times the number of days, which determines the lifetime maximum amount that the policy will pay
- Any optional benefits you choose, such as benefits that increase with inflation

If you are in poor health or already receiving long-term care services, you may not qualify for long-term care insurance, as most individual policies require medical underwriting. In some cases, you may be able to buy a limited amount of coverage or coverage at a higher "nonstandard" rate. Some group policies do not require underwriting.

Many long-term care insurance policies have limits on how long or how much they will pay. Some policies will pay the costs of your long-term care for two to five years. A few insurance companies offer policies that will pay your long-term care costs for as long as you live—no matter how much it costs.

...Life Insurance Policies

Some life insurance policies may allow you to tap into your life insurance benefit in the form of an accelerated death benefit (ADB). You may be able to use this if you are terminally ill or have a life-threatening diagnosis, need long-term care services for an extended amount of time, and/or are confined to a nursing home or incapable of performing ADLs independently. Typically this amount is capped at 1 percent of the death benefit per month for home care, 2 percent for nursing-home care, and 50 percent total.

Managing the Bills

No matter what kind of health-care coverage you have, if you have some responsibility for copays, co-insurance, or deductibles, keep track of your provider's medical bills and rectify them against the statements from your insurer (payer). This is no small task. I can see how people would give up and just write a check to pay the bill. But usually when someone hands me a bill, I look at what they are charging for. This is more important with medical care than with, say, the plumber, but it's also more complex. Here's how it works:

Billing codes. When you go to the doctor, they check boxes for the different procedures that occurred in that visit. Each procedure generates a medical billing code, called a CPT code. The doctor's billing department then assembles the codes into a claim form and submits it to the insurance company.

Some codes are for a procedure and some are time based for a procedure. For the time-based ones, you may see more than one unit or code for that procedure in that visit. The billing codes usually have five digits and may have a two-digit modifier at the end. For example, 97110 is the CPT code for a physical therapy therapeutic exercise, or 97110-59 is that same code with a 59 modifier. You may also see ICD-9 or ICD-10 codes on your statement. These relate to the diagnosis or condition treated—not the billed procedure.

Don't be afraid to look up a billing code to see what the provider is billing you for. You can try typing "CPT code" and the number into your search engine. If this proves frustrating, there are sites you can join at a pretty low cost that will give more results. https://www.findacode.com/ offers this service for a small monthly fee.

Multiple providers for a single appointment. In addition to the doctor's bill, the facility where you had the doctor's appointment may have its own charges, as may the lab or imaging center or what have you. Each provider will generate its own bills and submit them to your insurance provider (payer).

Insurance (payer) statements. The insurance provider will then process the bills through a clearinghouse. If the claim is "clean," it will be processed usually in 30 days. If there is anything that throws the claim out (a redundant claim or modifier that isn't accepted by the insurer for example), it is not a clean claim and will go back to the provider for revision.

If you have more than one insurer—say, Medicare and a Medicare Supplemental Insurance plan, the supplemental plan will get the bill after Medicare has fully processed and paid its portion. Then the process starts all over again with the supplemental plan. This can all take up to six months.

In the meantime, the provider's patient accounts office is generating and sending you bills, and your insurance company is generating and sending you "Explanation of Benefits" (EOB) statements with some kind of breakdown of what was charged and what was paid. For Medicare, these statements are called a Medicare summary notice (MSN). Don't pay until you get the EOB or MSN. That confirms that the provider's claim was submitted to the payer.

Yes, you will get multiple statements with multiple pieces of paper for each visit to a provider. It's hard to keep it all straight. Here are some tips to help:

Reconcile Provider Bills and Payer Statements

Keep track of your bills by each provider, arranged by date of service and then listed by each charge. Often you will see a write-off amount: the difference between the amount the provider has billed and the amount allowed by the payer—Medicare or private insurance. Then you will see your copay, percent pay, or remainder that you are being billed.

As the insurers' EOBs or Medicare's MSNs come in, check them off against the provider bills. The amount you are being billed should match the "your responsibility" amount shown on the EOB or MSN. Keep in mind that a provider's bill might not show a zero balance, due to write-off amounts, but the amount your insurance or Medicare says you owe should match the amount on the provider bills. If there are multiple payers wait until all payers give you an EOB or MSN before paying the bill. Also, reconciling bills and statements this way will help you keep an eye on the maximum out-of-pocket and benefit limits for each payer.

Sometimes you may need to create a spreadsheet for keeping track of provider bills and insurance statements. List the providers in rows, by date of service for each charge, and create a column for each payer (Medicare or private insurance), a column for your copay and your percent pay or remainder bill, and a column for the write-off amount.

Check for Mistakes

People make mistakes. Keep an eye out double billing and for what seems like an excessive charge. I once found a bill for a $10,000 scalpel, for example. If you find a bill that seems really out of line, contact the provider's patient accounts office first, and—this is very important!—record notes of all conversations: who you talked to, the date, and what they told you. If you must continue to follow up, do everything in writing, keep a copy in a file you make for this billing problem, and consider sending copies to your insurance payer and the office of your state's insurance commissioner. Exercise your patience muscles here. It took me over a year to resolve the scalpel issue, but because the case was "in discovery," I wasn't liable for a late charge on the bill.

Find Out Who Can Answer Billing Questions

Gain a relationship with your provider's patient accounts office and your payer's claims office early on. Try to identify a contact there—if not an individual person, at least a division with a contact number. You can start this process on admission to a provider's care. Doing this might not be so easy with Medicaid or Medicare, but remember that those who work for these agencies are people too.

If you contact the provider with a billing question and they stonewall or give you some other nasty treatment, **Medicare** invites you to file a complaint at https://www.medicare.gov/claims-and-appeals/file-a-complaint/complaint.html. Medicare also has a Medicare Ombudsman in many states. They can help tremendously with any problems you might have. Keep in mind that just whining doesn't help anyone—state the problem and how you think it should be resolved.

Paying the Bills

If you are facing a large bill and you have the means to pay it today, you might just contact the provider's business office. They want to be paid in full and close that claim. Ask if they might offer you a discount if you pay in full today. My physical therapy practice used to give a discount of up to 20 percent for same-day pay.

If you find that a hospital or nursing-home bill is going to be difficult to pay, ask your provider if they have a foundation or other charity-care organization. Their billing office may have more knowledge about what programs are available to help you pay a large medical bill.

Ask Someone to Help Manage the Bills

Managing the bills sounds like a lot of work. And it is. This may be something that you could hand off to your cousin in Rochester who really wants to help but cannot be there to help as a caregiver. Whoever you choose to take on this task will need to be detail oriented and persistent, with terrific "on-hold" skills. They will also need written or verbal authorization to talk with each party in your behalf.

...Appeals

Medicare, Medicaid, and most private insurance companies give you the right to appeal any decision they make, such as denial of coverage for a service or item, the amount they pay the provider, or the amount you must pay on a medical bill.

For Med A and B: To file an appeal with traditional Medicare, you have some options. One simple way is to circle the item on your Medicare summary notice (MSN) and on a separate piece of paper write an explanation of why you disagree with the decision. Copy both pieces of paper and send them to the company that handles the bills for Medicare, which is listed on the MSN. You could also use a CMS form 20027 (type the name of this form into your browser to get a PDF copy). You can also request any information from your health-care provider to support your appeal.

You must file an appeal within 120 days of getting the MSN. Medicare tries to give you a decision within 60 days. You can request a fast appeal with an independent reviewer, called a "beneficiary and family-centered care quality-improvement organization," if you feel you are being discharged from a facility such as a hospital, skilled-nursing facility, or outpatient facility because of loss of Medicare benefits.

You can contact your state health insurance program (SHIP; see Getting Help Navigating the System earlier in this chapter) for assistance with filing an appeal.

For Med C and private insurance: The procedure will differ company by company. Your policy papers should describe the procedure for appeal in the Benefits Booklet (contract).

For Med D: Contact your Medicare D plan administrator (the company that the plan is with) for a written "coverage determination." Or use their EOB statement and write on a separate piece of paper "Ask for exception"; you could do this to waive a coverage rule, request to include the drug you need on their formulary, or change the benefit amount you don't agree with. Copy both pieces of paper and send them to the plan administrator. You or your prescribing health-care provider can also call for an expedited determination for a drug that must be approved. You will need a medical reason from your doctor as to why your exception should be approved.

Provider Appeals

Appeals are often written in behalf of the patient by the provider. The provider needs to include accompanying documents with the appeal letter. In the appeal letter, they basically need to say that active treatment (a treatment plan) was in place and give solid reasons why the goals of treatment and end of the care episode were not met in the usual time, because payers usually have a set predicted time for care for a particular diagnosis code.

Here is an example: With a knee replacement, patients should be up and out of bed the next day and should be able to walk in the facility, get to the bathroom, etc., within a certain amount of time. If that person has a complicating problem such as arthritis in their shoulders that makes it very difficult to use a walker for weight bearing, they might not meet these time marks. This needs to be explained and supported with documentation from the doctor, the X-ray reports on their shoulders, and their physical therapist's notes.

What Medicare and all payers want to see is that a patient has real goals that will improve their function and their life and in the long run make them healthier—saving the payer money. What they don't want to see is the same treatment being done over and over without improvement and without good reassessment and justification for continuing this treatment. Because insurance provides coverage against something bad happening, a baseline level of health and function is usually what the payer wants to achieve. They are not pushing for better than baseline.

There is a secondary appeal process if the first appeal is denied. Contact the provider's patient accounts office to see if you might be responsible for any bills generated in the time that the secondary appeal is being considered if it gets denied too.

...Advance Beneficiary Notice (ABN) of Noncoverage

The advance beneficiary notice (ABN) of noncoverage is a form from a provider giving you notice that Medicare most likely, or definitely, won't cover a health-care service or item. The ABN isn't an official denial from Medicare. You could still ask the provider for the service and ask them to submit a claim to Medicare. If Medicare denies the claim, you could appeal it. If your appeal is denied, you will be responsible for the bill.

If your provider was supposed to give you an ABN and didn't, they may need to pay you back for the bill you paid. This is tricky, because it is sometimes questionable whether they were supposed to anticipate noncoverage or not. For more information, find "Medicare Appeals" at https://www.medicare.gov/claims-and-appeals/file-an-appeal/appeals.html .

...Grievances and More Help

For **grievances** and more assistance with billing and coverage issues, you have more options available. Each insurance company, Medicare, Medicaid, and the Department of Veterans Affairs all have offices and mechanisms to accept and resolve grievances. Your insurance policy's Benefits Booklet will have the contact method, as will the "Medicare and You" booklet and your state's Medicaid office. Usually each EOB statement has a contact number for questions and problems as well.

The Office of the Insurance Commissioner (OIC) is a state organization that can help sort out insurance problems and advocate for you in your complaint. They can help make sure that the insurance company followed the laws of the state in their dealings with you and advocate for you if they didn't. But they will not be your lawyer. They can't fact find, determine if someone is lying, or legally enforce a judgment. They can make the insurance company pay a claim or refund a premium. They may also have links to other organizations in your state that can help with more specific problems. Their office may support or link to other advocate organizations such as the Long-Term Care Ombudsman and the Statewide Health Insurance Benefits Advisors (SHIBA).

There are also attorneys who specialize in elder law. They can be tremendously helpful not just in resolving grievances, but in finding and straightening out resources and setting things up for the course of care down the road. The **National Academy of Elder Law Attorneys** https://www.naela.org/ can help you find one in your area. The **National Legal Resource Center** http://nlrc.acl.gov/Services_Providers/Index.aspx can help connect you with legal assistance and other resources on a state-by-state basis.

Interlude

Backflips

How does a person turn back flips with broken ribs and a shattered spine? It was Karen's back pain that brought us to the doctor. That back pain turned out to be fractures. The fractures began where cancerous breast cells had replaced healthy bone. Now Karen also faced treatment with aggressive radiation and toxic chemotherapies.

She didn't take chemo well. We dubbed her "Our Princess" as she absorbed her first emergency transfusion for medication toxicity and severe anemia. The therapy was effective initially, but as the cancer receded, her spine crumbled. Fractures appeared in her pelvis, middle spine, ribs, and neck. Tumors were everywhere.

This would take all the strength we had, and strength yet to be discovered. Is this what it means to live deeply?

Even with all the tumors in the depth of disease, the body clings to life. It struggles to repair and recover. The very same principles that carried Karen across triathlon finish lines were needed to carry her now. The first day she could walk, she began to do wobbly squats. She would grin that champion's grimace as we'd count them off: six, seven, eight. We would celebrate each victory, each step forward. She would collapse into my arms or we'd gently high-five or maybe just exchange a look and a smile. Then we would eat, rest, and fully enjoy each triumph.

Life itself became the challenge. How to walk a little easier, eat a little better, deal with … everything became our mountain to climb. The day she walked the three blocks to the beach, we had hope she could go to Canada. And so began our journeys. With love and care and work and a strong decision to live as fully as can be in that brief time between birth and death, we went to Paris to visit my sister and her family. We went to Norway to visit my family there and find Karen's long lost relatives. We went to Italy with our bike racing friends, and we went to Sweden to visit a friend we hadn't seen in years. All this we did while just walking was still difficult.

* * * * *

Physical strength might carry you out the door, but it is your heart that opens your eyes. Keeping your heart open means keeping your brain as healthy as can be. Karen's brain was under siege from the disease. Pain threatened to pull her into anxiety or shove her down into depression. The barrage of medications swirled inside her, warping her perceptions and causing more anxiety. The tumors as well were attacking her on multiple levels. There were tumors in her brain, near her spinal cord, and all over the front of her spine where the chain of ganglia (cell body groups) live that control many of the visceral parts of the fight-flight-freeze response. My mom suffered this and it was catastrophic for us all.

Karen began a meditative practice and gratefulness journaling. Through the contemplative practice, she actively strengthened her nervous system. She gained more self-control. She gained more Self. Her spirit seemed to grow larger. We didn't know at the time how immensely important this would become. We didn't know how this growth would change… everything. Even under the crush of disease she learned more, and we all learned and lived more in her final year than we had in the previous fifty.

*****

Whenever you begin on a journey, you can never fully know all of what the journey will show you. And whenever you choose to grow into a new challenge, you can never fully know all the gifts you might earn.

Your path might be different from ours.

Whatever it is for you, you will need to accept your fears. You will need to embrace the hardships. You will need to choose to live deeply.

The ground is coming.

Part 3. Caregiving Skills and Advice From the Field

You will find a tremendous amount of practical information in this long section. In this section we discuss how to help someone with many of the basic needs of life; eating, sleeping, getting around as well as and exercise, medication, and medical care. *Caregiving 101* was written by people who not only work in the field but also have lived it on a most personal level. You may search for the topics that apply to your loved one's needs right now and find the solutions that you need. For instance, if you wake up to find your grandmother out of bed and on the floor, you can simply turn to Fall Recovery in Chapter 15, Basic Mobility and Transfers for very usable descriptions of different ways to help someone off the floor.

If you haven't done so already I beg you to read Part I. Being a Caregiver and Taking Care of Yourself. It may save your life.

Chapter 9. Doctors

At some point you and/or your loved one may be sitting down with a doctor, social worker, or other health-care professional discussing care plans, levels of care, care facilities, specialists, rehabilitation and placement, and … well, it can make your head spin. There's enough at stake here emotionally without having to wrap your head around all these details at once.

In this chapter we hope to give a handy reference guide to managing medical appointments, what some of the letters behind health-care professionals' names mean, and a little bit about how to choose health-care providers. Knowing this little bit might help those decisions come a bit more smoothly. Let's talk about the appointments first.

Managing Medical Appointments
"Yes, got it … Now what was that middle part?"

I once had a calculus professor who would write equations on the board with his right hand while erasing them with his left hand. Sometimes he would lecture about something else at the same time. This was a "weed-out" class: a class designed to challenge you as a student more than teach you anything about math. We quickly learned to work in groups, with one person's job being simply to write everything down so we could make sense of it all later.

After the initial shock-and-awe appointment when we learned that Karen's cancer had returned, the lesson of the weed-out class came back in spades. Distraction is the brain's natural memory eraser. When you're trying to record things from short-term to long-term memory, distraction or fixation caused by the emotional intensity of the moment interrupts that recording process. It is like my calculus professor's left hand.

Karen and I quickly found that the emotional stress of these medical appointments was so high that we couldn't remember important details. Emotional support is crucial too, but it's hard to write when you're holding someone's hand. Be sure to take someone with you whose job is just to write everything down so you can make sense of it all later.

…What to Write Down During an Appointment
Things to have someone write down include:

- the doctor's name
- the current working diagnosis: what the doctor thinks is going on
- the doctor's plan of care: what additional tests or treatment plans they have
- what the benefits of those plans are
- what the risks and costs of those plans are
- any specific instructions or precautions (things your loved one shouldn't do)

Let your loved one lead the discussion and ask their own questions—it is their treatment, after all. However, if the discussion doesn't cover everything in the list above, you may want to ask these questions and have someone write down the answers. Use a pencil if writing overviews: things change.

...Calendars to Keep Track of Appointments

In today's busy world, most of us have gotten used to using some type of calendar system. If you haven't, you need to now. Your medical-appointments calendar could be your smartphone, a calendar book, or even something you got from the boy scout down the street.

Any calendar you use should allow you to see the whole week, and even the whole month, at once. It should allow you to record dates and times. It should have room for notes. And it should be something you can look back at a month from now, or even years from now. It is a good idea to cross-reference the date with the day of the week to help avoid the snafu of recording it in the wrong month or even the wrong year (don't laugh—I've seen that happen).

...Tips on Scheduling Appointments

Whatever appointment calendar you use, it needs to come with you to medical appointments. It needs to come out when you begin talking about treatment plans in the physician's room, before you talk with the doctor's scheduling department. The timing of appointments and treatment between different health-care providers is important. The physicians know this, but their schedulers don't always consider it fully when trying to squeeze you in.

Use your calendar to get an overview of the treatment plan and the interplay of the different health-care disciplines involved. As you schedule, make sure the appointments you make fit with the treatment plan as it was described by the physician.

Record the name and contact information of the physician *and* their contact staff member. This may help you speed through the phone tree if you need to contact them. You might want to record their health-care discipline or the procedure, just to keep it all straight.

As you schedule medical appointments, keep in mind that you still have a life outside of treatment. Try to allow the rest of life's obligations to fit as well as possible with the treatment schedule. You may not want to schedule radiation on the same day as nephew Johnny's bar mitzvah.

Plan for sick times and recovery times. For any surgery under general knock-you-out anesthesia, plan 24 hours of anesthesia hangover. For chemotherapy and radiation consider that the effects are cumulative over the course of treatment. The first few doses will most likely have only moderate effects, but you will take some time to recover following the last dose. Your physicians can help you with knowing what to expect for recovery. It might be good to have the calendar out when you ask about this.

...Help with Appointments

Most support websites have a calendar function that allows you to request help with appointments from your caregiver team. Please don't be afraid to ask. Remember all the Tupperware? People who love you want to help you. You just have to help them know how. Using an online appointment calendar is one way that helps family and friends know how they can help you, and it helps them deal with the illness as well. Here is a calendar page that we used https://www.mylifeline.org/gokaren/helpingcalendar/calendar/2013/1

Knowing What the Letters Behind Providers' Names Mean

This section gives you a handy reference guide to what some of the letters behind health-care professionals' names mean—the alphabet soup of medical terminology.

MD. This means doctor of medicine, a board-certified physician who went through pre-medicine training in college (usually a bachelor of science degree), then four years of medical school (a doctorate in medicine), then an internship, then a residency in their specialty. MDs can be general practitioners, or specialists. There are specialists for nearly every type of treatment and each system of the body. I counted more than a hundred in a simple web search. One that I should introduce to you here is called a **physiatrist.** This is a doctor who specializes in physical medicine and rehabilitation. If your loved one undergoes rehabilitation in a rehabilitation hospital setting, the physiatrist may become a key player.

DO. This means doctor of osteopathy. They also enjoy rigorous pre-medicine training, four years of medical school, internships, and residency just like MDs. In the osteopathic schools of medicine, they are also trained in a set of manual (hands-on) skills for joint manipulation or adjustment called *osteopathic method*. DOs tend to be more holistic in their approach and often are general practitioners, but there is no medical-school reason why they might not be orthopedic surgeons or any other specialty.

PCP. This stands for **primary-care physician.** This is your family doctor. They are usually internists, general practitioners, or family practice physicians—and yes, each of these is a special board certification and all are somewhat different. PCPs are the doctors you see for most medical issues, and they will often oversee your care, following your treatment through the hospital and visiting you there. It is important that your medical care have someone who oversees the whole case and all the different teams of specialists. Many health plans require your PCP's referral to cover any contact you have with other specialists. In this way, your PCP is sometimes the gatekeeper to your medical care. They may step aside if the bulk of your care falls to a particular specialist or team of specialists. For Karen, her oncologist took the lead role in coordinating her care.

PA. This means **physician assistant.** They complete premedical college courses plus work in the medical field, then attend two to three years of special physician assistant schooling and sit for licensing exams. They work under the direction MDs and DOs and are trained to examine, diagnose, and treat most medical problems.

NP. This stands for **nurse practitioner.** This is an advanced nursing degree that allows them to diagnose and treat patients, including prescribing medications. They also work with MDs and DOs much as PAs do, but they come from a nursing background. If you are seeing a PA or NP, don't fret: they are most likely quite knowledgeable and can help you.

RN. This means **registered nurse**. Some complete a bachelors degree and some a professional program. They can be generalists or specialists, such as emergency flight nurse or oncology nurse. They can give medications under a physician's prescription and often serve as the front line of care for patients.

LPN. This means **licensed practical nurse.** They complete a program that may consist of a year or more of coursework and practical training before they can sit for licensure exams. They work under the supervision of a doctor or registered nurse and can perform most of the practical nursing tasks such as giving medicines and caring for IV lines, but they cannot assess or diagnose.

CMA. This is a **certified medication aid.** They can give oral medications under the supervision of a registered nurse or physician but cannot give medication by central lines, IVs, injections, or any of the other myriad ways to introduce a medication directly into the body. They also cannot give certain types of medications such as barium or chemotherapy.

CNA. This is a **certified nurse's assistant.** They study basic nursing skills through a certificate program. They work under the supervision of a registered nurse and can help with the bulk of patient care but do not give medications. Most home care assistants are CNA certified. You may see the letters rearranged to NAC or NA-C in some states. If you see NA-R, this might mean they have taken the coursework and registered to become certified, but have not yet received their certification.

...Ancillary Service Providers

PT. This stands for **physical therapist.** They are absolutely the best people on the planet ... oh, uh, full disclosure: I'm a PT, so maybe that's just my opinion. They earn a bachelor of science degree in college, studying much of the same pre-medicine coursework as physicians, and attend a three- to four-year doctoral program. PTs use the body's ability to learn, heal, and adapt as medicine. They also can specialize and you may see other letters behind their names after PT or DPT. In hospital, rehabilitation, and skilled-nursing settings, they primarily focus on the basic functions of mobility. They help teach the body to stand, walk, and get from place to place again. They can help with mobility aids such as wheelchairs, walkers, special braces, and so on (see Chapter 15, Basic Mobility and Transfers).

OT. This means **occupational therapist.** They also use the body's ability to learn and adapt, but their role is slightly different from that of a PT. OTs are concerned more with activities of daily living (ADLs) such as dressing, basic hygiene, cooking, and so on. They often focus more on fine-motor skills (things done with the hands), while a PT focuses more on gross-motor skills (things done with the rest of the body). OTs are the best consults for adaptive equipment to make tasks of ADLs easier, such as sock aids to help one get dressed, special plates and silverware, and adaptive shower equipment (see Chapter 15, Basic Mobility and Transfers).

SLP. This means **speech language pathologist.** They do much more than help a person learn to communicate again. They can assess and help with swallowing and with preventing aspiration and pneumonia. They also assess and help with memory and cognition and design and implement specific therapies to help. Remember, the nervous system is our most adaptable tissue. It responds to training faster and better than muscles and joints. Everyone in ancillary services works on this system, and the SLP takes more specific training on this than PTs and OTs.

PTA, COTA, and SLPA. These are **assistants to PTs, OTs, and SLPs,** respectively. They have earned a profession-specific associate degree (two years of college). They work under the supervision of the PT, OT, or SLP and can perform most of the procedures that the primary service provider can. They do not perform evaluations and assessments for patients, and must consult with their primary service provider on any alterations of the plan of care.

PT and OT aides. These people are trained on the job and can help with basic tasks for their primary service providers. They may help with setups for modalities, help keep the work area functional, and help with the general flow of patient care. They generally do not directly assist patients or perform any skilled procedures.

...Other Providers

There are many other types of health-care providers you might meet: phlebotomists draw blood, X-ray technicians take X-rays and other images, and so on. There are far too many to mention them all here.

The one that I should mention is your **social worker (MSW, LICSW, or LCSW)**. They will be your key resource for deciphering your medical options and your medical coverage issues. If you find a good one, it might be helpful if you get their contact information and keep in touch with them as they guide you through this journey.

A social worker at the advanced level has a graduate degree Masters of Social Work (MSW) and completes a post-graduate period of 3 years before sitting for a licensing exam. The LICSW is an independent license. They may work at a hospital or agency and/or have a private therapy practice. **Medical Social Workers** most often work in hospitals or outpatient clinics and are specialized in emergency department care, medical specialty care, oncology, chronic illness, and other specialties. They are often holistic and trained in various psychotherapy models including cognitive behavioral therapy, mindfulness based therapy, and trauma informed therapy. They often run patient and caregiver support groups.

Each medical facility may have its own team of social workers. They will know the ins and outs of that particular stage in your care. Still, it may help to put them in touch with the one social worker you identify as really helpful to you, the one who knows who you are and your whole case.

The other providers you may want to know more about are the people who have varying levels of caregiving skills, especially the folks who might help in the home. We have described these people in Selecting the Right Professional in Chapter 2, Calling in the Pros.

Finding a Good Doctor

No matter what the letters are behind their names, if health-care providers are there to care for you or your loved one, they should do just that. The clinician should walk in well versed with your case, they should be prepared for the encounter, and you should be able to get the follow-up care they recommend in the time frame that they recommend it. In your interaction with the providers, you should feel heard, the diagnosis and plan of care should make sense, and your concerns should be addressed.

The provider should *listen* to you. They should be aware of what you're telling them, both verbally and nonverbally. They need to be able to convey back to you that they are hearing you and that they "get it."

Their diagnosis and plan of care should make sense. Your doctor should know, and be able to explain, why they are telling you whatever they are telling you. They should be able to give you their reasoning both for the diagnosis and for the plan of care they are proposing.

They should be able to answer your questions. Their answers should make sense. Doctors are people too. They can't and don't know everything. "I don't know" is a perfectly reasonable answer, and I honor the doctor who has the honesty to say just that. Remember, it is not a sign of a bad clinician if they tell you that they don't know. They are just trying to do their best for you.

...When and How to Fire Your Doctor

According to a good friend of mine, the esteemed Dr. Samuel P. Martin III was fond of saying, "Don't get crosswise with your doctor. You'll put them off their game and they'll make the mistakes you're afraid of." That said, you do need to be your own best advocate, and that includes getting another opinion or even switching providers.

In advocating for yourself or your loved one, try not to second-guess the provider in their office. Try never to argue, but do keep your eyes open. You are most likely not a specialist in whatever field your provider is practicing in. They have studied and worked in this field for years and you probably haven't, so it is difficult to know what your open eyes are seeing. However, below are some things that should raise concerns.

Problems with their office. A poorly functioning support staff may indicate problems with the office. If the provider has trouble getting notes, either their own or from other providers, then they have to rely more on immediate impressions and snap decisions. If appointments are nearly impossible to get and do not coincide with the plan of care, the care is compromised. If the office is always frantic or the doctor seems off balance, it might have more to do with the office but is still a bad sign. Long times in the waiting room and short visit times are unfortunately pretty normal now, but the visit should not be frantic.

Indications of poor "bedside manner." If the provider is not fully listening to you, they are probably missing clinically valuable cues about your case. If they cannot convey back to you that they "get it," then their bedside-manner skills are lacking. You can double-check whether you're being heard by simply asking the provider simple questions about aspects of your case that should be part of the medical record, or ask them about something you have already told them.

In some cases, surgeons or other practitioners have poor bedside skills but otherwise have excellent technical skills. If you suspect this, it's probably OK to work with them as long as you don't need to make any difficult medical decisions with them. If you do need to make any difficult medical decisions, the provider's bedside manner is important and should be a deal breaker for continuing under their care. Recheck their reputation and success record. It should be exceptional. If it is only average, there are plenty of average providers with better bedside manners.

Questions about the medical care they provide. Educate yourself as best you are able about what the provider is telling you. This might be easier than you think. For most cases, simply typing the name of the procedure and/or the diagnosis into your search engine will yield plenty of information about what is more-or-less standard care. Wikipedia is a good place to start, mainly for the listed references at the bottom of the articles, which are often primary sources. Sites like Web MD also tend to offer some ideas of standard care. If you can read scientific journals, seek compilation articles that examine a broad group of literature; most of the time, a single study is not powerful enough to change clinical practice standards. You can probably throw out "miracle cures" and "magic treatments" with "amazing results." You can also probably throw out pieces that assure you that "scientists confirm ..."

Based on your research, if you suspect your provider might be making a significant medical mistake, seek a second opinion prior to consenting to the plan of care. Do try to avoid providers who offer something that is far different from standard care, regardless of how much they promise a cure or regardless of how much you might like them.

...What to Do If You Have Concerns

If you do see enough of the aforementioned warning signs, do not get mad, but do begin to research other providers as soon as possible. Use these other providers initially for second opinions.

If the interaction with them is much better than with your current provider, you can switch to working with them instead of your current provider. Don't forget to check with your insurance company or payer to be sure the new provider is covered under your plan. Then request that the pertinent medical records be sent to the new provider. Be sure to contact the entire care team, including all the other providers on your case as well as your primary-care or family physician, and tell them of the new provider. Give your care team the new provider's contact information and a signed consent for release of medical records. Most medical offices have such a form; simply ask for it at the front desk, fill it out, and hand it back.

Don't worry too much about hurting your former doctor's feelings. Having an unhappy patient who doesn't trust your judgment is way more hurtful than having a patient who transfers to care they are happy with. Simply inform their office staff and be sure any follow-up appointments are cancelled.

Chapter 10.
Hospitals and Other Medical Facilities

This book is written with caring for your loved one at home in mind, but this is not always possible. And, if it's terribly isolating for your loved one, it might not be the best choice, even if you and your team can provide the care needed. Hospitals and other kinds of medical-care facilities may have special facilities, even whole buildings for specific conditions or types of treatments. In this chapter you will learn about most of the facilities out there, how to choose between them, and how better to manage it all.

Short-Term Medical Facilities (Hospitals)

We all know of hospitals. Different areas of **larger hospitals are now much more specialized.** They may have separate wings for orthopedics (bone and joint issues), cardiac care (heart issues), and general medical services. There is often an emergency room (ER), an intensive care unit (ICU), and a critical care unit (CCU). Usually the larger the hospital and the larger the metropolitan area, the more specialized each of these hospital areas can be. For a more complete listing of them, type "parts of a hospital" into your browser and see what pops up.

It's probably best to choose a hospital because they have the services and medical professionals your loved one needs, but once they are admitted, you may have little choice over the parts of the hospital they will see. That will be determined mostly by the care team there, depending on what type of care is needed and sometimes by the availability of a bed or room.

Having all these specialty areas doesn't necessarily mean that the hospital's care is better. Many small hospitals have excellent staff and give wonderful care. You might get a general idea of some of the good and bad experiences people you know have had in different hospitals near you. There are several **hospital rating systems**, but at the time of this writing, unfortunately, there is very little agreement about a particular hospital according to the ratings. A hospital might get a good rating from Consumer Reports and only one bar from the Leapfrog Group. This poor inter-rater reliability is because each system looks at different measures and does so in different ways. I'm sorry we can't be more helpful here. Maybe by the time you read this, it will be better.

Helping Your Loved One During a Hospitalization

As a caregiver, there may be things you can do to help your loved one during a hospital stay. **Visiting** is powerful medicine. It can keep hospital shock from setting in, can distract the person from pain and boredom, and can help their will to recover.

Bringing in familiar pictures and articles from home can also help with hospital shock (see Delirium in Chapter 18, Managing Discomforts). **Asking if there are chores at home** that need attention, especially if their home is left unattended, can relieve their worries.

Being with your loved one during physician rounds is often helpful. Sometimes the hospital staff will have a rough schedule for this. Take notes if possible. Things to write down include:

- the doctor's name
- the current working diagnosis: what they think is going on
- their plan of care: what additional tests or treatment plans they have
- what the benefits of those plans are
- what the risks and costs of those plans are

Let your loved one lead the discussion and ask their own questions; it is their treatment after all. If any of the above questions don't come out in the discussion, you may want to ask about them. If this list looks exactly like the notes of what to write down during an appointment with doctors outside the hospital, it's because it *is* the same (see Chapter 9, Doctors).

Sometimes the hospital staff may have ways to keep notes for you or for the doctor to communicate with you if you are not able to be there directly. Ask the attending nurses about this, as it differs from facility to facility. Remember that you need to have medical power of attorney or be the caregiving family member for the hospital staff to share with you this otherwise private medical information.

Talking to the hospital social worker can help you understand the financial issues. The social worker and/or discharge planner can help you plan for what you will need when your loved one leaves the hospital and where they might go from there.

Having patients transfer out of the hospital as soon as the tests and treatments there are finished and they are medically stable enough to do so is best for the patients and for the medical system. If your loved one still requires more care and treatment than they can get at home, there are several options for continued care or rehabilitation, depending on what is needed and available.

Rehabilitation Facilities

A **rehabilitation hospital** or **inpatient hospital rehab,** or simply **rehab**, is no cushy vacation for the patient. They are there to work hard to regain their basic functions. They need to be able to participate in at least three hours of therapy per day, five to seven days per week. The rehab team is often led by a physiatrist, includes daily round-the-clock access to physicians and nursing staff, and may include any or all of the ancillary service providers listed in Chapter 9, Doctors, plus other rehabilitation specialists.

These settings are also very expensive, so payers have laid down somewhat complex decision-making criteria to determine whether this type of treatment is warranted and beneficial. The basics of these criteria are that the patient needs to:

- **be medically stable** enough for their care to be managed in this setting, yet still needs close medical supervision by a physiatrist or other qualified physician and needs 24-hour availability of skilled nursing.
- **be able to participate** in the therapies (greater than three hours per day five days per week) and to benefit from those therapies significantly more than they could a lesser amount of therapy. They may also need the access to the specialized equipment in the facility.
- **have clear, realistic, functional goals** that they are expected to achieve in a reasonable time frame. In most circumstances those goals need to help them be able to go home or to some other community-based environment.

That's where you and your caregiver team come in. You will most likely work with the rehab team to help determine what's possible and what's needed, and you'll help to make those goals a reality.

The things you can do listed above under Helping Your Loved One During a Hospitalization also apply during rehab, except you might not want to overwhelm them with too many daytime visits. They are there to work. Visiting still helps, but keep in mind that they will need their energy for rehabilitation.

Transitional Care Units (TCUs)

TCUs are somewhat less therapy-intense than a rehab facility and less medically intense than a hospital. TCUs still provide daily round-the-clock nursing and therapies five to six days per week, but do not have the three-hour-per-day therapy minimum.

Don't worry; it is still intense for most patients, but patients in a TCU don't need to have as much endurance and can be more medically involved. The intended stay in a TCU is relatively short, usually between 5 and 30 days, and TCUs have more of a home environment. Patients may be expected to wear their own street clothes, eat in the dining room, and participate in the therapies in their care plan.

A TCU also has more flexibility in discharging patients, so discharge options may include nursing homes, assisted-living facilities, or other settings. As in a rehab facility, you and your caregiving team should work with the TCU team to help determine what aftercare is needed and make it a reality.

Subacute Care Facilities

This is another rehabilitation setting available in some states that is much like a TCU with relatively shorter stays. General subacute care facilities may serve patients who are more medically stable but cannot tolerate or benefit from the high amount of rehabilitation therapies at a rehab facility or a TCU. They provide therapies three to five days per week, less than three hours per day on average. Nursing may not be available 24 hours per day, but these facilities are staffed round the clock and can help people who may still need a lot of assistance eating, dressing, toileting, and moving around. Like a TCU, general subacute care service may be located within another setting such as a nursing home.

Care Centers

These are illness-specific facilities for conditions such as multiple sclerosis (MS), stroke, spinal cord injuries, and Parkinson's Disease. They can be inpatient or outpatient facilities. They often provide more specialized services and equipment for the problems people have with a specific illness. Most care centers are located within larger cities and are attached to hospitals or other types of care facilities. You may ask your social worker if such a facility is available in your area, or type the diagnosis, the word "facility," and your city into your search engine for a good start on locating options near you.

Comfort Care, Hospice, and Home Health Care

Comfort care is more of a concept than any kind of facility. The concept is simple and wonderful: provide medical care intended to make someone's life better. The focus is to help relieve symptoms, to help people have less pain, less swelling, less breathing problems, better emotional and social lives—in short, to help them be more comfortable.

Comfort care is a wraparound service. Many hospitals now have comfort care teams with doctors, nurses, and other professionals. It is not necessarily associated with end of life or withdrawal of medical treatments meant to prolong life. Services can be in a hospital or other inpatient setting or at home, and services are billed much like the rest of medical care, with each procedure, service, or prescription billed separately. Medicare and private medical insurance usually cover comfort care services.

Hospice is a comfort care model applied to end-of-life care. Typically a hospice organization is contacted when the doctor has given the patient a prognosis of six months or less of life. Like comfort care, hospice provides a wraparound, team approach to care, offering visiting home nurses, access to ancillary services such as PT and SLP, chaplain or counseling, and many other services. We even had the most wonderful harpist come to our house during Karen's hospice. Hospice does not usually provide in-home caregivers for attendant care, but some hospice services have inpatient facilities that can be used for respite or when the needs of the patient are beyond what can be done at home.

Deciding to contact hospice is not a death sentence. Usually treatments whose goal is trying to "beat the disease," such as chemotherapy, are discontinued but you can change your mind about treatments at any time. Though life-saving, life-prolonging treatments are not typical while someone is in hospice care, they can be used to make the patient more comfortable.

Financially, hospice is an all-in-one service. Medication, equipment, supplies, and all the tremendous services from the professionals who helped us were all under one umbrella. Medicare, Medicaid, and private health insurance have provisions for hospice care. Be sure to check your particular policy contract.

Home health care is the term for the services of certain health professionals (PTs, OTs, SLPs, RNs and social workers) that are available to (and may be financially covered for) people who cannot reasonably get to an outpatient facility. These providers usually come in for one or two hours one to three times per week for specific treatments. Services need to be ordered by the doctor, and, like rehab, treatments need to address clear, realistic goals.

There are also caregivers who come to your home to help with basic things like bathing, getting dressed, cooking and eating, and just to provide supervision and companionship. The term "home health care" does not refer to these folks however. These good folks may be called caregivers or home health aides (see Chapter 2, Calling in the Pros).

Longer-Term Medical and Residential Facilities

There are a host of other options for longer-term care, depending on what your loved one needs. You might not think that you will need these options, but it's a good idea to look around anyway to find a few good places that would work if your loved one does end up needing longer-term care. If you take a little time now to plan ahead, you won't be caught flat-footed in a medical emergency. This section covers some of these options.

Skilled Nursing Facilities (SNFs)

Nursing homes may also be referred to in the medical profession as skilled nursing facilities (SNFs). They may act as a bridge between a hospital and the home or other place, or may be used for long-term care. SNFs can help care for people when they are quite medically involved but stable enough to be out of the hospital. Patients of an SNF are referred to as "residents." They have access to daily round-the-clock nursing and oversight by physicians. SNFs offer rehab services (PT, OT, SLP) but often at a lower level of intensity than a rehab facility or TCU. Depending on the SNF, much of the day-to-day care is provided by CNAs, rehabilitation aids, and other helping staff.

Alternatives to the Traditional Nursing Home

All over this country, and in many other countries, people have worked to provide a better vision of care for people who might otherwise need a nursing home. There is no one nationwide project to refer you to, but below are a couple you might look into for ideas of where to look in your area:

Eden Alternative www.Edenalt.org is a nonprofit working to uninstitutionalize the care institution culture. Children visit; residents have pets and houseplants. On the Eden Alternative website member facilities that hold the organization's values and methods are shown on a map. If you are lucky, there may be one near you. At the time of this writing, there were none in my state, Washington, but the neighboring state of Oregon and Canadian province of British Columbia had some.

The Green House Project www.Thegreenhouseproject.org is a nonprofit franchise with affiliates throughout North America. Their goal is to foster relationships. The six to ten residents in a home have private rooms but share open living and dining areas. This organization also has a map of their affiliates which can be found on their website.

Memory-Care Facilities

Memory care usually consists of a wing or floor within a nursing home or assisted-living facility dedicated to people with marked difficulty making new memories who may have difficulty with wandering off (exit seeking) or have behaviors that may be difficult for the residents of the regular wings or floors to deal with. Memory-care units usually have special training for the staff and more staff per patient. They should also be set up more specifically for these patients with secure doors, secure outside areas, special amenities such as music, furniture, and other items from earlier decades, and activities and special environments to help these people be happy and calm.

Geropsych units, which are a little different from a memory-care unit, are more geared to treat and manage older people with mental illness. These gerontology psychiatric units may be located in a hospital, SNF, or stand-alone facility.

Assisted-Living and Independent-Living Facilities

Assisted-living facilities (ALFs) provide housing for people who can't live independently but don't need skilled nursing care. Assistance depends on what the person needs. It may include bathing, dressing, laundry, housekeeping, medication management, and safety checks. Meals are usually provided in a community dining room or café, and these facilities usually have activities and recreation opportunities too. Costs vary from place to place and may depend on what assistance your loved one needs. These facilities may also be associated with a nursing home or TCU so residents may be able to more seamlessly transition between these levels of care as situations change.

Continuing-care retirement communities offer facilities from independent retirement living to assisted living and nursing home care, even memory-care, depending on what the person needs at the time. These places offer to care for the person in one place for most everything they would need for the rest of their lives. They are usually paid for out of pocket and are more expensive. They may charge an entrance fee ranging from one thousand to several thousand dollars plus a monthly rental, or have the entrance fee include the purchase of a home there, which can cost $100,000 to $1,000,000. The home can be sold again later. They will also have monthly charges of $3,000 to $10,000. Their charges may vary greatly depending on the services your loved one needs. Be very careful reading and signing any contracts for these facilities, especially regarding the pricing and payment for additional services and how much discretion the facility has to determine the person's needed level of service and conditions regarding discharge.

Retirement communities can be a range of residence options, from age-targeted leisure communities like the famous Sun City in Arizona, to independent-living facilities that usually offer community dining rooms and some home services such as housekeeping, linen service, and transportation, to continuing-care facilities (discussed above). The homes, which can be apartments or single-family homes, are usually designed to be easier to get around in but are not medical facilities. These communities do not tend to be licensed and are not regulated or paid for by Medicaid. They offer cohort companionship and a lifestyle that may fit with many adults.

Adult Family Homes and Other Private In-Home Options

Adult family homes (AFHs) and **board-and-care homes** provide housing and meals and assume responsibility for the safety and care of the residents. Both types may differ from home to home regarding what other care they may provide and how independent the residents need to be. They may help with intermittent nursing, handling medications, and ADLs such as dressing, bathing, and mobility assistance, as well as recreation activities and outings, etc. Most states require a facility license, but the agency that licenses them and the terms may vary from state to state.

AFHs are generally smaller, with six residents or fewer, and are usually located in a regular single-family home in a regular urban or suburban neighborhood. They are often owned and run by a family or individual, but may be a business partnership and may hire help. Board-and-care homes have more than six residents and may look more like a facility than a home.

Adult foster care can be much like an AFH in its mission and the living environment. The definition varies state by state, but usually they are smaller, with one to four residents. The licensing requirements vary state by state as well.

Home sharing is basically renting a room. Let's say your parent now has a bigger house than they can handle and wants more income and/or help with chores, plus companionship. Arrangements could be made to rent rooms to your parent's friends, other adults of their generation, or younger people. This is simply a private rental agreement based on local rental laws.

Home sharing may also work in a situation where your loved one moves in with someone else and rents a room in their home. I even have a friend who arranged for his mother and father to share a home near him, even though they had been divorced and lived apart for many years. I thought it was a pretty risky move, but it did in fact work out.

It is crucially important that your loved one actually wants to do home sharing and that the arrangements are well spelled out in advance. There are a lot of potential problems, including elder abuse, theft, and just plain not working out—like any home-sharing situation (remember your college roommates?). If you are considering this option, I encourage you to at least look at the links below.

Home sharing may make all the difference in allowing someone to stay in their home, but you and your loved one shouldn't expect a renter or a landlord to become a caregiver. There are local agencies to help find potential home-share situations for both renters and homes; here are some good links to check out:

Basic Definition https://www.caring.com/articles/home-sharing

Questions to consider https://www.caring.com/articles/planning-to-share-a-home

Finding and arranging https://www.caring.com/articles/arranging-home-share

Adult Day Services

Adult day-care centers operate during daytime hours, Monday through Friday, enabling people to socialize and participate in activities while still receiving needed care and supervision. They also give caregivers a much-needed respite in which to attend to personal needs or simply rest and relax while knowing that their loved one is in good hands. There are three basic types:

- **Social:** provides meals, supervision, and activities
- **Adult day health care (ADHC):** usually staffed with an RN and CNAs and may have PTs, OTs, and SPLs
- **Dementia-specific:** care centers that usually provide more specially trained staff, a higher ratio of staff to participants, and activities to help people stay more engaged, interested, and happy. They usually have systems to prevent wandering as well.

The average cost is $64 per day, but many factors can affect this. Medicaid and many locally based resources can help cover some if not all of the costs. To find centers in your area, visit http://www.eldercare.gov/Eldercare.NET/Public/Index.aspx. Be sure to ask about financial assistance and possible scholarships. Private medical insurance policies sometimes cover a portion of adult day-care center costs when licensed medical professionals are involved in the care. Long-term care insurance may also pay for adult day-care services, depending on the policy. Additionally, dependent-care tax credits may be available to you as caregiver.

Choosing a Long-Term or Residential Care Facility

So now you know a little more about what's out there and the care they offer. How do you choose? You will need to consider how this type of facility will be paid for. Your medical care providers, especially your social worker, can help you in this discussion. **Note:** Medicare can pay for 100 days in nursing homes following a medically related three-night hospitalization. They will pay the first 20 days in full, then require a copay for the next 80 days. In 2016 the copay amount was $161 per day. This is still less than the full costs, but it adds up quickly. The following link gives a good rundown of costs and benefits https://www.medicare.gov/your-medicare-costs/costs-at-a-glance/costs-at-glance.html#collapse-4808. If your loved one qualifies for Medicaid, they do not have a time limit for assistance, and a caseworker can help immensely. For more on this, see Chapter 8, Medicare, Medicaid, and Private Insurance.

Make a List of Places to Consider

Make a generous list of the places you are considering. I like to pin-drop them on a map program just to make it easier to keep track of it all. Your social worker or caseworker can be your best resource in this. If your neighbors and friends have experience with any of the places, they can help with local knowledge and personal experience. Medicare keeps a list of all the certified nursing homes by Zip Code at https://www.medicare.gov/nursinghomecompare/search.html. Your state Medicaid office may also keep a list of facilities by region. In many states this includes assisted-living facilities, adult family homes, board-and-care homes, and adult foster care (if they use that term). Your state's Medicaid office or Long-Term Care Ombudsman's office may generate a list. Try http://theconsumervoice.org/get_help to find your states office. You may also search "Medicaid" and the name of your state.

There are **private referral services**, which may be easier to use than doing it yourself. A Place for Mom www.aplaceformom.com is a pretty good service for this. Keep in mind that "free" placement agencies may require membership of the facilities they list, and thus their lists may not be complete. Many charge a fee to the facility when your loved one is admitted, often your first month's payment. There have been problems. If the facility wasn't a good fit, the resident could not get a refund of the first month's payment, because that money went to the placement agency. This could be several thousand dollars.

Each facility's website will most likely be promotional, but they should give some view into the location, size, services offered, and overarching vision or mission.

Now let's narrow the list. As you look through the facility websites, consider what your loved one's goals are and what their needs are now and may be in the future:

- **What care is needed or will be needed?** Consider the level of medical attention, assistance, rehabilitation, and any special services or equipment.
- **What is the length of time that is or will be needed?** Will this be temporary or long term?
- **Is the location close to loved ones, friends, and caregivers?** If your loved one is mobile, is it a location they are used to or could get used to and like?
- **Where will your loved one find comfort, purpose, and fulfillment?** Will they find companionship and social connection there?

- **If the facility is inpatient, are visiting hours important?** Can your loved one go on day trips with the facility or with you?
- **Are there cultural and/or language considerations?**

This should narrow your list to those facilities that are appropriate for your loved one. The order in which you do the following steps may vary depending on how long your list is and how easy it is for you to drop by versus do desktop research. I think you'll see a natural sequence that works for you. Any way you go about it, don't skip steps, especially reading the contracts.

Research Reports on the Facility

For **nursing homes**, the Medicare website has a function called "Nursing Home Compare", which publishes their annual inspection results and any complaints that required action or "letters." The site also has a five-star rating system, which seems simple enough, but at the time of this writing, it did not seem representative of people's experiences or reports of problems.

For assisted-living facilities, adult family homes, and **other long-term care facilities** with a state license, Washington State's Medicaid agency, the Department of Social and Health Services, maintains a complete list on their website. Under the tab "letters," you will find letters regarding enforcement actions against the facility in the past year. This type of reporting varies state by state, but it is worth a telephone call or look at your state's Medicaid website.

The state ombudsman's office http://theconsumervoice.org/get_help may be allowed to give you information regarding care-based complaints for a specific facility you might be interested in. They may also be able to steer you to the best local resources in your state for information on particular facilities. It's worth a call or a look at your state's website.

Call the Facility

If you haven't yet, consider the questions and the priorities you might ask a long-term care (LTC) facility. Again, look at the questions listed above under "Make a List of Places to Consider" to help you write specific questions. Create a question page for each place you will call. Record who you talked to, their contact information and job title, their answers, and how you felt about the conversation. You might use this conversation to arrange a visit.

Make an Arranged Visit

Chances are, if you arrange a visit, you will get a tour. If the arranged visit is your second-to-last step, you might do this with your loved one. This visit also gives you more time to ask more-direct questions, such as:

- **Who draws up the resident's service plan?** How involved is the resident and their family in this process?
- **How often is the service plan or plan of care reassessed?** Are fees based on this?
- **How much advanced notice does the resident have if fees will rise?**

- **How does the facility manage changes in the resident's needs?** Does the facility have access to higher levels of care, like an attached nursing home or rehab facility?
- **What would make the facility need to transfer a resident out?** How is that handled? If the resident's transfer is temporary, do they save the resident's living unit for them?
- **How does the facility handle a medical emergency?**
- **Do they have a waiting list?**
- **Is there a probationary period?**
- **How are grievances handled?**
- **Is there a family or resident council?** When do they meet?

Take home a copy of the Resident's Rights, the facility's rules, the price list, a floor plan if you think that location within the building is important, and any contracts or other documents that will need to be signed. This can all go in a folder for each facility that you visit.

Explain the specific needs and preferences of your loved one: "My mom's situation is …" Ask real questions: "What if she needs this? What if she needs that?" If they have difficulty accommodating your loved one's individual needs, maybe you should consider somewhere else.

Make More than One Drop-in Visit

An unscheduled visit gives you a chance to talk candidly with the rest of the staff, other residents, and their families. Try for a mealtime. Try for a resident council or family council meeting. Keep in mind that it will be busy at mealtimes and in the morning, and it may feel unorganized at shift changes.

Read the Contracts

Yes, read the contracts and all that other paperwork. Are there discrepancies between what they have promised, what their brochures and/or website say, and what the contract says? Other red flags include "responsible party" provisions that make family members or loved ones liable for expenses, claims that injury or harm is common or unavoidable, or provisions that give unauthorized justifications for eviction or that limit arbitration. Assisted-living facilities' contracts might also include red-flag provisions such as pricing of additional services that can be exorbitant or claims that residents can agree to accept a lower level of care than they actually need. A facility might also cloak eviction in terms of not being able to meet the care needs of the resident, so they might write themselves a lot of leeway in their contract for this.

Other Options

If you are in a long-distance caregiving situation, **care management companies** can help with selecting, vetting, and monitoring placement in LTC facilities. Ask directly if they physically visit or just talk with the facility on the phone. **Aging Life Care Association** https://www.aginglifecare.org/ is the professional association of care managers. They have a referral service to local care managers.

Good, you've done your homework and you now have a list of a few good LTC facilities where your loved one can be comfortable if it's needed. You can put these files away and perhaps you won't need them. But it sure is nice to know you have a plan, if you need it.

...Helping Your Loved One After They Move into a Long-Term Care Facility

If your loved one does move into a long-term care facility, you can still be tremendously helpful for them. See Helping Your Loved One During Hospitalization earlier in this chapter: you can do much the same if they are in an LTC facility.

Visit often. A regular visit schedule helps give your loved one structure and lets them plan their time. I remember our neighbor Bea was so gregarious she needed some help to manage her social calendar while she was in a nursing home.

Go on outings. Take your loved one on outings if possible. Life is short. There is no good reason not to live it as well as you can.

Help them remain engaged in activities they enjoy and find meaning in. See how many ways you can encourage favorite activities. They may start new meaningful projects such as creating a memoir or visiting their friends, who may have their own health problems. Can they help make a care package for a friend? Do they like to work in the garden? Often, LTC facilities have one for residents who garden. Often people find terrific relationships with pets. Can their pet join them there? Some facilities have "therapy animals" that live at the facility.

Attend care meetings. As with the hospital rounds described earlier in this chapter, let your loved one lead the discussion with the facility's health-care providers if possible. Ask what is missed. Take notes. Consider well the risks, costs, and benefits of any changes or of not making changes. Talk to staff about any changes you observe in your loved one's behavior or condition. Chances are that they have noted these too, but it doesn't hurt for them to hear it from you as well.

...Addressing Problems in a Long-Term Care Facility

There will most likely be some things that you and your loved one won't like about a move into an LTC facility. For instance, moving into most long-term care facilities does come with some loss of personal freedom. But you don't need to accept everything passively, especially if it is something the facility promised but is not delivering.

You and your loved one's first venue for addressing grievances is the **Residents Council** or the **Family Council**. This is a formal meeting of the residents to voice concerns and help direct the staff and their policies to address such issues. The Family Council is a similar body for family members. By law, nursing homes have to allow a space and time for these meetings. The Missouri Ombudsman Program developed this document to describe better what a Resident Council is and how to set one up http://health.mo.gov/seniors/ombudsman/pdf/HowToOrganizeAnd_DirectAnEffectiveResidentCouncil.pdf. These councils can approach the facility directly, or they may file formal complaints to the state Long-Term Care Ombudsman.

Each state has a **Long-Term Care Ombudsman Office.** The ombudsman advocates for people regarding long-term care in the state, fielding complaints and solving problems. They also monitor the licensing agencies and inspections, publish reports like those you might have reviewed when looking for a place, and act as your advocate in addressing lawmakers regarding regulation of these facilities. To find the Long-Term Care Ombudsman in your state, search "Long-Term Care Ombudsman" and the name of your state, or check into the Consumer Voice http://theconsumervoice.org/get_help.

Most grievances can be solved through the council's or the ombudsman's office. Unfortunately, sometimes it is indeed a matter of law and you may need a good lawyer. The **National Academy of Elder Law Attorneys'** website https://www.naela.org/ has links to attorneys who specialize in elder law by region. For public-assistance lawyers, the **National Legal Resource Center** (NLRC) publishes a map by state that links to legal resources by state http://nlrc.acl.gov/Services_Providers/Index.aspx.

The best publication on this I have come across concerning resolving problems in long-term care is "20 Common Nursing Home Problems and How to Resolve Them," published by **Justice in Aging**, a legal advocacy group focused on laws and issues affecting seniors http://www.justiceinaging.org/20-common-nursing-home-problems/.

...Moving Out of a Long-Term Care Facility

Moving out of a long-term care facility may be nearly as traumatic as moving in. Chances are, some type of medical emergency brought your loved one to the facility. Now, if they're moving back home, they may have needs that may require getting new care systems in place. They might even be moving to a new home or facility altogether.

Chances are, the LTC facility took care of medications, meals, laundry, housekeeping, medical appointments, transportation and provided supervision, structure, routine, and help with ADLs. How much of these things can they do for themselves now? How much assistance will they need? This book can help you with each realm they may need help with. Here is where to look for what:

Medication: Nursing homes and other LTC facilities that provide medication management should give your loved one a 30-day supply on discharge. See Chapter 11, Medications.

Meals: See Meals on Wheels in Volunteer Organizations in Chapter 1, Building a Caregiving Team, and Chapter 12, Food and Nutrition.

Laundry and housekeeping: Your team might be able to help here (see Chapter 1, Building a Caregiving Team), or you might hire in-home help (see Chapter 2, Calling in the Pros).

Switching medical providers: If they are moving to a different home, will they need a new doctor? See Chapter 9, Doctors.

Transportation: Will they be able to get in and out of your car? See Physically Helping Your Loved One Move in Chapter 15, Basic Mobility and Transfers). Will they be able to drive? Have you considered public transportation options such as Paratransit or Access?

Supervision: See Chapter 1, Building a Caregiving Team; Chapter 2, Calling in the Pros; and Medical Alert Systems in Chapter 15, Basic Mobility and Transfers.

Mobility: If they are moving to a different home or their mobility has changed, will they need new modifications, adaptive equipment, or furniture? See Fall Prevention, Mobility Aids and Adaptive Equipment, Physically Helping Your Loved One Move, and Positioning for Comfort in Chapter 15, Basic Mobility and Transfers.

Hygiene: For help with bathing, toileting, and oral care, see Chapter 16, Hygiene, Bathing, and Toileting.

Other services: What other services will they need? Have you considered adult day-care services?

As soon as you start thinking about moving your loved one out of an LTC facility, begin to consider a target date. The social worker or discharge planner can help immensely through the whole process. They may also help connect you with the resources that help; https://www.benefitscheckup.org/ offers a very nice search function to locate local resources. You'll also need to arrange for transitions that are a part of any kind of move:

Budget. Research how your loved one will pay for mobility devices and home caregivers. See Chapter 8, Medicare, Medicaid, and Private Insurance.

Important documents. Make sure that your loved one or you take their important documents—medical and/or durable power of attorney, advance directives, etc.—with them when they move. Will they need to move their financial account(s) to another institution? See Chapter 6, The Notebook of Important Papers.

Contact information. Do they need to change their address with the post office? Will they have new phone or Internet service?

I like this nice simple document with a timeline spreadsheet to help you through the process of moving your loved one out of an LTC facility http://theconsumervoice.org/uploads/files/general/consumer-tips-for-nh-transition.pdf.

Chapter 11. Medications

By the time you find yourself in a caregiver role, your loved one probably takes more than a few medications. Their med lists may seem daunting, and they may need help keeping it all straight, taking the right medications at the right times, and refilling prescriptions before they run out.

You may wonder if all those pills and such are causing some of their struggles. We caregivers are not the prescribing doctors, and it's not usually a good idea to try to be, but we *are* on the front line, spending the most time with that doctor's patient, helping them take their regular medications, and helping make decisions about the ones that are to be taken as needed.

You can help your loved one and their doctors if you have a better idea of what each drug is taken for, a little about how it works, and what to watch out for regarding side effects, bad interactions, and overmedication. This powerful information might be easier to collect and organize than you think.

Making a Medications List

Start by making a medication list. List the **regular medications** first. Note the dosage, the time it should be taken, and any notes about taking it, such as "take with food" or "don't take if …" I found it was a good idea to use a heading with the general reason a drug is taken, for example, "chemotherapy" or "for nausea." Include medication creams, patches, liquids, and inhalers. These are all drugs and can have an effect.

Include **over-the-counter (OTC) drugs** such as aspirin or antacids. Include **herbal supplements;** the chemicals in herbs are drugs, too; many of the pharmaceutical drugs on the market are synthetic versions of herbal chemicals. Include **nutritional supplements and vitamins**. These all can have an effect and are also pills that you will need to count when you're laying the meds out.

There are plenty of **tools for creating this medication list**; you can find one at http://www.drugs.com/. We initially used an Excel spreadsheet, but then settled on a word document template with hand-writing out parts on a simple white sheet of paper.

Here is one of the simple med lists we used:

Date: _____

Karen's Medication List

MANDATORY-should not skip these! If unable to take, talk to Dave or Hospice

	morning	noon	eve.	bed
Morphine ER (extended release) 30mg+ Morphine ER 15mg every 6 to 8 hours			☒	
Methylphenidate 5mg morning & noon			—	—
Citalopram 10mg daily at bedtime	—	—	—	
Senna 1 daily (with dinner)	—	—		
Lidoderm patch on back in the morning, take off in the evening	On	—	—	OFF

OPTIONAL MEDICATIONS (can skip if nauseated)

	morning	noon	eve.	bed
Ibuprofen 200mg, 2 pills twice daily (must be taken with food)	—			—
Acyclovir 500mg 1 daily at noon	—		—	—
Multivitamin 1 daily at noon with food	—		—	—

AS NEEDED MEDICATIONS (found in blue medication bag)

	M	12 pm	E.	BED
Morphine IR (immediate release) 15mg every 4 hours as needed for pain.				
Lorazepam (Ativan) ¼ of a pill every 4 hours may repeat once if symptoms not relieved after 1 hour.				
Zofran 10mg every 6 to 8 hours as needed for nausea.				
Docusate Sodium 100mg daily as needed for constipation				
Marijuana (¼ a Fuber) as needed for pain, anxiety or nausea (there is also a pill form of this (Dronabinol) available				

Keep it current. Change it whenever the dose or prescriptions change. This is also discussed in Creating a Carebook in Chapter 1, Building a Caregiving Team.

Keep pharmacy information sheets behind the med list. When you pick up a new prescription at the pharmacy, the pharmacist will provide information about the indications, actions, and possible side effects of each drug they provide. They will often give you a brief verbal rundown and hand you several pages of information.

Don't just toss the information. You might take a moment to read it through, taking note of interactions, the more common side effects, and how the drug is eliminated from the body. We kept those sheets in a section of the carebook.

There also are several websites that provide good information on most medications; http://www.drugs.com/ works well. It has a handy reference by drug name, an interaction checker, and a tool that allows you to identify unknown pills by shape, color, and marking. We also were good about culling out information for meds that were no longer used so the carebook didn't just become a big mess.

Take the meds list to doctor appointments. When your loved one visits the doctor, or the nurses visit you, bring the medications list. People can become overmedicated by too much and too many prescriptions and prescriptions that interact. Some drugs might affect how another drug works or how it is eliminated. Drugs are usually eliminated by being broken down and/or filtered out by the liver or kidneys, or both. Anything that affects these organs will affect how a drug is eliminated. If someone's liver function is slow, you might expect them to more slowly eliminate a drug processed by the liver, so more of the drug will be circulating in the body. If they are dehydrated, the kidneys will filter more slowly too. Problems with elimination are the most common way for someone to become overmedicated.

In this day of brief appointment times, it's far too common for a health-care provider to add another drug to address a symptom rather than to thoughtfully tease through the patient's entire history to eliminate drugs and habits that might be causing the problem. If someone's care is compartmentalized between different teams of specialists, it's far too easy for a clinician to look only at their own records and not see the whole picture.

Your loved one's prescribing doctors should know *all* the medications they are on before they add another medication to the list. Your med list can really help make it clear for them. It also might help them, your loved one, and you consider why a drug is being prescribed. It might make it a bit clearer about how and why it should be taken and help everyone be more aware of possible drug interactions.

A thoughtful pharmacist can help screen out possible interacting drugs too. Sticking with one pharmacy, especially a pharmacist who knows your loved one, is a good idea. I believe that much can be gained from periodically giving a good thoughtful review of the entire health history and medications list.

Now that I've scared the bejeezus out of you and encouraged you to read through long lists of symptoms and side effects, I'd better tell you about the worst side effect: Med Student Syndrome. Most of the severe side effects and interactions are rare, but simply reading about all those symptoms might make you think your loved one has them. You don't want to be like John, a second-year med student who was thrown into a panic after too much pondering over the lists of clinical presentations: "Oh my God!" he screamed out. "That's it, I must be pregnant!"

Giving and Storing Medications

How hard is it to count out a few pills and take them as directed? If you give a research subject a very simple task—say, to hit the red button when the screen turns red and the green button when the screen turns green—and enough trials at it, they will make mistakes. That's why hospitals, air traffic controllers, and mountain climbers all develop very simple systems with double-checks to minimize these simple, avoidable errors. Just being careful isn't enough.

The pill caddy. This is a little (usually plastic) box with separate compartments for each day's worth of medicines. The best pill caddy has a sealed compartment for each dosage time in the day—such as morning, noon, evening, and bedtime—for an extended period such as a week. This allows you to lay out all the pills once in a week. The fewer times you have to perform a task, the fewer chances you have to make a mistake, the fewer mistakes you will make. A comfort-care nurse on our care team introduced us to the Cadillac of all pill caddies, and originally I thought, "We don't need that," but then I thought of the simple red-green studies and thought, "Yes, of course." It helped immeasurably.

Filling the pill caddy. Keep all the regularly scheduled medicines in one container (such as a large resealable bag for all the pill bottles). While you are reviewing the medication list, bring out each pill bottle, double-check the label on each pill bottle against the med list, take a handful of the pills, and place them in the caddy at their assigned times of day. Do this for each pill bottle until the bag is empty. Then go back and count the pills in each compartment to double-check that the number is correct. If there are more than just a few pills, try pulling the larger pills aside to make your count.

Having the pills laid out for the week makes it easier for other caregivers because they don't have to count pills out of bottles. The pill caddy also gives everyone a double-check against the med list to see if meds were taken or not. Just one more added benefit: It helps you to see if you are running out of a medication within one week of actually running out, so you have time to refill that prescription.

Storing the medications. So how do you store the medications before you dole them out into the pill caddy? We kept pills in their bottles until it was time to lay out the supply in the pill caddy for the day or week. You can keep all the pill bottles in a clear food storage bag or Tupperware container. Be sure to mark it clearly, and if more than one person (or a pet) in a house has medications, mark it with their name ("Bowser's meds") and keep it separate. We also could keep our current medication list inside the bag if we wanted, but we chose to keep that in our carebook.

Where do you store the bag of meds? Most medicines are fairly reactive chemicals. They need to be protected from exposure to excessive light and humidity and kept at or below room temperature. They also should be kept out of reach of pets and children and never taken by anyone else.

We were blessed with a little cancer swag from the first chemo drug Karen was on, a blue neoprene bag with the logo of Xeloda uncomfortably silk-screened across the front. This bag was dark, resistant to temperature change, and very obviously not candy or food. We could keep the bag in a drawer, away from where we showered (humidity) and out of reach of kids and adults who might behave as kids. This also kept any medications in tubes or any topicals away from the toothpaste. Imagine a late-night mistake there. Yuck.

We found it best (and it is recommended) to keep all the medications for a particular person in one place as much as we could. However, there were certain liquids that had to be refrigerated. These we kept each in their original box in their own special place in the upper back corner of the fridge.

Keeping a Medication Log

You can make and keep a **daily log of medicines** in the carebook (see Chapter 1, Building a Caregiving Team). This med log will let you know at a glance what med was given and when. The boxes in our example above are big enough to record the time for as-needed medicines.

If you have room on the page, a few lines for **notes on changes or reactions to meds** might be very useful. You could also use the back of the previous page, so that when the book is open you can see the list and the notes page at once. If the issue is more complex, you can break out a separate tab in the book for a notes section. At various times we had sections on pain, diet, and bowel and bladder. You might have a section on anything that is an issue currently requiring a close watch. Other sections you might consider include anxiety, nausea, and breathing. Try to keep it to three or fewer sections at any one time, as recording in many sections is cumbersome and information will get lost.

Using Basic Charting Techniques

Keeping accurate, useful, medical-style records in a private setting like your home is much easier than you might think. You are not bound by all the insurance and legal requirements that the clinicians are, so you can focus on recording just the useful factual information. Do this in a consistent way so it is easy to understand when you look back at it. These records can live in the Carebook Chapter 1, Building a Caregiving Team.

...What to Include

Begin with the **date and time**. Record **what your loved one said** and/or **what you saw**. Record **what you did,** if you did anything, and **how your loved one responded.** If you have some great idea or observation about what happened, record **what you thought,** and if you **plan to change something,** record that too. There—you just created the basic medical SOAP note:

> **S = Subjective:** what they said
> **O = Objective:** what you saw, measured, and did
> **A = Assessment:** what you thought about it
> **P = Plan:** what you're going to do in the future about it

As a private citizen caregiver just making notes for you and your caregiving team, you don't need to record something for each letter in the SOAP model, only what is important for the current concern.

...Examples

Here is an example of a note that has too much writing but is missing some key information:

> *3:30 She's really feeling bad, lots of pain in her back and legs. I think the cat has been bothering her making it worse. I gave her morphine.*
>
> *6:00 Pain is coming back again. I hate this.*

I think you can see where the TMI (too much information) is, but can you see where there is not enough information? Was the time a.m. or p.m.? Care is 24 hours. There is no dosage recorded. How much morphine did we give her? How did she do with that dose? There is no follow-up note on its effectiveness 30-60 minutes later. Now, with all that extra information, as well as missing information, think how cumbersome it will be to look back and read a week's worth of entries.

Here's how to do it better:

3:30 p.m. Pain level 4. Gave 15 mg morphine IR.—Dave

4:15 p.m. Pain level 2. Alert. Dose effective but not too much.—Dave

For pain, the pain number system works well. If your loved one is nonverbal, record things such as "grimacing," "agitated," or "elevated heart rate."

For anxiety, record heart rate, emotional outbursts, or specific things they say or do.

For diet, record what they ate and drank and about how much. Also, record if they became nauseated or add special notes such as "really liked that" or "difficult to swallow, aspirated."

For bowel, record whether the voided amount was large, medium, or small, and maybe note consistency, such as loose or firm. Unusual color might be important too, such as yellow or black.

For breathing, note shortness of breath (SOB) and/or oxygen saturation (O2 sat) if you are using an oximeter (a little meter with a red light they stick on the end of your finger), if your loved one is using oxygen or if they just used a nebulizer or inhaler. You might also record productive or unproductive coughing and sounds from their breathing such as crackling or wheezing.

...How the Charting Notes Help

Within a few days of recording these charting notes, patterns will emerge and be easily recognized by you, the nurses, and the doctors. This will make adjusting the medicines and treatments much easier and more effective.

An example of this might be that you notice your loved one's pain ramp up each afternoon. You could look in the notes for causes, and you could increase the longer-acting regular dosing of pain medications at noon or in the morning. If bowel function is a problem, a quick check in those notes will let the prescribing physician know how the bowel program needs to be adjusted, especially if the pain medicine is to be adjusted.

Once an issue is under control and stabilized, you and the caregiving team may discontinue noting on it. This will save you time and make looking back on it easier. You can leave the notes in place in the carebook. We did write a brief dated "last entry" that stated that we discontinued note taking and why.

Taking notes in this way, creating a useful home medical record, makes you a valuable part of the care team and helps coordinate the care your loved one receives from everyone involved. It takes only a few minutes here and there during the day and helps keep everyone on the same page.

Paying for the Pills

Drugs can be ridiculously expensive. The particular rules of the US insurance system change over time and are beyond the scope of this book. That said, there are a few things we can say here to help.

Most insurance providers maintain an ever-changing list of drugs they pay for and the amount they will pay. This is their **formulary**, and the list is available from your insurance carrier.

Depending on your loved one's insurance plan, the carrier can help pay part or all the cost for the prescriptions. There may be a **copay** (fixed cost to you) or a **percent pay** (you pay a percentage of the cost) for a drug.

They also may contract with certain pharmacies or pharmacy networks to pay only a certain amount for the drugs on their formulary. When they do this, the insurance company usually will try to encourage you to use their "**in-network providers**" by making you pay more if you use someone else.

Most formularies will cover more of the cost for a **generic drug** than for a **name-brand drug**. This usually isn't a bad thing. The cost of developing a new drug is very high and the chance of success is very low, so when a new drug is produced, that company will charge a lot for it. Often when a drug comes off patent protection, another company will produce a drug using the same active compound but charge much less for it. It makes sense that your loved one's insurance will opt for the less-expensive version of the same drug on their formulary.

Under the rules at the time of this writing, any carrier must provide at least 60 days' notice of **any change in the formulary** that affects any drug your loved one is taking and allow a 60-day supply before the change takes effect, so you have some protection against the seemingly random changes in the formulary.

There are many **charity programs** to help people pay for medications. Your loved one's **social worker** can also help identify programs that might help. This very nice search function helps locate local resources https://www.benefitscheckup.org/. Here is one list of charities that was valid at the time of this writing http://www.medicarerights.org/pdf/copay_charities.pdf. You can see from this list that loving people often create charity programs around specific conditions or diseases. You might search for more resources under whatever condition has brought you to caregiving.

Hospice and Medicaid programs tend to cover all the prescription costs but may limit what is available on their formulary. **Medicare** now has a prescription drug plan called **Medicare part D.** This is a voluntary program that your loved one must opt in for and pay an insurance premium too. It is less expensive if they opt in on their first availability to Medicare, and the overall cost is hugely subsidized by our taxes. For more information on these programs, and Medicare in general, look into your regional **State Health Insurance Program** (SHIP) http://www.seniorsresourceguide.com/directories/National/SHIP/.

With the Affordable Care Act (ACA, or Obamacare), private insurance and Medicare also come with a **maximum out-of-pocket clause**. This means that policies are no longer written as a maximum benefit (insurance covers only so much, then you're on your own) but instead are written that your loved one will pay only so much, usually only a few thousand dollars per year, then they will cover the rest. This helps keep people from medical bankruptcy and helps providers get paid for their services.

See Chapter 8, Medicare, Medicaid, and Private Insurance for more on Medicare parts C and D and private insurance and drug coverage.

Disposing of Unused Medication the Right Way

What the heck do you do with all those unused pills and patches? Can you just throw them in the trash or dump them in the toilet? Well, some, but not all.

Some of those medications don't break down fully in the wastewater treatment system and end up with the fish. Some of those medications, if taken by someone who doesn't have the illness or the "experience" with them, could be fatal. In the United States we have several **prescription take-back programs** hosted through local law enforcement agencies. This link will help you find one in your area http://www.deadiversion.usdoj.gov/drug_disposal/takeback/index.html.

If there is no program near you, most medicines can be **disposed of in the trash** with a little extra care: Mix, but don't crush, the medicines with kitty litter, dirt, or used coffee grounds (this prevents animals and human animals from eating it). Place the mixture in a sealed plastic bag and throw that bag in the trash.

Opiates (pain meds), benzodiazepines (Diazepam and Ativan), and a few others should be **flushed down the toilet or rinsed down the sink.**

For a more complete list, check this FDA Web page http://www.fda.gov/Drugs/ResourcesForYou/Consumers/BuyingUsingMedicineSafely/EnsuringSafeUseofMedicine/SafeDisposalofMedicines/ucm186187.htm. You can also look at the **drug information sheet** your loved one's pharmacist gave you with the prescription for disposal recommendations.

Before throwing the pill bottles out, it is a good idea to scratch names and personal information off the labels. In some places they can also be recycled. Check with your local recycling recommendations.

Chapter 12.
Food and Nutrition

Our food is more than sustenance or fuel. It is an integral part of our society. We gather together around our meals. We give food to say "be happy" and "I love you". We toast to life and to health. As a person is going through illness, incapacity, and treatment, many factors can affect the delicate interplay that makes food feel good to us. This can cause a dilemma because your loved one may not feel like eating despite knowing they should or may feel like eating things that are not necessarily good for them.

Karen lived life to the fullest, and this included the enjoyment of a good meal, especially when enjoyed with friends. As her health began to fail, eating became a struggle. This became one of the challenges she and her loved ones tried to keep in perspective so she could continue to revel in the enjoyment of a good meal. To navigate this ever-changing and sometimes difficult terrain, we used common sense, read up on the issues, consulted several times with dietitians (very helpful), and paid close attention to Karen.

This chapter begins with a list of factors you may encounter that affect your loved one's intake of food, then some specific conditions and how they affect a person's eating. *Bon appétit.*

Weight Loss

Many factors can decrease intake of food and lead to weight loss when someone is ill. The most common factors are discussed in this chapter, each with their own heading. Page down to Changing Food Preferences, Changes Involving the Tongue and Olfactory Sense, Early Satiation, Nausea, Sore Mouth and Throat, and Swallowing Issues.

In addition, some health conditions increase caloric needs so that even if your loved one is not eating less than usual, they can still lose weight. Some of the more common conditions that affect diet and weight are discussed in this chapter as well. See Eating and Depression, Eating and Cancer, Eating and the Aging, Eating and Dementia, Eating and Stroke, and Eating and the End of Life.

Tips to help prevent weight loss include the following:

- **offering small, frequent meals**
- **creating a calm environment** for eating
- **keeping portions small** so as to not overwhelm them, which might affect their appetite
- **adding calorie-dense ingredients** such as fats to meals

Healthy fats include olive oil, canola oil, sesame oil, and walnut oil. For packing in calories when that is difficult to do, coconut milk works well too. There are also diet supplement drinks such as Ensure, which are easy to serve and drink. I preferred creating our own shakes and smoothies, which can be supplemented with protein and calorie- and nutrition-dense ingredients. Recipes for shakes and smoothies are at the end of this chapter. If possible, shakes should supplement meals rather than replace them.

Weight Gain

Though it's not usually expected, it is possible to gain weight during illnesses. Beverages with calories (juice, pop, milk, alcohol) can quickly increase caloric intake without affecting appetite, so people will still eat the same amount of calories from food. Thus, drinking your calories can lead to weight gain. Often, people crave sweets and refined carbohydrates, which may be a side effect of depression or an alteration in taste buds.

It is important to make sure the foods you offer to your loved one are nutritionally dense, low in fat, and low in refined carbohydrates (sugar and white flour). Consider stocking your pantry and fridge with fresh or frozen fruits, vegetables, whole grains, lean protein, low-fat dairy, and noncaloric drinks—water being the healthiest choice. Allowing for favorite treat foods on occasion will help prevent your labeling foods as good or bad as well as avoiding your being labeled "the food police."

Pushing Too Hard to Get Them to Eat

Even if you have the best intentions, pushing your loved one to eat and/or eat certain foods can backfire. No one likes to be told what to do, and when your loved one is ill and possibly losing their independence, food may be one of the only areas in life they are still able to control. **Ellyn Satter** http://ellynsatterinstitute.org/index.php has many books and resources on how to get children to eat a healthy diet without causing food and eating to become a battle zone. You may find that some of the same suggestions work for you.

Briefly, try to offer several healthy options at meals and snacks so you will be comfortable with whatever your loved one decides to eat—then eat together and create a tranquil environment for the meal. Please, avoid linking your loved one's consumption of food to your approval or happiness.

Factors that Affect Food Intake

This section covers reasons your loved one might not be able to eat like they used to. The services of a nutritionist are usually recommended. They can guide you to a number of tricks specific to certain types of treatments, such as using a wooden spoon to avoid the metallic taste some treatments can give or "magic mouthwash" to numb the mouth before eating.

...Changing Food Preferences

With many conditions, the very appetite and the types of food a person enjoys might change as they go through illness. About midway in her illness, Karen developed a taste for comfort foods. Mac 'n' cheese was king on the list. We always kept several boxes of easy-to-prepare mac 'n' cheese. We often had the ingredients to make a special batch from scratch. Once word got out, our friends who could cook prepared pans of the most wonderful deluxe mac 'n' cheese with fine cheeses, fresh macaroni, and baked bread-crumb toppings so we could slice out a small portion of this love for Karen whenever the craving arose.

We kept other comfort foods as well, in easy-to-prepare, pre-prepared, and ready-to-prepare forms. We kept soups, mashed potatoes with savory meaty gravy, *lefsa* (she is half Norwegian), and this funky dish that my mom used to make with Campbell's mushroom soup (she was Norwegian too). Still, with all this comfort food, we made a point to not let "Karen food" take over the whole pantry and refrigerator. We lived there too and could not continue to stay healthy if we didn't keep our diets healthy. Please see Eat Right in Chapter 4, Dancing in the Rain: Healthy Habits for Caregivers.

Your loved one is not Karen. Their tastes might very well change, but they might not turn to comfort food. However they turn, try to **keep easily prepared and deluxe versions of the dishes they now prefer**. Try to avoid relying on only the easily prepared processed versions. These versions lack much of the nutrition and the nuance of flavor that make the meal healthy. Also, try to avoid letting your loved one's changing preferences take over your diet as well. Their needs and tastes now are probably not the same as yours. It is a little more effort to prepare two meals simultaneously, but if you can, try to do so. A meal is better when enjoyed together.

...Changes Involving the Tongue and Olfactory Sense

The flavor and desirability of our food is one of the most complex sensations in the body. It involves not just the tongue, but also the nose, the palate, the stomach, the eyes, and the mind. The sense of smell in both the nose and the palate (olfactory sense) may give foods a slightly different flavor for your loved one than what you or I would taste in the same foods. Oftentimes we naturally adjust for this in how we prepare food. If you have ever tasted the food in a nursing home, you might remember it was very salty. This helps make up for the lack of flavor many of the elderly patrons perceive as their olfactory sense has dulled with age.

Adding a little salt may be OK. Salt, for most people, is not unhealthy. The reason why salt gets a bad rap in our culture is that it increases the fluid volume of the blood. If the person has any problem with high blood pressure, vascular disease, or edema, excess salt should definitely be avoided. Other conditions for which salt should be avoided include congestive heart failure, certain urinary diseases, and Menier's disease (a condition of the inner ear affecting balance) https://en.wikipedia.org/wiki/M%C3%A9ni%C3%A8re%27s_disease. Also, if your loved one's mouth is tender, salty foods may make this worse. Their primary-care physician should be able to tell you if salt or high sodium should be avoided.

Many medications, especially chemotherapies, may give a metallic taste sensation. This is only made worse by nausea and the loss of appetite that accompanies chemotherapy. One trick is to avoid using metallic eating utensils. Try wood or plastic.

A little spice or sweetener may also give food more flavor when sensation from the tongue or smell is different. The processed-food industry knows this very well. Just read the label from those processed foods you find in the middle of the grocery store and you will find added sugar or sweeteners in foods you might not think of as sugary. Everything comes with a trade-off, and this is true with adding sugar or spice. Sugar and other sweeteners, including the zero-calorie kinds, change our sensation of hunger and satiety, change our appetite, and cause an insulin response leading to the sugar crash, fat storage, and, in extreme cases, insulin resistance (type II diabetes). Excessive spice is difficult for people with any problems in their mouth or the rest of their gastrointestinal (GI) tract (that's everything between the lips and the anus).

I'm not saying that you shouldn't add any sugar or spice to make food taste better, but it helps to know what it does and how to be more careful with using that approach. Adding a pinch or two of salt, a half-teaspoon of sugar, and/or a savory spice such as Spike or Dash may help make the meal more flavorful for your loved one. Before flavoring the entire meal, try offering a little bit of the added flavoring on a bite of their portion and see whether they like it. You might not like it added to your meal.

Also, **ask your loved one's doctor about checking their zinc levels**. If this micronutrient is low, it may be affecting your loved one's sense of taste. This is especially important if diarrhea is an issue, as this can lead to zinc deficiency. If their zinc levels are low, you can ask their provider about supplementation. *It is always important to ask their doctor before adding supplements of any kind, as they may affect the efficacy of the medications being prescribed.*

...Early Satiation

When a person requires very little food to feel full, that is called early satiation. This can happen if the stomach lining is tender, as with advanced age or chemotherapies. It can also happen if your loved one hasn't been eating much for a while and their stomach has shrunk. Please do not channel my grandmother by saying, "Eat, eat, you're going to blow away if you don't eat."

To avoid the food battle, try instead to **offer small portions of food frequently**, up to every two hours.

Keep healthier snack foods in easy-to-access places: for example, a bag of washed and cut carrots in plain sight in the fridge.

Keep fluids separate from meals so your loved one doesn't fill up on liquids. If you are struggling to provide enough calories, choose liquids with calories and protein (milk, soy milk, smoothies). I have included some recipes for smoothies and shakes at the end of this chapter. You may add greens and other nutrient-rich foods to shakes and smoothies, too.

You may **add fats to foods to increase calories** without increasing the volume of food. Healthy fats include olive oil, canola oil, sesame oil, and walnut oil. It is important to add protein powders or other-protein rich foods, such as egg beaters (*never* add raw eggs), cottage cheese, tofu, or Greek yogurt to smoothies to make sure their protein intake meets their needs. The **National Cancer Institute** has snack ideas, recipes for drinks, and information about adding calories http://www.cancer.gov/cancertopics/coping/eatinghints/page1.

...Nausea

Recall for a moment any time when you felt nauseated. Maybe you were seasick or just had a few too many martinis the night before. Do you remember how hard it was to face that bowl of oatmeal? Your loved one may be going through the same thing.

Again, it's helpful to **offer small portions.** Just looking at the plate of food is difficult, so use small plates or bowls and don't fill them. Make a date to go out for a snack instead of a meal. This might help quell the anxiety your loved one associates with eating that only makes nausea worse. Here are some other tips:

- **Give them something to eat within one hour after they have woken up.**
  Allowing them to get hungry can worsen nausea.

- **Offer room-temperature foods** to prevent nausea, since the aroma of food can make nausea worse.
- **Limit the use of spices and fats**, since rich, spicy foods are usually not well tolerated by someone who's nauseated.

If your loved one does throw up, don't try to have them eat or drink until vomiting has stopped for at least half an hour. Then try small amounts of clear liquids first, such as water or bouillon. Once they can keep clear liquids down, try a full liquid such as soup. For a list of foods that are easy on the stomach, see http://www.cancer.gov/cancertopics/coping/eatinghints/page7#list3.

It's most likely your loved one has medications to take. Have them **take their meds with meals** to prevent the stomach upset the meds might cause if they try to digest the pills on an empty stomach. Check with the instructions on the medication, however: Some should be taken with food, some before meals, and some on an empty stomach.

Save favorite foods for days when your loved one feels good so they don't associate these foods with feeling sick. Again, avoid the food battle. Look again at this section's second paragraph, above: Think "small portions, full liquids, and clear liquids." Also see the advice in Early Satiation above: readily available snacks, smoothies and shakes, protein, and calories.

...Sore Mouth and Throat

If it is painful or difficult to swallow, eating can be a chore. Think of the last time your mouth was sore from the dentist or you had a very sore throat. What kinds of foods could you eat most comfortably? Avoid the corn nuts and probably the carrots. This is one time you probably want to cook the vegetables soft or use the blender. Applesauce, ice cream, cooked or canned peaches in yogurt, even baby food all work better than anything crunchy or chewy.

Cut food up small for your loved one so they can take smaller bites and have to chew less. A smaller utensil works well to encourage small bites; sometimes Karen would use chopsticks or the little silver baby spoon we got from her mother. Utensils got smaller, bites got smaller, and meals got smaller but more frequent. A hobbit would be proud, as we could have breakfast, second breakfast, lunch, afternoon snack, supper, and dinner.

You also can **supplement with shakes and smoothies.** A straw worked well for drinks. We are lucky to have Asian markets in Seattle, where we could find the superfat straws they use in bubble tea. These worked well.

Hot or very cold foods; spicy, salty, or acidic foods such as orange juice or tomatoes; and anything with alcohol all needed to go away. The Listerine went away too.

To help create a more pH-tolerant mouth and help with the sores, consider rinsing the mouth with a **weak baking-soda mouthwash.** Try mixing together 1/8 teaspoon baking soda, 1/2 cup lukewarm water, and a pinch salt and having your loved one rinse their mouth with it several times per day. A lidocaine mouthwash may be available on prescription from a formulating pharmacy to help numb the mouth before meals. For more information, see Oral Care in Chapter 16, Hygiene, Bathing, and Toileting.

Oh, yes—and just in case you have not figured this out with common sense, smoking with a sore mouth and throat is just plain silly.

...Swallowing Issues

If a person is having difficulty swallowing to the extent that they are letting food or fluids into their windpipe more than just rarely, the first thing they need is a **swallowing evaluation with a speech language pathologist (SLP)**. This requires a referral from your loved one's primary-care physician or through hospice. The speech pathologist will make an assessment and give you recommendations for what types of foods and fluids will work best, especially regarding thickness and softness of the food. They also will have specific tips for feeding that may help tremendously. Here is a video we produced with the speech pathologist for our care team. https://youtu.be/Yugl6aqlAa4

Swallowing is a complex motor (muscle-activation) reflex involving the muscles and tissues of the throat. Anything that disrupts this reflex can lead to a **swallowing accident**. Most of us have experienced swallowing something "the wrong way." We cough and cough and usually end up with teary eyes and a glass of water. Someone inevitably wants to slap us on the back, as they think this will help. Please don't slap your loved one's back. It usually just hurts and can lodge the obstruction farther down the windpipe. The last time that swallowing the wrong way happened to you, you were probably distracted or tired, or both. Usually having the person alert in a calm environment where they can focus helps.

The type of foods matters too. **Thick, smooth foods that hold together well are easiest to swallow**. Thin fluids and foods that crumble into little bits are most difficult. Large things like tougher meats are harder to swallow too. The speech pathologist might describe the softness and thickness of foods that they recommend, such as "honey thick" or "fork soft" (you can cut it with a fork). They also can give you products such as "Thick It" http://thickit.com/ to adjust the thickness of fluids.

They may discuss environment, certain cues that work best, and even utensils that work best. For us it was a quiet room, one-on-one meals, and a baby spoon so Karen could not take too big a bite. The recommendations are very individualized. The evaluation is important.

For someone with a swallowing issue, it might be a large piece that goes the wrong way, but it might also be a **trickle of fluid down the windpipe** that gradually builds up. This can even happen when they are sleeping. The speech pathologist or your loved one's nurse may have recommendations for sleeping and resting positions to help address this, such as when positioned on the back, use a slightly larger pillow or remain slightly propped up.

Way back when dinosaurs roamed the earth and I went to physical therapy school, part of the curriculum included **positional drainage** and something called tapotement (percussion of the body) to help with draining the lungs and airway. No one expects you to learn those techniques, but do consider that fluid drains down with gravity, and the bronchi expand from the middle of the lungs outward to the various lobes of the lungs http://en.wikipedia.org/wiki/Bronchi.

Put the heel of your palm on the center of your chest, thumb up and spread your fingers out. Imagine your windpipe as a tube going upward along the line of your thumb, and imagine the bronchi tubes traveling outward in 3D to the lobes of the lungs kind of the way your fingers are pointing. The other hand positioned in the opposite direction would be the other lung.

In the video we made, you will see us having Karen bend over a pillow to clear her airway. She did this to help the fluid in her windpipe drain outward so she could cough it out easier. Likewise, lying on the left side helps parts of the right lung drain, and vice versa. For more on this, see http://www.nlm.nih.gov/medlineplus/ency/patientinstructions/000051.htm.

Swallowing can get better with practice. While swallowing is poor, a one-on-one eating environment helps, especially if your loved one is impulsive or their focus wanders. Stay vigilant and enjoy this intimate time—and good luck.

Techniques for Physically Helping Your Loved One Eat

Eating is such a personal task. Some of us like to mix foods; others eat each food one at a time. Some cannot stand to have foods touching. And the pace of fork to mouth, chewing, swallowing, and drinking are all unique. When experiencing an illness or injury, a person has lost control over their body and the course of their life. Eating is one of the few areas of control that may be left to them, so the caregiver who is physically helping them to eat has to be sensitive to their wants and needs.

...Feeding a Person Who Has a Disability

It is a tricky business to help your loved one eat. For some, it signifies a loss of dignity, so do stay focused on respect and compassion. Here is a training video showing preparation for feeding an adult: https://www.youtube.com/watch?v=TFhbmeS3FZc . This training video is not quite real life—did you notice the mannequin in the next bed and the person with the clipboard? Still, note a few things that the caregiver should do:

1. **Wash the patient's hands** even though the patient might not use their hands to eat with.
2. **Wash your own hands** too.
3. **Position the person to be sitting up,** which makes swallowing easier.
4. **Sit in front of the patient** so the patient doesn't have to turn their head to eat.
5. **Talk with the patient,** asking what they want, making some small talk, being as natural as possible.
6. **Watch the patient's eyes if they are nonverbal,** as they may look to the next item of food they want from the plate.
7. **Observe that the patient chews and swallows food successfully** before offering the next bite.

Some neurological disorders or complications can cause a person to reflexively bite down on a spoon or fork, so be aware of this and move to vinyl-covered utensils as needed.

...Using Specialized Dishes and Silverware

Sometimes it's not just the foods someone eats, but the physical act of eating that is difficult. We are clever creatures, however, and people have come up with many creative ideas for specialized plates, cups, utensils, and a host of other products to help with eating difficulties.

Utensils with wide, soft, or angled grip may help the troubled hand grasp more easily. A hand or wrist brace may be fitted with a pocket to hold the handle of a fork or spoon. A dish with a scooped side allows someone to get a good scoop of food with one hand. A grip surface (on a plate, placemat, or table) keeps the plate from sliding. We found that extra-wide straws helped when Karen's lips were a mess, but straws can be terrible for someone with difficulty swallowing properly. Occupational therapists are the masters at choosing the right eating utensils and teaching someone how to use them. Here is a link to **some of the utensils that are out there**, with pictures http://www.elderstore.com/kitchen-and-dining_51.aspx

How to Use Nutrition to Keep the Gut Balanced and Moving

The balance that the body normally keeps as it processes food into fuel and waste can be easily upset by disease and medicines—and the complex emotions accompanying them. The combinations of things that can go awry with the digestive tract is complex, but the basic concepts for management are simple. "Squish, gush, and push" are the main factors we were told as we received our first lessons in this. In other words, the food mass needs to be soft enough but not too soft, moist enough, but not too moist, and the smooth muscle that surrounds the intestine needs to contract in a strong and coordinated way to move things along. If things stay in there too long they tend to dry out, get hard, and get stuck. If they don't stay in long enough we call it diarrhea. Fiber and fluids keep the consistency, exercise and movement of the intestines keep things moving. Once the food mass reaches the large intestine bacteria and other microbes finish the digestion process. Each of these can be adjusted with what one eats and drinks. Still, getting it just right may seem like trying to adjust the computer with a hammer. Your loved one's nurse, pain doctor, dietitian, or pharmacist may be able to help with both a diet program and a bowel medication program.

Let's discuss each dietary factor in more detail so you may better understand how to make adjustments to prevent constipation or treat mild constipation (no movement for two days. If your loved one is eating and the bowel has stopped for more than three days this is now acute constipation. The strategy needs to change. For this see Treating Constipation in Chapter 18 Managing Discomforts.

Fiber

Fiber is all that roughage that the body does not digest in the small intestine. **Soluble fiber**, which dissolves in water, acts like a sponge: absorbing water, adding bulk, and softening the food and waste mass. Soluble fiber is good medicine for somewhat loose stools as well as for hard or dry stools and difficult bowel movements. The fiber will draw water from the body, so drink an extra glass or two of water each day when increasing the intake of soluble fiber.

Soluble fiber is found in large amounts in fruits and vegetables such as apples, bran, barley, and beans. For a more complete list, see http://www.livestrong.com/article/28882-list-foods-high-soluble-fiber/ and http://www.mayoclinic.org/healthy-living/nutrition-and-healthy-eating/in-depth/high-fiber-foods/art-20050948. Be careful with bananas, especially green ones, as they tend to slow things down, causing constipation.

A few of the over-the-counter-supplement sources of soluble fiber, including Metamucil, Heathers Tummy Care http://www.heatherstummycare.com/heatherstummycare.asp, Arlamucil, Hydrocil, and Serutan, along with over 20 prescription supplements, all use seeds of the psyllium plant. For a more complete list, see http://www.drugs.com/condition/dietary-fiber-supplementation.html.

Insoluble fiber does not dissolve in water. It adds substance to the food and waste mass and helps move things along. Increasing insoluble fiber in the diet is good for someone with infrequent or small bowel movements and is a good part of a regular regimen for tummy health. If your loved one is experiencing diarrhea, avoid sources of insoluble fiber and return to it slowly after the diarrhea subsides.

Natural sources of insoluble fiber include the bran portion of whole grains, all the stringy and peely bits of fruits and nuts, and the chewy parts of raw vegetables. The highest amounts are in apple skin, carrots, cabbage, and beets. Over-the-counter supplements and prescription insoluble fiber laxatives include psyllium husk, wheat dextrim, methylcellulose, and inulin. For a good chart listing some brands, see http://www.nationalfibercouncil.org/supplement_chart.shtml.

Be careful with rapidly increasing the amount of soluble and insoluble fiber your loved one eats or takes. Fiber literally ferments in the large intestine, feeding the normal bacteria there. Any rapid change to their world can cause diarrhea, gas, and tummy upset. Ever eat too many beans?

Fluids

Water or fluids that aren't too sweet or salty soften the food and waste mass. Fats tend to lubricate the mass a little but can end up in larger amounts in the large intestine, especially if there are liver or gallbladder problems. The kidney affects the balance of fluids in the body. If your loved one is dehydrated, or the food and waste mass stays in the intestines too long, it can become very hard to move. In several places in this chapter we recommend drinking more than a quart (five 8-ounce glasses) of fluids per day. Consider that soups and other foods with high liquid content can also count.

Movement

Moving the body—that is, exercise—can help to more gently and naturally get the gut moving and keep it moving. Walking is the best, most natural exercise. More-augmented motions include squatting or sit-to-stands coupled with standing knee lifts. If these exercises are something that your loved one can do, try to have them do two to three rounds of 6 to 10 squats followed by 6 to 10 knee lifts, like marching in place.

Opiate-based pain medication also slows and weakens the normal contractions of the digestive tract, increasing transit time and making the food and waste mass drier and harder as well as reducing the strength of the digestive-tract muscles that are used to make the final big push of bowel movements. Said more simply, opiate-based pain medication causes constipation. If your loved one is using opiate medications regularly, some type of bowel program that may include exercise will be needed to maintain regularity.

Stimulating Peristalsis

Natural **peristalsis stimulants** can be used if mild constipation occurs. They might also be used as part of a daily regimen, especially when medications that decrease peristalsis are prescribed. **Caffeine** is a natural stimulant for the bowel. **Prunes and**

plums contain dihydroxyphenyl isatin, another natural stimulant. These fruits are also loaded with both soluble and insoluble fiber and contain the natural stool softener sorbitol, which works by drawing water into the intestines. Prunes or prune juice can be used daily as part of the bowel-maintenance program. For more on peristalsis stimulants, see Constipation in Chapter 18, Managing Discomforts.

Balancing Intestinal Flora

Healthy people normally have hundreds of different types of microbes living symbiotically in their large intestine. The microbes help us digest our food, produce certain vitamins like vitamin K, and help protect our intestinal lining from our own gastric juices and from other possibly harmful microbe colonies. Microbes also may play a role in our immune system function. If your loved one has had a bout of severe diarrhea, a round of antibiotics, or treatments such as radiation to the abdominal region—all of which might change their intestinal flora—they may need to help their intestinal flora recolonize.

Probiotics, which means ingesting certain live microbes, can help to change our normal intestinal flora. In addition to live-culture yogurt and acidophilus milk, kimchi, *kombucha*, and all those other foods with live microbes, there are many foods and supplements to help with balancing the intestinal flora. Your dietitian and most good pharmacies can help you there.

Prebiotics means choosing certain foods or supplements that can help the microbes already in our intestine to grow and thrive. This is pretty much the same as fiber, but can be selected for certain strains of microbes. For more on this see https://en.wikipedia.org/wiki/Prebiotic_(nutrition). Also there is small but growing evidence that it may be helpful to induce more-helpful microbe strains to fight other strains that may be giving a person intestinal difficulties.

Relaxing the Pelvic-floor Muscles

Relaxation helps mild constipation quite a bit. This is one more instance in which relaxation breathing exercises and/or meditation is very useful. For more on these, see Mindfulness Meditation in Chapter 4, Dancing in the Rain: Healthy Habits for Caregivers.

Finding What Works

Getting your loved one's intestinal tract working just right might take adjusting one or more of the approaches listed above. Keeping their intestinal health working right can be somewhat of a moving target, and the results often somewhat lag the adjustments you make using the above approaches. Any rapid adjusting, such as eating that huge bowl of baked beans, will almost always create havoc as their natural flora take time to adjust to what they eat and what other measures they take. Try to keep the adjustments small and incremental. You may need to record their bowel results as part of their daily log, see using basic charting techniques (see Chapter 11, Medications) to learn more about keeping daily logs.

...Eating to Treat Mild Constipation (Two Days)

If the bowel has stopped for more than a couple days, your loved one is mildly constipated. Adding fiber may only add more bulk to an already stopped-up digestive tract. Change your strategy from prevention to gentle measures that will **generate peristalsis, add water and/or lubrication** to the food and waste mass, and **relax the pelvic-floor muscles.** Five dried prunes with two glasses of water can be a very effective and gentle way to add fiber and fluid as well as a peristalsis stimulant. The exercises and relaxation breathing described above can also help. If these methods don't work in one more day, your loved one is officially constipated; for a more complete discussion of treatment, see Constipation in Chapter 18, Managing Discomforts.

...Eating and Diarrhea

If your loved one has loose or watery stools three or more times per day, you might need to **back off on their fiber intake**; it's good for loose stools but bad for full-on diarrhea. Do take care to **help them stay hydrated**. Have them drink a cup of clear liquid after each run to the bathroom, or try for 8 to 10 glasses per day. Also take care to **keep their electrolytes in balance**. Salty snacks like saltines, pretzels, and soups work well and can provide some easily digested calories. Hydration drinks like sports drinks or Pedialyte can also be a lifesaver.

Try to **offer small meals at first**, focusing on the easiest foods to digest: clear soups, white bread, skinned cooked potatoes, and maybe fruit juices. Protein sources that are low-fat may be more easily tolerated. Baked or broiled meat or cooked eggs may be added if the white bread and such are tolerated OK. Avoid offering milk products, as they are mostly digested in the large intestine. If the person was recently on antibiotics, an opportunistic infection may be the problem. Consult their doctor.

A couple of **green bananas** will slow the intestine quite a bit and also provide potassium. There are also several over-the-counter and prescription **medications for diarrhea**. However, giving your loved one immodium (or even green bananas) to stop up something that their body is trying to get rid of can cause severe problems.

If diarrhea lasts more than three days or is severe or violent, consult your loved one's doctors. For a more compete discussion on treating severe diarrhea, see Diarrhea in Chapter 18, Managing Discomforts.

Approaches for Diseases and Conditions

This section describes approaches for responding to eating problems associated with specific conditions and diseases. First we will consider with the commonly overlooked condition of depression, as it can be a part of so many other conditions.

...Eating and Depression

Depression is a neurological disorder; it is a malfunction of the brain that affects the whole body. The sadness that often comes from profound illness, end of life, and all its losses, prolonged physical pain, and sleep issues, can each cause enough changes to the architecture and chemistry of the nervous system to cause the disorder. This list is far from complete and description too simple, but dietary problems are also on this list. Depression may affect eating habits and the desire for food, and it is affected by the food one eats.

Change in Eating Habits

Depression interrupts decision making and suppresses motivation. Often people who are depressed end up eating the same simple meal over and over, such as a bowl of cold cereal for breakfast, lunch, and dinner. Often they skip breakfast because mornings are just plain difficult anyway. Sometimes they skip meals all together.

You can help by preparing food for them, creating a menu with them and posting it on the fridge, making food with them in a large enough amount that they might have another meal from the leftovers, and taking them out for snacks or a meal. There are many services that bring meals into the home, such as <u>Meals on Wheels</u> (see Volunteer Organizations in Chapter 1, Building a Caregiving Team), but companionship is probably more important than the food.

Loss of Appetite

Depression can suppress the appetite, making getting enough calories more difficult. If your loved one suffers from depression and weight loss is a problem, see <u>Weight Loss</u> earlier in this chapter.

Craving for "Comfort" Foods

Sweet, starchy, and fatty foods are called comfort foods because they temporarily raise serotonin levels, giving a mild "cared-for" feeling. Just reaching for these kinds of foods and putting them in the mouth often gives a small dopamine and endorphin release as well. Unfortunately, as with most substances associated with dopamine and/or endorphin release, they are addictive and do require more and more to get the same release. Also, the good feelings from the serotonin release are temporary.

Often the lack of nutritional value, the sugar crash, and the weight gain associated with eating these foods lead to more bad feelings in the longer term. The longer-term hormonal effects also lead to more bad feelings and further distort the sense of hunger and satiety and a person's food cravings. If the answer to the ugly and distorted feelings is to dose again with those comfort foods, a vicious cycle begins.

To curb this cycle, **take sugary, starchy snacks out of sight** and perhaps make them more difficult to reach. Food cravings may be triggered by seeing the snack. Try placing them in a low or high cupboard or in a room not associated with food, like the garage. Junk-food cravings are usually short-lived and shallow. The brain quickly weighs the reward of the cookie versus the effort. The little bit of time and effort may be all it takes to make finding and eating the cookie not worth it.

Replace the cookies with something more healthful (see Eat a Balanced Diet in Chapter 4, Dancing in the Rain: Healthy Habits for Caregivers). **Avoid giving cookies and such things as rewards or comforts.** This fosters an association of food and reward. Give something else, like a hug or a flower. It's just as rewarding without the bad feelings later.

Treating the Depression

Helping address the depression directly is best. The same healthy habits outlined for the caregiver will help your loved one (see Chapter 4, Dancing in the Rain: Healthy Habits for Caregivers). Social time, good rest and sleep, relaxation and meditation, pain control, exercise, activities, and a sense of purpose all help stem depression. In addition, consider helping them join a support group, seek counseling, and get medication support. For more ways to help, see Chapter 5, A Brief About Grief.

For more information on depression and chronic illness: https://www.nimh.nih.gov/health/publications/chronic-illness-mental-health/index.shtml

...Eating and Cancer

Many chemotherapy treatments target cells with high metabolism. Not only does this include the one most of us associate with cancer treatments—hair cells—it also includes the linings of the mouth, the stomach, and much of the intestine. This can cause sores on the lips and in the mouth and throat, nausea, and difficulty digesting more-complex or rich foods and fiber. To address these issues, please see Sore Mouth and Throat, Nausea, and Fiber earlier in this chapter. Report any mouth sores to your loved one's oncologist, as they are a sign of the patient's tolerance of the treatment.

Chemotherapy can also change the taste of foods. Most common is a metallic taste. See Changes Involving the Tongue and Olfactory Sense earlier in this chapter, but be very gentle when considering adding any extra salt or spice.

More advanced cancer can be a very heavy metabolic load on the body, requiring more protein and calories. See the later part of Early Satiation earlier in this chapter regarding getting more calories and protein. We used shakes and smoothies to augment Karen's diet. The protein she tolerated best changed over time, from whey to rice to hemp. If one form of protein is difficult for them, try another. Some protein supplement powders come in single-serving packets, making it easier to give them a test run.

With more advanced disease, your loved one might be on opiate-based pain medications such as Vicodin or morphine. These medicines slow the movement of the gut, causing constipation. This can be a terrible combination: poor gut motility and poor tolerance for fiber. For help, see How to Use Nutrition to Keep the Gut Balanced and Moving earlier in this chapter.

For more information on eating and cancer, including recipes and many links to other good information, try http://www.cancer.gov/cancertopics/coping/eatinghints/page1.

...Eating and Aging

Age in itself is not a disease. We all, if we're lucky enough, will get there. However, as we get there, our cells will tend to slow down and most of us will become less physically active. Our body's **need for calories, as well as hunger and thirst, may also slow down**, but our nutrition needs and hydration needs remain the same. This means we want less food and fluids, but need the same amount of vitamins, nutrients, and water—so the foods we eat need to be more nutrient dense and we need extra encouragement to take fluids. All of this is true even if there are no other health or life concerns.

Many of our nation's elderly are also taking **multiple medications, which may affect their thirst, hunger, and digestion**. They may have a change in tastes as the receptors in the nose become less sensitive, diminishing the subtle flavors of foods. For more on this, see Changes Involving the Tongue and Olfactory Sense earlier in this chapter.

They may have difficulties with short- to long-term memory processing, depression, or cognition that make it **difficult to remember to eat or be motivated to eat**. See Eating and Depression and Eating and Dementia in this chapter, as well as Chapter 19, Dementia.

They may have **difficulty with their digestion** as those cells slow down and they move around less, giving less exercise stimulus to the intestines. For more on this, see How to Use Nutrition to Keep the Gut Balanced and Moving earlier in this chapter, and look at the issues with and solutions for nausea earlier in this chapter, as some of those are similar for the elderly too.

Before they eat, you may need to cue them to better affix dentures or **take care of other issues in the mouth and throat**. For more see Oral Care in Chapter 16, Hygiene.

As we age, we tend to collect **multiple other health concerns** too varied to mention specifically here. Please check the table of contents, as many health concerns are addressed elsewhere in this book. You can also search online and/or ask your loved one's health-care providers, especially the dietitian, for help with specific difficulties.

Living Alone

Perhaps the largest factor affecting eating for the elderly is that many live alone. Preparing meals for oneself and eating alone doesn't encourage much in the way of preparing something nice and enjoying it fully.

About the best thing you can do is to **help your older loved one with shopping, preparing meals, and eating together**. The time you take with this might be some of the best time you share together, so this is a terrific place to be a little more generous with your time.

When **shopping with or for your older loved one**, consider that what you bring into the house is what will make it to the table. Avoid large amounts sugars, starchy foods, and fats that are very calorie-dense. This may be especially challenging, as the palate of the elderly often turns toward salty, starchy, or sweeter foods. Consider much more deeply colored fruits like berries and peaches and brightly colored vegetables such as carrots and kale as alternatives to muffins and potatoes. Consider leaner meats, fish, nuts, beans, and dairy in moderate amounts to obtain sufficient complete proteins. Consider lighter oils such as olive oil rather than Crisco or margarine.

When **helping your loved one to prepare meals**, consider making enough to leave them meal-ready leftovers both in the refrigerator and in the freezer. Consider preparing (and also storing meals) in smaller portion sizes. Large portions are often daunting for anyone having trouble with eating or digestion. They can always have two portions if their appetite is good. Most elderly people have a microwave and are familiar with using it. They may think of you as they enjoy again the leftovers from meal you prepared together.

Include plenty of liquids; more than a quart per day is recommended. This may be in the form of just water or may be soups, smoothies, tea, or coffee (yes, tea and coffee do make you pee, but it is still water intake). Having tasty, ready-to-drink liquids available help to cue the person to drink more. Consider having a water bottle handy for them in the house. I like mixing a little juice in the water to make it tastier.

When **eating out with your older loved one**, you may call ahead to the restaurant or hosts to be sure they can accommodate any special needs, be it a wheelchair ramp or a quiet corner. **Volunteers of America** http://www.voa.org/Get-Help/National-Network-of-Services/Senior_Services/Senior-Center--Meal-Programs offers meal services at community dining sites, so your loved one may be able to go out to dinner a bit more often than you can take them.

For many of us, our days seem too short and we can't be there enough. There are services to help. **Meals on Wheels** http://www.mowaa.org/ is one of the largest volunteer organizations in the United States that helps with providing meals and safety checks for homebound seniors. Yes, these volunteers are heroes. Look at their national website to find links to local chapters.

Tufts University has created a terrific "plate" model to further discuss nutrition tips for the elderly http://now.tufts.edu/news-releases/tufts-university-nutrition-scientists-unveil-.

...Eating and Dementia

When the brain is involved in an illness, any function of it-including seeing, thinking, or moving—can be affected. Though Alzheimer's Disease is the most talked-about kind of dementia, there are many types, each affecting the brain in different ways. Consider the parts of the brain that work well and how to maximize those functions while compensating for the functions that are difficult, be it new-memory creation, movement initiation, attention, or anything else. Some of the more common concerns are discussed in Chapter 19, Dementia.

Early Stages

In the early stages of dementia, many of the issues and strategies discussed in Eating and Aging, earlier in this chapter, apply. Someone with dementia may have more **trouble with shopping and preparing meals** and is at risk of leaving the stove on. Helping them shop, making small, ready-to-eat microwave meals, and calling in Meals on Wheels may be important. When you're helping them shop or prepare meals, exercise your patience muscles and try to give them the power of simple choices and self-direction. Again, all the same strategies and methods discussed in Eating and Aging work here.

People with dementia may have more **difficulty with appetite**, similar to or related to the symptoms of depression that often accompany dementia. See Eating and Depression earlier in this chapter.

People with dementia may also **forget to eat or drink** or may misremember yesterday's lunch as having happened today. Giving them a call before mealtimes may be one good way to check up or cue them to eat: "How was that pickled herring and *lefsa* we made yesterday? Did the second day improve that flavor?"

Weight loss is very common in dementia and may precede the diagnosable onset by several years. If you are noticing weight loss in your loved one, please get them to their doctor. In the meantime, you may help augment their food intake. Weight Loss, earlier in this chapter, has good suggestions.

Someone with dementia may have **changing food preferences** (see earlier in this chapter). They may have changes in their perception of foods (taste, look, smell). Again, let them be as self-directive as is reasonable. It's OK to try something new. A little added sugar now may help make things more palatable.

Be sure that they are taking enough **fluids**: a quart or five 8-ounce glasses per day is recommended. Dehydration can cause confusion, dizziness, headaches, and, ironically, loss of appetite and loss of thirst. In addition, have their thiamine, B6, and niacin levels checked because deficiencies in these vitamins can mimic the symptoms of dementia.

Middle and Late Stages

In the middle and late stages of dementia, the breaking of bread becomes even more important as a social and temporal (time-of-day) anchor. It offers you and your loved one a chance for intimacy that may be more and more rare as the well-functioning parts of their mind have more difficulty connecting with the outside world. If your care team includes professional or volunteer help, be sure to cue them to your loved one's preferences around meals and food. Remember, there may be cultural differences you take for granted that an outside caregiver is unaware of. If you set the stage well, problems will be minimized. If you observe well and listen with your heart as to what they might be experiencing, you can make everything easier for everyone and help them get the most out of these moments. Here are some tips:

Cue the appetite. Preparing meals together is an excellent source of connection and helps get the body ready to eat. Even in the later stages, you may be surprised how they can help if given a simple task. Can they butter the bread or wash the vegetables? Even being close to food preparation with all its sounds and smells helps cue the appetite. Creating attractive yet simple dishes also helps tremendously. A plate that has color and an attractive arrangement is so much more appetizing that that blob of gruel.

Minimize distractions. Serve one dish at a time with only the silverware needed. Shut off the television and remove that annoying brother-in-law (having people around they like helps minimize agitation). Make sure the room is bright enough and without glare.

Consider whether their brain is having difficulties assembling the lines and colors the eye sees into images and objects. Consider minimizing visual distraction and giving better contrasts; brightly colored foods within a different-colored dish help make food attractive and easier to see. Minimize background visual noise like placemats or patterned tablecloths. Have both hot and cool liquid available in clear or bright cups to cue drinking, and give more choices.

Allow plenty of time. No one wants to be rushed through a meal. If their attention drifts it is OK to cue them that they are eating. Consider saying "How is that pea soup treating you?" rather than my grandmother's "Eat, eat, you're going to blow away." Check to be sure the dish has not gotten cold and unappetizing. If you heat it up, be sure it's not too hot. They may have trouble discerning too hot or too cold for themselves.

They might not be eating the volume of food in a meal that they used to or that you are used to. Multiple small yet nutritious snacks or mini-meals might work much better than trying to do a big dinner. Also, they might not be at their best at your standard mealtimes. It will probably be better if they have their dinner when they are most awake and alert rather than at 6:00 p.m. like you do.

Make the meal easy to eat. Make sure any dentures or bridgework is in place and secure. If they have difficulty handling food, cups and bowls work better than plates. Spoons are easier than forks and knives. Spill-resistant cups, like coffee travel cups, work well. An occupational therapist can help a lot with techniques and tools to make eating easier. Cut foods up, serve softer foods, or make it finger-ready, such as little sandwiches and pieces of fruit. Have you ever fed a toddler? What worked there? Oh yes, and don't be afraid to let them make a mess. It's part of the fun. A bib napkin and a hard-surface floor can help a lot.

Help them eat if necessary. If they have trouble feeling their mouth, you may check at the end of the meal to be sure they aren't pocketing food in their cheeks. If they are having trouble swallowing, please see Swallowing Issues earlier in this chapter. If they have difficulty with initiating the action of bringing the spoon to their mouth, you might physically help them one or two times to help kick-start the motion. If they still have trouble beyond one or two times, they might need you to do it for them; see Techniques for Physically Helping Your Loved One Eat earlier in this chapter. Again, eating with them might be the best thing you can do. It helps cue them that it's mealtime, helps them model you in how to eat, and, mostly, it's connection.

They may become agitated, angry, or frightened or just refuse food. Please do not take this personally. It is just plain ridiculous to get into a battle of wills with someone with a brain disease. Most likely they are uncomfortable about something. It may be internal or external. They might have a very difficult time communicating with you or knowing what they need themselves. If you really observe and think about what may be happening with all of their senses, you may be able to figure it out and solve it for them.

Watch for weight loss. Supplementing with shakes and smoothies helps quite a bit if they are losing weight; see Weight Loss earlier in this chapter and the recipes for shakes and smoothies near the end of this chapter. If they are having trouble with weight loss, changes in food preferences, digestion problems (diarrhea, constipation, nausea), or other problems such as fluid retention, consider keeping a food log. See Creating a Carebook in Chapter 1, Building a Caregiving Team, and Using Basic Charting Techniques in Chapter 11, Medications.

...Eating and Stroke

A stroke can happen anywhere in the brain, but the most common places affect the regions involving sensation and movement on one side of the body or the other (*hemiplegia*). This can affect the muscles of the throat as well. Make sure to have your loved one's **ability to swallow evaluated**. See Swallowing Issues earlier in this chapter.

One-sided weakness or discoordination may affect how they sit and/or the use of their arm and hand. Have you ever tried to eat with one hand? It is not easy. They **may need help with food preparation and eating**. Techniques and special utensils and dishware are available to assist the person in being able to feed themselves. See Using Specialized Dishes and Silverware earlier in this chapter. Occupational therapists can help immensely here with both techniques and tools.

The one-sided loss may affect their vision and attention. In more-severe hemiplegia, the person may neglect one side as if it isn't here. You may find that rotating the plate or bringing it a little toward their strong side brings it back into their awareness. Because eating is such a basic function in our lives, the occupational therapist may also be able to help **make the simple act of eating a key part of their recovery**.

Strokes may also affect their motivation, emotions, and/or sensations of taste, texture, and smell. It **may change their desire to eat and the foods they prefer**. There are some cues in Changes Involving the Tongue and Olfactory Sense, Eating and Depression, and Early Satiation—all earlier in this chapter—that may help here. Also look at Weight Loss earlier in this chapter if getting enough food is a problem.

They might do much better with company for regular meals to help with motivation and remembering to eat and to reestablish the habit of eating at regular meal times. However, the difficulties around eating that a person with a stroke experiences can make them shy about eating with others. They **may avoid eating out or social situations**. A little preparation can help. Call ahead to restaurants or hosts to be sure they have what your loved one needs to be comfortable, be it a quieter corner or wheelchair access. Go to places that are familiar, at least initially.

Be aware of **dietary needs for the conditions that may have led to the stroke**, such as high blood pressure or diabetes. If high blood pressure is part of what led to the stroke, avoid adding salt, as this increases blood volume in the body and, thus, blood pressure. Your dietitian can help with food choices, nutrition, and meal planning. Good professional help, a little planning, and a lot of love may help ensure not just that food is adequate, but also help return mealtime to its place of sharing and love in our lives. For a terrific document on eating and stroke, see http://www.stroke.org/site/DocServer/NSAFactSheet_Eating.pdf?docID=987.

...Eating and the End of Life

As the body starts to shut down, many people begin to lose the desire for food and, later, no longer take fluids. Initially they may want only small portions of their favorite foods, usually something home cooked. I well remember Karen taking little straw sips of Marc's coffee and little bits of mac 'n' cheese a few days before she passed.

As the intestine, liver, and kidney shut down, **eating and drinking may actually be more painful and somewhat more dangerous for them**. If the body does not process stomach contents, it may cause nausea or cramping or be coughed up and aspirated into the lungs, where excessive fluid not processed by the body may cause congestion or increase the load on their weakening heart. Eventually Karen wanted nothing. This might be especially hard for family members, as we associate food with caring, with life, and with health.

Withdrawing from food and hydration seems to be a natural part of the body's shutting-down process. It is not starvation. Starvation is when an otherwise healthy person is hungry and there is no food. In the dying process, people do not report feelings of hunger. It is usually not painful. It's usually associated with an increase in the body's natural pain-relieving endorphins, and people often report being more comfortable than when they were taking nutrition.

Ease restrictions and be aware of the cues that they don't want anything. Give them whatever they want, but be aware that they might not want it. They might turn away, spit things out, or bite the straw to shut it off. Have you ever fed a small child? Think of all the ways they told you when they'd had enough. Make food available, but do not push. Do not put them in the position of making you feel better by eating. Simply honor their refusal at that time. You may offer again later, as things might change over time, but again, do not push.

If they are not taking fluids, you might take a little more care to **help them keep their lips and mouth moist**. It is common to use a device consisting of a small sponge on a stick to wet the lips and mouth.

For more on end-of-life care, see Chapter 20, Near the End, or, http://hospicefoundation.org/hfa/media/Files/Hospice_TheDyingProcess_Docutech-READERSPREADS.pdf and http://passageseducation.org/images/top_ten_myths_about_dying.pdf.

The Brief Summary

...For Weight Loss, Early Satiation, or Increased Calorie Needs
- Keep healthy snack foods in easy-to-access places.
- Keep fluids separate from meals so they don't fill up on liquids.
- If your loved one is struggling to eat enough calories, offer liquids with calories and protein (milk, soy milk, smoothies). Here are more recipes for high calorie drinks from Virginia Hospital's Health Library http://www.vhcphysiciangroup.com/health-library/nutrition-and-cancer-recipes-for-high-calorie-drinks
- Add fats to foods to increase calories without increasing the volume of food. Healthy fats include olive oil, canola oil, sesame oil, and walnut oil.

...For Weight Gain
- Remove sweetened drinks and high-calorie drinks. This includes sports drinks.
- Remove junk foods and snacks.
- Measure and record your loved one's intake of foods and drinks.
- Avoid simple carbohydrates and sugars if they are not exercising vigorously.
- Don't let them skip breakfast, and encourage them to have regular meals but avoid snacks.
- Encourage them to eat if they're hungry, not because they're sad or bored, and remind them to eat only until they are not hungry.
- Use a smaller dish.
- Remind them to chew their food.

...For Nausea
- Use small dishes and don't fill the plate or bowl, so portions do not seem overwhelming.
- Offer small portions of foods frequently—up to every two hours.
- Try room-temperature foods to prevent nausea, since the aroma of warmed foods can make nausea worse.
- Offer them something to eat within one hour of getting up. Allowing them to get hungry can worsen nausea.
- Limit use of spices and fat since rich, spicy foods are not as well tolerated.
- Save favorite foods for days when they feel good so they don't associate these foods with being sick.
- If they are able to exercise, encourage them to! This can improve their appetite.

...For Soreness in the Mouth or Throat
- Have them take small bites of soft foods.
- Offer small, frequent meals.
- Avoid extremes of hot, cold, spicy, salty, and acidic.
- Try a weak baking-soda mouthwash.
- Try a lidocaine mouthwash.

...For Swallowing Issues
- Get a speech pathology evaluation for your loved one.
- Create a peaceful, quiet environment for meals to make it easier for them to focus on eating.

- Be cautious with offering thin liquids, hard or crumbly solid foods, and large bites.
- Consider postural drainage to help them clear their lungs and bronchi.

...For Constipation
- Gradually adjust their intake of soluble and insoluble fiber: soluble fiber pulls water in, insoluble fiber adds bulk.
- Help them stay hydrated.
- Encourage them to stay as physically active as possible.
- Help them maintain a bowel program if they're on medications that affect the bowel.
- Keep a log if they're having problems, and make small adjustments to the treatment measures accordingly.
- Once constipation occurs, focus on treatments that stimulate bowel movement, rather than on increasing fiber. Here is a list in increasing order of strength:
    - Exercise and relaxation breathing
    - Three to five prunes and two glasses of water
    - Polyethylene glycol (Miralax)
    - Senokot (senna)
    - Stool softeners (Doss, Surfak)
    - Saline laxatives such as magnesium citrate
    - Enemas

If these are not effective within 24 hours, consult their doctor.

...For Diarrhea
- Help them stay hydrated: 8 to 10 cups of clear liquid per day.
- Keep their electrolytes balanced; salt and potassium are key.
- Give them the BRAT diet: bananas, rice, applesauce, and toast.
- Add lean meats after simple starches are tolerated.
- Avoid milk products.
- Begin with small, frequent meals rather than large ones.
- Fiber is OK for loose stools but not for diarrhea (loose or watery stools three or more times per day).
- Consult their doctor if they have recently had a course of antibiotics or if their diarrhea lasts more than three days.
- Keep the buttock area clean and protect the skin.

Recipes for Shakes, Smoothies, and the Best Comfort Food Ever

These recipes are just to give you an idea of some ways to offer nutritious foods to your loved one when eating is difficult.

...Shakes and Smoothies

Shakes and smoothies are a terrific way to add good, nutritious calories to the diet in a way that is easy to chew, easy to digest and absorb, and delicious. What is the difference between the two? According to the Reluctant Foodie blog, shakes are diary based and smoothies are usually fruit based. They both can be thick and delicious. It is easy to supplement either with protein powder; greens such as spinach, mint, and parsley; or other vitamin- or nutrient-rich foods such as blueberries or ground chia seeds. If your loved one has trouble with air in the tummy, let the smoothie settle for five minutes before serving it. Here are a few favorite recipes:

Banana Shake. Blend 2 bananas, 1/2 cup vanilla yogurt, 1/2 cup milk, 2 teaspoons honey, a pinch of cinnamon, and 1 cup ice.

Strawberry-Banana Shake. Blend 1 banana, 1 cup strawberries, 1/2 cup vanilla yogurt, 1/2 cup milk, 2 teaspoons honey, a pinch of cinnamon, and 1 cup ice.

Parsley, Kale, and Berry Smoothie. Blend 1/2 cup parsley, 4 kale leaves (with the center ribs cut out), 1 cup strawberries or raspberries (frozen works well), 1 banana, and 1 teaspoon ground flaxseed (optional). Add about 1 cup water and 1/2 cup ice for liquid and to help it blend.

Kale and Ginger Smoothie. Blend 1 banana, 1/2 cup blueberries, 2 teaspoons peeled grated gingerroot, 1 cup kale leaves (with the center ribs cut out), 1 cup unsweetened almond milk, 1/8 teaspoon cinnamon, and 1/2 to 1 tablespoon honey. Add more almond milk or ice if too thick.

You can add small amounts (1 teaspoon) of oils that have little flavor such as flaxseed oil, canola oil, or walnut oil. You can add dense protein-oil sources such as peanut butter or almond butter. Be careful when adding a strong taste. Adding fish oil might work on the Norwegians in my family, but it's probably not for everyone. You can also experiment with your own combinations. It's fun. I like adding about half a can of coconut milk for added flavor and calories. For more recipes, see https://www.pinterest.com/pin/38351034298973553/

...James's Most Wonderful Mac 'n' Cheese
This was one of Karen's favorites. It took only a couple years of cajoling to get James to make his recipe public. I hope it brings the joy into your home that it did for us.

3 slices bread (I use Dave's Bread)
6 tablespoons butter, divided
½ cup grated Parmesan cheese
1 pound dried pasta (penne, elbows, or rigatoni work best)
6 tablespoons all-purpose flour
1½ teaspoons dry mustard
¼ teaspoon cayenne pepper
5 cups whole milk (don't use skim)
4 cups (about 16 ounces) shredded cheese (a mixture of cheeses works best; I usually use 2 cups sharp cheddar, 1 cup swiss, and 1 cup smoked cheddar)
1 teaspoon salt

1. Lightly toast bread slices and let cool, then pulse in blender or food processor to make bread crumbs.
2. Melt 2 tablespoons butter and toss with bread crumbs and Parmesan cheese. Set aside.
3. Preheat oven to 400°F. Cook pasta in boiling water until tender. Drain and set aside.

4. Heat remaining 4 tablespoons butter over medium-high heat until foaming subsides. Add flour, mustard, and cayenne. Whisk constantly until mixture deepens in color, about 3–4 minutes.
5. Add milk, whisking constantly, until mixture comes to a boil. Reduce heat and simmer until thickened, about 5 minutes. Remove from heat.
6. Add shredded cheese to milk mixture 1 cup at a time, whisking each time until cheese is fully melted. Whisk in salt.
7. Combine pasta and cheese sauce in large bowl. Transfer pasta to buttered 9-inch-by-13-inch baking dish. Spread bread crumbs on top.
8. Bake until cheese is bubbling and bread crumbs are brown, about 20 minutes.

The Link Between Exercise, Hunger, Satiety, and Diet

Exercise? Wait, isn't this whole chapter about food? How did exercise sneak its way into this chapter? **Answer:** Physical activity changes and helps so many of the factors that affect eating that are discussed in this chapter that it simply has to be discussed here. And besides, I'm a physical therapist. We just can't stop talking about it!

Exercise, and movement in general, stimulates and regulates appetite, lessening anorexia and nausea and making the emotional eater more likely to crave something that their body actually needs. Movement of the body stimulates the digestive tract and helps move the bowel. The left-right reciprocal movement of most exercises such as walking stimulates right-left cross talk in the brain, stimulates more normal stress-rest cycles associated with day and night, and helps with appetite and restful sleep. Stage three and four sleep help with human growth hormone production and, again, help with appetite. Movement, especially of the head, with a left-right rhythm—or any rhythm, for that matter—stimulates the vestibular system, which is also soothing. Have you ever noticed how rocking a baby seems to help soothe them and make them ready to sleep or eat?

The bottom line is that if your loved one can get up and move, or move in any way, encourage it. Going for a walk is most always good, but not if it is a source of pain. Try doing things with a purpose, like going outside to water the flowers, going on outings, or helping with straightening up the house. Try working a little exercise into things they do regularly. A favorite lower-body strengthener of mine is to ask the person if they can do 6 to 10 sit-to-stands (sit down and get back up again) every time they use the toilet. Work with what they can do. Ask their physical therapist, nurse, or doctor about an exercise prescription, about bed exercises, and about getting some resistance tubing or light weights to make this easier.

Exercise well, and *bon appétit*.

Chapter 13. Exercise

Many people believe that if someone is ill or frail, exercising is simply out of the question. But exercise doesn't need to conjure images of Cross Fit or a young Arnold Schwarzenegger. It can be any movement of the body, any subtle challenge. It's all relative to the condition your loved one is in now. If they haven't been out of bed for a week, a really big exercise day might be walking to the bathroom.

Exercise also doesn't necessarily need to be boxed into a workout session or be a bunch of otherwise purposeless repetitive movements. It's simply a matter of getting the body moving, getting the body's systems up and running, and perhaps challenging the body a little.

This chapter discusses some of the basic exercise concepts and the elements of an exercise program, and it maps out a basic exercise program. It also gives you links to other exercise programs and discusses special considerations for various diagnoses and problems.

You might notice extra passion written about this subject—not only in this chapter, but sprinkled throughout the book. If you find that I get a bit into the terminology too much for you, don't worry about it. Please read through the precautions and guidelines, but otherwise, you don't need terminology to get moving or for movement to help.

...Important Precautions

- **Keep any doctors' precautions in mind.** See Special Considerations later in this chapter for diagnosis-specific recommendations.
- **Make sure they do not get heart symptoms:** chest, face, or shoulder pain or pressure, lightheadedness, paleness or faintness, or markedly short of breath. Stop if they get any of those symptoms. Check their pulse for normal rate and rhythm. Be ready to call 9-1-1, especially if their heart rhythm is abnormal or if the symptoms persist longer than two minutes. If they are only short of breath, allow two minutes for them to recover before starting again at a lower rate.
- **Stop the exercise if they have any marked change in symptoms:** nauseated, dizzy, or lightheaded; feeling markedly weak or having blurred vision, muscle cramps, unusual sweating, undue pain, or any other change that you wouldn't expect with a little exercise.

...Basic Guidelines

Warm them up a little first with gentle movement and breathing.

Encourage basic natural body movements such as going from sitting to standing, pushing, or pulling. Movements should be in your loved one's normal range of motion and generally pain free. A little muscle burn and exertion is OK.

Try for a bit of exercise in each of the realms—endurance, strength, skill and balance, and flexibility—with strength exercise for a particular muscle group or movement being done every other to every third day.

Consider what they have done in the past for exercise and activity. They know these activities and probably like them. Can you modify the movements so they are able to do them in some way now?

Consider any physical activity as part of their exercise. Movement and exertion is movement and exertion, whether it is as "exercise" or just doing something fun or useful.

Set attainable goals. This helps inspire and mark progress. Track milestones such as distance walked or weight lifted so they may better feel their progress.

Encourage them to do what they can, not what they cannot. If your loved one is very weak and just starting out, try for something easy at first, like exercises in bed and sitting up at the edge of the bed. Let them do only what they can with moderate exertion. If they haven't been exercising for a while, you may expect their ability to exercise to double every three or four days. If they have been exercising, you might expect 10 percent gains every week or two. Try not to let them go beyond doubling their prior performance. Generally it is safe to try for a 10 percent gain if the prior session didn't make them sore or overly tired the next day.

Expect good strong days, relative rest days, and medium days. Shoot for a strong day every third day or so, and expect them to maybe be a bit more tired and sore the day after. On relative rest days, still get them moving a bit. This will help with any soreness. We usually shoot for 30–50 percent less on a rest day than on a strong day.

Expect declines or step-downs as part of the process if they have a progressive disease. It's best to try to return to exercising and making gains between the step-downs. You might switch the exercises and goals as your loved one adapts to their new level, but still they can start to make gains again. Getting back up and keeping going after a step-down is the very definition of resilience.

Don't demand or nag. Exercise should generally feel good and be fun, and most people want to move if they're given half a chance. It might be helpful for you to do the exercises with them, both for the connection of it and so they can mirror your movements.

Exercise Concepts (More Information Than You Want)

At the start of this chapter, I mentioned exercising in different *realms*. This means endurance, strength, skill and balance, and flexibility—and combined or functional exercise. The body adapts to the stresses you put it through very specifically, so it will get stronger in the realm or type of exercise you do, but not necessarily in the other realms. The techniques to train in each realm are somewhat different, but all adhere to the "overload principle": it takes stressing the body a little to stimulate it to make gains.

...Endurance

Cardiovascular or endurance exercise usually involves a repetitive movement using multiple and large-muscle groups, such as walking or riding a bike over a period of time. Any time over two minutes is enough to get the body's energy systems up and running. Over 20 minutes brings the energy system into full function. Endurance exercise can be done daily, with one or two days off per week.

Walking is the king of moderate-level endurance exercise, but it can be anything your loved one likes to do. Consider what they've done in the past and enjoyed when they were healthy—tennis, dancing, bicycling? How can you adapt these passions and the skills they developed into something they can do now? Tennis—can you play seated with a balloon and maybe a badminton racquet? Dancing is very nice. It allows you to be close yet supportive and it allows you to regulate the intensity to their needs.

Intensity

Intensity is usually described as training in a "zone" related to a percentage of our maximal energy-system function (or VO2 max). Zone 1 is 50–60 percent, zone 2 is 60–70 percent, zone 3 is 70–80 percent, and so on. We can get a rough estimate of our zones by taking our heart rate in beats per minute and applying this simple formula: 220 minus your age, multiplied by the zone percentage you want to work in. Expressed mathematically, the formula would look like this:

(220 – age) x target %

The zone concept and formula aren't quite set in stone, as different authors describe different zone levels and different numbers of zones, but you get the idea.

Another way to look at it is as a perceived level of exertion, where 10 is very hard (for example, a sprint), 5 is hard but sustainable (for example, a jog), and 0 is resting. Usually exertion level 5 is equivalent to zone 3. Exertion level 2 is equivalent to zone 1. For our purposes, we will consider staying between zone 1 and 3, or light to moderate work.

Another simple way to look at intensity is the talk test. If someone with normal lungs can still talk without panting, they are usually in or below zone 3. If they can breathe in a relaxed way through their nose, that's usually zone 1.

...Strength

Exercising for strength means strongly contracting the muscles. This is what we usually are doing with weight lifting. Most weight-lifting movements can be broken into variations of the basic movements of going from a squat to standing, pushing, and pulling.

If your loved one has experience with weight lifting or other strength exercise, such as from the military or sports, they may know some basic lifting technique. Oftentimes we can just put weight in their hands and they know what to do. Otherwise, see these video and websites for more specifics of basic lifts and modifications:

The exercise video series we made and described below:

Exercise Program Day 1 Leg Day https://youtu.be/2fwmWxC8UuU
Exercise Program Day 2 Balance Day https://youtu.be/3Ra1SiX_mr8
Exercise Program Day 3 Upper Body Day https://youtu.be/05AGnwj2lv4

The Eldergym has produced basic exercises for frail people with discussion and videos:

https://eldergym.com/hip-exercises.html
https://eldergym.com/elderly-flexibility.html
https://eldergym.com/elderly-endurance.html
https://eldergym.com/elderly-balance.html.

The Mayo Clinic produced these basic exercise videos and discussion http://www.mayoclinic.org/healthy-lifestyle/fitness/in-depth/strength-training/art-20046031.

This is an article on how to find the right exercise video for you http://www.webmd.com/fitness-exercise/features/12-best-exercise-videos-beginners#1.

I love the original Jack Lalane show. This also has continuation to later shows https://www.youtube.com/watch?v=y4A3mdG5zbQ.

Strength-building exercises can attempt to isolate muscles, such as a biceps curl, or can use many muscles at once, such as a squat. The benefit of **muscle isolation** is to be able to focus on one movement or muscle group. This allows one to train something that may be weak. A **mass-muscle exercise** like a squat activates many muscles in concert to produce a larger, more functional movement. This is a more efficient and functional way to strengthen, but it can allow for weak areas to be avoided. You can emphasize different aspects with any lift or movement. The movement can be altered to emphasize one muscle group over another, or part of the movement can be emphasized to gain different training effects.

Let's consider a push-up. Bringing the hands closer together emphasizes the back of the upper arm, while having the hands wide apart emphasizes the chest and front of the upper arm. The **concentric** part of the movement would be the *up* part of the push-up, shortening the muscles as they contract. This part of the movement tends to be safe and well tolerated. It can help with tight muscles or aches if done with moderate loads and through the middle part of the motion only.

The **eccentric** part of the movement would be the part where you *lower* your chest back down to the floor, lengthening the muscle under load. To emphasize the eccentric movement, we have you lower slowly and may add resistance. This demands more from the muscle and the nervous system and tends to build more strength as a result. It can be done with more resistance than someone can push in the concentric phase (overload), getting yet a stronger response. This part of the contraction also can cause more soreness and can more easily cause injury, so it's best to work for several weeks with a movement before trying eccentrics or eccentric overloads.

An **isometric** contraction means "no motion"; this would be like holding a push-up halfway up. This is very safe for joints but still is work for the muscles and tendons. It can be easily done with one muscle working against another by simply "making a muscle": for example, tighten your thigh muscles and hold for 5–10 seconds until it burns a little.

...Repetitions (Reps) and Rep Max

When considering strength-training movements, the resistance (weight) and repetitions (reps) make a big difference. *Reps* means the number of times you do the movement without rest. The number of sets of reps, the length of rest periods, and the overall exercise volume also make a difference. *Sets* are the number of groups of reps with rest in between, such as three sets of 15 reps of push-ups. *Volume* is the overall amount of exercises in a session or in a day. It can also refer to the overall amount over any period of time, like a week or a month. Working to maximum, or failure, means you give maximal effort but cannot perform another repetition. A *rep max*, such as a 10-rep max, means the weight at which you achieve failure at 10 reps. More weight usually means a lower rep max.

A **lower rep max**, such as 1–3 reps, allows for maximal efforts that drive the nervous system to recruit a lot of muscle all at once. This is terrific at gaining strength and for gaining function, but it's hard on the joints and connective tissue, so we usually work up to this over a period of time with lighter-weight exercises. Sometimes, with the sick and frail, we need to perform a low rep max for function, like one rep of getting up to standing so they can get from a bed to a chair or commode. A 3- to 6-rep max still allows a very strong muscle contraction, gaining much of the benefits of a 1- to 3-rep max, but is a bit lighter and thus safer than the higher load.

Moderate rep max—and **submax** lifts, like 10–15 reps to "I feel it work but I could do a few more"—uses the energy stored in the muscles, builds the connective tissue and muscle some, and often helps with tight, achy muscles. This is what you will usually use for most exercise bouts with people who are frail or sick, especially starting out.

High rep max like 20–30 or more reps uses the energy stored in the muscles, builds the body's energy systems, builds endurance, and helps stimulate the system and lubricate the joints. It is pretty safe for joints and tendons, but it doesn't give as much strength gain—and it is kind of boring and takes a lot of time.

Sets

The standard for most training is 2–3 sets. Often we begin with a set of moderate reps at submax to lubricate the joints and get the system up and running. We allow 1–2 minutes of rest but usually not more than 2 minutes. We then try for a higher weight at a lower rep max such as 8–12 reps. The higher weight can be repeated once or twice more to use up the energy stored in the muscles so the body is stimulated to make and store more.

Volume

Volume is the amount of exercises over any period of time. The exercise volume can be calculated but, for our purposes, needs only to be roughly considered by keeping in mind the overall amount your loved one is doing. Consider the amount of weight and the overall number of reps all together. Try to keep the overall amount within their usual range. You can expect it to double every three to four days if they are new to exercising. If they are used to it, expect it might go up 10 percent every one to two weeks. The big early gains happen because their body, especially their nervous system, is becoming more efficient in how it contracts and relaxes muscle and uses energy. Also consider that if they do give any maximal efforts, that will tax their system much more than a submaximal effort, even though the weight and reps might be only a little more.

Building Strength

The body gets stronger two ways: by building more muscle, bone, cartilage, tendon, etc., and by learning to contract muscle and move the body more efficiently. Normally, for strength training, those muscles and that movement will need one to three days of relative rest (working the muscle at 30–50 percent less than their maximum) to allow it to recover and rebuild before attempting a maximal effort with that muscle again. After three days of rest, the body will begin to get weaker again and so the exercise should be done again to continue strengthening.

You can expect a little muscle soreness after the max effort, and a little light exercise is the best cure for that. If they do the maximal effort and don't get a little sore, it's time to try for a 10 percent increase on the next strong day. If the soreness lasts longer than two days, back the max down by 10–20 percent.

In learning to contract and relax muscle more efficiently, strength gains can come during the exercise. To emphasize this we can, after a good warmup and on their strong set, increase the resistance every three reps in rapid succession until it gets too difficult. This often results in a rapid increase in strength. We then can cut that maximum weight by 10–25 percent for their next set. This is usually much more, double to triple, of what they were doing prior to the "three rep ladder." This now becomes their new strong-set weight. This can be done a couple times about two weeks into their exercise program to greatly increase strength.

...Skill

Skill exercises focus on a particular skill or movement pattern. It may be as simple as asking your loved one to take big strides while walking or having them step over a visual line such as a crack in the sidewalk. Physical therapists have quite a bit of training in what all the body's systems are, how they work together, and how to train them. A PT might give very specific assignments to work on balance, postural integration, muscle timing and initiation, or movement patterning. The exercises they give should be done with great attention to doing the movement right to build the skill or movement correctly. Once the skill is mastered and the movement pattern integrated into the person's normal movements, the exercise can be discontinued.

Without knowing all these systems, you can use common sense to help you design some basic skill exercises. If your loved one has a problem with a movement or system, try to simplify the movement into something their body can do but that challenges that skill just a little. Try to have them **centered in their balance** and to **have their posture as good as possible**. Have them pay attention to their balance: the sensations they get from their feet, their hips, their back and trunk, and their shoulders are cues to build a good base and awareness with which to practice from. Have them practice as best they can, focusing on doing it right.

Usually it takes many repetitions of practice, about 1000 reps, to learn or alter a movement pattern. As they learn, they can try things that challenge their skill a little more. You can try making it a little faster or a larger movement. You can try adding another component to the motion, making it more like the functional task they are trying to learn. For it all to work, it's best if they are paying close attention to what they are doing and getting as much feedback from their body and from you as they can process. To get 1000 repetitions, we try for 3 sets of 30–35 reps twice per day. In five days you have close to 1000. You get to count only the ones done right.

Practicing a skill or movement in the imagination can be almost as good (and sometimes better) than practicing in real life. The brain still works through it all even if the body doesn't actually do the movement, and in the imagination there is no limitation or pain from the body or risk of injury. If the body can do the movement on one side but not the other, they can use the well side to teach the affected side. Perform the motion with the side that works well, do 10–20 repetitions, then ask them to imagine the motion on the well side 10–20 times. Now ask them to switch sides in their imagination and perform another 10–20 repetitions. Now try it with the body, on the affected side. Again, lots of repetitions done well grooves in the skill.

...Flexibility

Stretching, or flexibility exercises, should feel good. We are basically taking the body through its normal anatomical movement, asking the muscles to relax and lengthening the tissues. The movement should be natural, full, and easy. As with strength training, we can get very specific with isolating the motions, stretching a specific muscle or tissue, or we can be general, moving across many joints at once in a more natural functional movement.

If you don't know a large repertoire of specific stretches, using the natural movements of the body that make sense will work just fine. Here are basic stretches from the **Arthritis Foundation,** with a video to help you http://www.arthritis.org/living-with-arthritis/exercise/videos/stretches/.

Classic Stretching

In classic stretching, we bring the movement to its first barrier—the point when we feel resistance from the tissue—then gently breathe and, as the body naturally relaxes on the exhale, move into the motion that gives us. Thirty seconds, or three full breaths, is enough time to reach into each movement. Usually we go through each movement twice: the first time gently and the second time more fully, bringing the movement past the first barrier into the second, the firmer tightness that you feel past the first barrier, and continue for two to three breaths. Again, we can stretch into the motion the body gives us as we relax with the exhale.

Stretching is usually best done when the body is warmed up, either internally with a bit of exercise or externally as with a warm bath or shower. It is not usually done as a warmup to exercise unless your loved one's movement is restricted so much that they couldn't do the motions of the exercise. In warming up prior to exercise, we may use a shorter, easier style: dynamic stretching.

Dynamic Stretching

In dynamic stretching, we go through motions relatively quickly, not holding at the end, but into the first barrier 6–10 times, not pushing or bouncing hard but simply reaching into the end of the motion. Again, the motions should be natural and feel good.

...Functional Exercise

Exercise that puts together all these exercise realms is called functional exercise, because it becomes a functional task using multiple joints and many muscles in a skilled way to get something done. Usually these exercises mimic something someone does in real life, such as standing up from a chair or reaching down to get something off the floor. Walking is the king of functional exercise, with squats a close second. These basic movements can be altered to make them more challenging for strength, flexibility, balance, and skill.

About Walking

Our bodies are made to walk, and for many of us a bit of walking would help us stay much more healthy than we are right now. Every system in the body gets involved and feels the benefits. Not only do our heart and lungs pump a bit more blood as our muscles work and our energy systems kick in, walking also demands a bit from our balance and coordination systems. The movement helps lubricate our joints and pump fresh nutritious fluids through our cartilage. It also helps our guts and bowel move, regulates appetite, and resets our normal stress-rest cycle, making for better sleep. It helps process stress hormones, regulates mood, and improves our general sense of well-being. If done with other people, it helps our social connections and bonding too. It is *eustress*—good stress—and it's good medicine for the body, mind, and spirit, even for the very sick or frail.

Building a Basic Exercise Program

This section describes a sample exercise program designed to improve your loved one's mobility. This program might be used by someone who is sedentary and frail enough to need caregiving. This is one example of an exercise program, but keep in mind that there are many ways to design a program. You may use this program or consider it a template to build your own. As you look through it, consider these things about your loved one:

- **their current level of activity and ability:** the exercises should be possible but challenge them just a bit
- **their goals:** in this example, mobility
- **what they are used to and what they enjoy:** in this example, walking and classic exercise

Your loved one can begin this—or any—exercise program on any day. It is laid out beginning with the big leg-strength day so it's easier to see the cycle. Note that the program describes the exercises from the point of view of the person doing them: your loved one. Also look at these elements in the design of this sample program:

- **It is divided into different days:** we don't do the same thing every day.
- **We have big strength days** for different muscle groups, **relative rest days, and skill-emphasis** (balance and coordination) **days.**
- **We do something almost every day.**
- **Each day begins with an easy warmup,** then a walk.

We produced short videos of each exercise day to help you. The days each show a different way to do the warm up: lying down, sitting, and standing. Please use whichever way works best for you and modify the exercises as you need to make the program comfortable yet challenging.

...Day 1: Leg Strength
https://youtu.be/2fwmWxC8UuU

Warmup and Flexibility

These can be done lying down, sitting, or standing.

- **Reaching up:** With deep breaths, inhale, **lifting your hands in front of you** then as far overhead as is comfortable, expanding your chest. Exhale, folding your elbows down and in, compressing your chest. **Repeat 3x**
- **Reaching wide:** With deep breaths, inhale, **reaching your arms wide**, opening your chest and expanding your shoulders. Exhale, bringing your elbows and hands together. **Repeat 3x**
- **One arm up, one arm down:** Inhale, reaching **one arm up**, opening the ribs on that side, while reaching the **other hand down**. Exhale, bringing your hands together in front of the chest. **Repeat 2x each side**
- **Gentle trunk twist:** Lying down or sitting, bring your hands and knees together in front of you. Gently swing your hands to the right, knees to the left giving a mild twist in your trunk as you exhale. Inhale back to center, and continue to the other side. **Repeat 6–10x**
- **Knee to chest:** Pull one knee gently toward your chest while with the opposite leg reaching down and straightening your knee. **Repeat 3x each side**
- **Knee swings:** (Sitting up or standing) Swing feet, allowing your knees to bend and straighten gently. **Repeat 6-10x**
- **Quad sets:** As you're letting your feet swing, try straightening one knee fully, pushing your heel down and away to tighten your thigh. Hold 1to 6 seconds to feel your thigh muscle work, then return to swinging the feet. **Repeat 3x each side**
- **Ankle circles:** Make circles with your big toe, moving through the ankle first clockwise, then counterclockwise. This can also be done with the quad sets. **Repeat 6–10x each side**
- **Hip abduction/adduction:** Push the knees apart and together, resisting with your hands to feel the warmth of work in the inner thighs and buttocks. **Repeat 6–10x**

Endurance

- **Go for a walk,** about as far as you can do easily with moderate effort. If you are doing well at two-thirds through the expected distance, speed up for 20–100 feet. Return to your regular pace for 20 steps. Repeat the interval speed-up 2–3 times.

Strength

Try for 1 to 3 sets of each exercise. Rest 1–2 minutes between sets.

- **Sidestep 20 steps each side.** For more of a challenge, you can add resistance to this motion by placing a belt around your hips and having your caregiver gently pull back against your movement.

- **Walk forward,** pushing against resistance, 20 steps.
- **Sit-to-stand:** Go from sitting to standing once, or from squatting to standing once. Do 6–15 reps.
- If you can do the above exercise to 15 reps on the first set, try it with small weights in your hands for 6–12 reps.

Cool-down

- **Go for a walk** of half to one-fourth of the distance you did during the endurance phase.

...Day 2: Balance and Walking Skill
https://youtu.be/3Ra1SiX_mr8

Warmup and Flexibility

Same as for Day 1.

Endurance

- **Go for a walk.** If you are tired from Day 1, skip the speed intervals.

Skill

This should be done with your caregiver guarding you with a gait belt. See Chapter 15, Basic Mobility and Transfers, and Contact Guard: Catching a Fall
https://youtu.be/KziiwT8VVCM

- **Tandem walking:** This is walking a line, like a cop's drunk test. Try for a length of 10–20 feet. Rest for 1 minute between reps. For increased challenge, touch your heel to your opposite toe as you walk the line. **Repeat 2–3x**
- **Walking with head turns:** Walk while you look left at an object such as a picture on the wall, then walk while you look right at another object in that direction. Repeat 10 times each side. **Repeat 3x** Rest for 1 minute between sets
- **Toe targets:** Place tape 6–10 inches in front of each foot and another piece out to the side from your little toe. Balance on one foot (using hands on a walker or cane if needed). Then reach out with one foot to tap the piece of tape with your big toe. Do this 3-6 times than repeat this with the other foot. **Repeat 3x each side**

Cool-down

- **Go for a walk,** about half the distance you did during the endurance phase.

...Day 3: Upper-body and Trunk Strength
https://youtu.be/05AGnwj2lv4

Warmup and Flexibility

Same as for Day 1.

Endurance

- **Go for a walk.** Try for the same or slightly greater distance than yesterday. If you feel good, repeat the intervals of Day 1.
- **Try some of the balance games** from Day 2 at about half the volume.

Strength

Rest 1–2 minutes between sets.

- **Half-depth push-ups:** Push-ups can be done against a wall, countertop, or tabletop—the more upright you are, the lighter the weight you'll push. Do 10–15 reps, one set.
- **Half- to three-quarters-depth push-ups** (needs to be pain free) at the next level—if you did the wall the first time, try the countertop—for resistance. Do 6–10 reps, 1 to 2 sets.
- **Seated rows:** Seated and holding a rope, towel, or bedsheet, have your caregiver hold the other end to provide resistance as you go through a rowing motion, like rowing a boat. Expand your chest as you pull your elbows back. Your caregiver should provide gentle, smooth resistance so that you can do 10–15 reps, 1 set with a mild "I feel my muscles work" response.
- **Seated rows with more resistance:** Do seated rows as above, but with your caregiver providing a little more resistance, so you can do only 6–12 reps for 1 to 2 sets.
- **Dips:** Place your hands on the armrests of a chair or walker grips and push down to lift yourself up with your arms. To make it easier, sit on pillows in the pan of the chair to raise you so you start higher and don't go back down so far. If you are standing, use your legs as much as needed so you can do 6-12 reps. Try for 2 to 3 sets.

Cool-down

- **Go for an easy walk.** Try for a quarter to one half of the endurance phase distance.

...Day 4: Rest Day

Warmup and Flexibility

Same as for Day 1.

Endurance

- **Do an easy walk.** Make this short, about as much as your prior warm down distance.
- **Try to do some of the balance exercises** from Day 2.

...Day 5: Start the Cycle Over

Repeat Day 1. If you feel OK, try to increase the strength and/or the walk. You should plan to increase by 10% every second time through the cycle, and more, up to 50% if you have not been exercising for a while.

Exercise Throughout the Day

For many people it works better to do a little, as they can, throughout the day. You still follow the basic principles, but take the exercises out of the "box" of a workout session and distribute them throughout the day as you can. Here are some ideas of things that can be done throughout the day:

- Do the warmup and flexibility described for Day 1 above.
- Go for a walk.
- Work on stairs, going up and down smoothly and safely.
- Work on balance—try the balance exercises from Day 2 above.
- Whenever you go to the bathroom, do the sit-to-stand motion several times (see Strength under Day 1, above).
- Play volleyball with a balloon. This can be done sitting or standing. You may need someone holding on, guarding you with a gait belt.
- Dance.
- Pull or push on a rubber band and light dumbbells by your bed or favorite chair several times per day.

Following a workout, take time to enjoy relaxing. Eat and drink soon after, within 45 minutes is best. Laugh, share, relax, and recover. Bask in the good feelings of exertion and recovery.

Special Considerations

This section discusses exercise programs specific to various conditions and diseases, as well as diagnosis-specific considerations for functional exercise; again, it addresses the person doing the exercises: your loved one.

...Exercise and Arthritis

With arthritis, it is usually best to warm up by moving gently without weight on the joint. Use small movements at first. After 10–30 gentle movements through one joint (such as flexing and extending the knee) or multiple joints (for example, pulling the knee toward the chest, then straightening the leg out), you can progress into fuller motions, perhaps with a strong isometric muscle contraction at the end of the motion (such as straightening the knee and contracting the thigh).

The small, easy motions help to lubricate the joint surfaces and warm up the tissues. Pushing at the end of the motion with a strong muscle contraction helps to stimulate the joint surfaces involved in the end of the joint motion and stretch the linings of the joint. It also helps keep the muscles around the joint strong and relaxed with the proper resting tension. I'm always amazed at how some joints that look terrible on X-rays can actually function very well if the muscles around the joint are strong and supple and the tissues in the joint keep their ability to move.

If the arthritic joint is not red and warm to the touch, a moist hot pack before and/or after exercise might help tremendously. Also, getting the joints and muscles on either side of the arthritic joint warmed up and moving makes function of the affected joint easier.

Once the affected joints are warmed up and the muscles supple and active, you may do well with exercises like those in the Basic Exercise Program earlier in this chapter.

Exercising without much load on the joints works well for arthritis. There are probably warm-water pools in your community that host exercise classes specific to arthritis. These are listed locally. To search for them, type "Arthritis Aquatic Program" and the name of your town.

Here are some specifics for joints affected by arthritis.

Knees: Before standing up with arthritic knees, wrap a moist hot pack or rice bag around the joint for 15–20 minutes. Then gently swing the feet 20–30 times before trying to straighten the knees all the way and tighten the thighs. For the knees, straightening is more important than bending, and getting the knees to go all the way straight will make the knees work much better. Stretching and making circles with the ankle, wiggling the toes, tightening the thighs and buttocks, and pushing down to extend the hip a few times will help the legs work best despite the knees.

Hands: A hot pack or warm soak for the hands works wonders. Follow this with gently opening and closing the fingers, working up to fully open and spread them, then pulling them closed into a fist.

Spine: Gently work flexion of the spine gradually at first. Be careful that the spine doesn't push into rotation or extension (arching backward), as this narrows the holes where the nerves exit the spine. Avoid activities that cause aches, tingling, or numbness down a limb or around the chest. Stretch into flexion, bringing the knees gently up to the chest. Stretch the hip flexors, perhaps lying down flat, reaching down with the feet while tightening the buttocks. Give gentle rotary motions to the back by lying with the knees up and gently rocking the knees back and forth, only about 30 degrees, as big twists might aggravate joints and nerves. Warm up the hips by pushing the knees apart and together 6–15 times. Doing all this before getting up might make getting up much easier.

Low back: For the arthritic low back, particularly with *stenosis* (narrowing of the holes where the nerves exit), walking might be very difficult and make symptoms worse. If your hips are tight, you will have to extend the low back to stand up and extend it more to take a step. Stretching the flexors of the hips, activating the buttocks, and relaxing the back muscles helps. If this isn't enough, using a cane or walker allows you to walk with your back flexed forward. It might be best to limit walking and choose another form of exercise. For many people, a recumbent bike or water exercises work well.

Shoulders: Supple muscles in the upper back, neck, and chest help the shoulder blades move properly, which makes movement much easier for the shoulders. Gentle shoulder shrugs, circles (up-back-down-forward), massage and moist heat, and gentle stretches of the chest all help. The warmup is designed to help with this. Avoid motions that are sharply painful, especially at the crown of the shoulder, or that give an ache down the back of the upper arm. Usually reaching far overhead or outward, especially with palms down or thumbs down, gives impingement and pain. Reaching far back stretches the biceps and can also be painful. Keep movements in the pain-free range and you'll probably be OK.

Rheumatic arthritis and the other rheumatic variants tend to have periods of exacerbation and remission. It is important to go easy, very easy, during a flare-up. Perhaps do only the warmups and flexibility as listed under the Basic Exercise Program earlier in this chapter. Usually gentle motion is still best. Also, do not heat a joint that is red and warm to the touch.

...Exercise and Orthopedic Precautions

These are the things that your surgeon or doctor said "don't do," like putting weight on broken bones or flexing a new hip replacement beyond 90 degrees. Be aware of these precautions and follow them. Exercise sessions are a terrific time for caregivers to remind their loved one of these precautions. Be creative on how to exercise and still honor the letter and intent of the precautions.

...Exercise and Heart and Vascular Conditions

Many people with heart and vascular problems are afraid to exercise. This is understandable, but it is unfortunate because 30–60 minutes of moderate exercise 4–5 times per week, with gradual increases, is one of the most effective treatments for most heart and vascular conditions. The strength of the heart muscle, the capacity of the blood vessels and their ability to regulate blood pressure, and the health of the blood itself all improve in response to exercise stress. Not only that, people who exercise tend to have better emotional balance and a better outlook (a very important factor for heart and vessel health) and better appetite regulation. They are also more likely to smoke less or give it up all together. Below are special considerations regarding exercising with heart and blood-vessel conditions.

Coronary Artery Disease (CAD)

Also called *coronary heart disease* (CHD), CAD is a disease of the vessels that feed the heart. At worst it can starve the heart muscle of blood and oxygen. This is often more related to spasm in the artery coupled with restriction, more than simple restriction. It is felt as angina or chest pain but may have other symptoms. Remember these precautions from the start of this chapter:

- **Make sure you do not get heart symptoms:** chest, face, or shoulder pain or pressure, lightheadedness, paleness or feeling faint, or marked shortness of breath. Stop if you get any of those symptoms. Check your pulse for normal rate and rhythm. Be ready to call 9-1-1, especially if your heart rhythm is abnormal or if the symptoms persist longer than 2 minutes. If you are only short of breath, allow 2 minutes to recover before starting again at a lower rate.
- **Stop the exercise if you have any marked change in symptoms:** nausea, feeling markedly weak, dizziness or lightheadedness, blurred vision, muscle cramps, unusual sweating, undue pain, or any other marked change that you wouldn't expect with a little exercise.

It is recommended that you consult your cardiologist or primary-care physician before beginning an exercise program if you have CAD. The doctor can give you a better idea of what is safe and what is too much. They may have specific recommendations for a program or may refer you to a supervised cardiac rehabilitation program. A supervised cardiac rehab program will monitor the heart closely and exercise at a higher intensity (70–85 percent VO2 max) than we do for unsupervised home programs (60–75 percent). They usually also prescribe a strength program much like the one in the Basic Exercise Program earlier in this chapter. Prescription and insurance coverage for supervised cardiac rehab programs varies. Check with the Medicare administrator or the insurance contract.

At home we usually recommend a program including a gradual warmup, a session of brisk walking (keeping it within the talk test—see Endurance earlier in this chapter), light weight lifting, and a cool-down. We avoid squats and other "big exercises" that demand strong work of many big muscles at once. We keep an eye out for the symptoms listed above. We try for 4–6 days per week of activity. This may include exercise sessions and activities such as gardening, going on outings that require brisk walking, and housework done at an intensity similar to the Basic Exercise Program listed earlier in this chapter.

That 30–60 minutes does not need to happen all at once. You may start with 3 sessions of 10 minutes in a day and work up by 2–5 minutes per day until you reach 30 minutes. Once you reach 30 minutes, you don't need to stop there; a little more is a little better. Do incorporate rest days, 1–2 per week, where you take it much lighter but still do something.

Congestive Heart Failure (CHF)

CHF happens when the heart cannot manage the load of the returning blood that the veins bring to it. This blood may stretch and distend the heart and/or press fluid into the lungs as the heart backs up. Believe it or not, exercise helps here too and can also be fairly safe. Again, check with your cardiologist or primary-care physician for recommendations. And again, look at the precautions regarding heart symptoms listed above.

With CHF, some of the key symptoms involve the lungs. It might present as heaviness in the chest or other signs of fluid in the lungs such as shortness of breath, coughing, gurgling on exhale, or crackling on inhale. If you have edema (see later in this chapter) in the legs, be careful as you get moving that you aren't pumping that fluid back into the system faster than it can handle. Also, as you lie down and your legs are elevated, more fluid will drain back toward the heart. Elevating the head and chest and using "pursed lip" or breathing with back pressure on exhale will help clear the lungs.

Begin with a warmup as described in the Basic Exercise Program earlier in this chapter. I recommend that after the initial minute of exercise, you stop for about 1 minute to allow the heart to catch up to the load. As you start again, the heart and energy systems will already be up and running and most likely caught up to the initial demand. You can then continue through the flexibility and endurance exercises. Otherwise, the exercise program is similar to the one described above for coronary artery disease.

Orthostatic Hypotension

Also known as low blood pressure, this condition occurs when the blood pressure to the head drops as you change position quickly or change the amount of exertion, which changes the demand for blood elsewhere in the body. This is usually associated with a brief period of wooziness when you get up too quickly or after some bit of strain. It can also show as foggy thinking, blurred vision, sweating, nausea, or even fainting if it's severe. If your caregiver takes your blood pressure, they may find the systolic reading (the first, larger number) is below 90 mmHg. If this happens, don't panic. This usually passes with a few minutes of rest.

If this condition is a problem, you can and should still exercise; you just need to begin things more gradually to allow the heart and blood vessels time to adjust. Allow time and get up in stages when switching to positions that elevate the head or put the feet down. Also be careful as you start and immediately after exercises that work a lot of large muscles, like squats. For most people, staying hydrated helps. If the symptoms don't fade after 15 minutes, then there may be a problem and it's time to call your health-care team for help. For more on this, see Dizziness and Wooziness in Chapter 18, Managing Discomforts.

Note that many people who experience low blood pressure (90 percent of early onset hypotension and 50 percent of delayed onset) have significant coronary artery disease.

Claudication

Artery disease in the limbs is called *claudication*. It usually affects the legs but can be in the arms, especially after injury, surgery, or radiation that disrupts the arteries. The hallmark symptom is a nasty ache in the limbs with exercise. It makes exercise difficult, but exercise usually results in vessel building, so it is also part of the cure. To help, I recommend beginning your exercise session by working limbs that aren't affected. This will increase blood flow in general without placing a demand on the affected limb. After 10–20 minutes, you can begin to work the affected limbs. If the ache begins, rest those limbs for 1–2 minutes.

One example of exercise for claudication in the legs is to use an arm bike or upper-body weights after the warmup and before the walk. During the walk, take a seat with you, such as a cane that folds out into a stool or a four-wheel walker with a fold-down seat. If you do big exercise (squats) for the affected limb, do it after such a warmup and be ready for the ache. It will pass in a few minutes. Try to keep the ache minimal. With a month or so of consistent workouts you should notice that it gradually takes more activity to bring the ache on.

Edema

Edema is swelling caused by excess fluid in the tissue. Exercising with it can be tricky. While movement and exercise helps pump fluid up out of the limbs, it will cause increased blood flow down into the limbs both during and after exercise. If the balance between out and back ends up being more out, it can make edema worse. Still, exercise stress builds vessels, so overall it can greatly help edema in the longer run. The trick is balance. Any demand for more blood into the affected limb must be balanced with increased drainage. Strategies for this are discussed in Swelling and Edema in Chapter 18, Managing Discomforts. **Warning:** Allowing the edema to get out of control stretches out the tissue, making more edema more likely. You can exercise, but be careful to keep it in control.

...Exercise with COPD and other Lung Disease

If you're reading this section, you probably know what COPD means (Chronic Obstructive Pulmonary Disease). You also probably know that exercising is the last thing someone wants to do when they have trouble getting air into and out of their lungs. Usually they're just trying to catch their breath and are quite anxious about the next time when that breath is just too short. The unfortunate cascade of avoiding activity, so becoming weaker and more deconditioned, thus doing even less activity, and becoming still weaker is the usual path this disease takes as the person spirals down.

The body needs some stress to stay as strong and healthy as possible. Exercise remains the most important part of every pulmonary rehab program. These guidelines will help make it possible and safe.

Here are some tips for preventing shortness of breath (SOB) from happening during exercise:

- If you use an **inhaler**, use it before exercising.
- If you use **supplemental oxygen**, use it during exercise.
- Start off with a **gentle warmup**, which loosens up the upper trunk and shoulders. You can use the warmup listed in the Basic Exercise Program listed earlier in this chapter or one you got from your pulmonary rehab or physical therapist. You may also look at these classic exercises for posture and breathing from Eldergym.com: https://eldergym.com/elderly-breathing.html and https://eldergym.com/elderly-posture.html.
- Learn **pursed-lip breathing** and **positioning for maximum airflow** for use during rest periods. See the end of this section for instructions.
- After the warmup, allow a **1-minute rest** for your breathing to catch up. After the first 1–2 minutes of cardiovascular exercise, rest again for 1–2 minutes. This allows your body to pay back the oxygen debt that developed during the startup phase. Don't rest for much more than 2 minutes, as this allows your energy systems to go back to sleep.

Use Caution with Endurance and Strength Exercises

Pulmonary rehab programs almost always include both cardiovascular and strength exercises. You can also include both, but be careful with strength exercises that use lots of big muscles, like squats, as these place a large demand on your system. We usually focus on the upper body, lifting the arms and chest together. Then allow the chest and shoulders to come down fully again as you return to the start position. The full movement, making the chest "proud," then compressing down again, stretches and opens the chest cavity and strengthens the muscles that help with breathing. In cardiovascular exercise, you can use intervals (like the periods of fast walking in the exercise program) but keep it at a level where your blood oxygen saturation is 90 percent or above. It's better to avoid episodes of SOB (Short Of Breath) than to go into an episode of SOB and then try to treat it.

Treat Shortness of Breath Before It Occurs

It's best to know how to treat SOB before it occurs:

- If you have **supplemental oxygen**, use it. You can turn it up 25–50 percent during an SOB episode to help get over it. Oxygen is usually delivered by a tube into the nostrils, but this helps only if you can breathe through your nose. If you just can't, you can place the tubes on your lower lip, mixing the oxygen with the air going into your mouth.

- Use **pursed-lip breathing** and **positioning for maximum airflow**. See below.
- Try to **relax.** Yeah, this might seem impossible, but it can help tremendously. Check out the section on Anxiety in Chapter 18, Managing Discomforts, for more information and techniques.
- Read more about **treating Shortness of Breath: Dyspnea** in Chapter 18, Managing the Discomforts.

Pursed-lip breathing: Breathe in somewhat deeply, about three-quarters of a full breath, through your nose if you can in a relaxed way, as if you are smelling a rose. On exhale, draw your lips close together, like you might to blow out a candle. You can let your cheeks relax like Dizzy Gillespie. As the air leaks out, allow the air in your lungs to rest against the back pressure your pursed lips provide, which gently stretches and opens the lungs. That's right: "smell the roses, blow out the candles." Here is a video from the American Lung Association https://www.youtube.com/watch?v=7kpJ0QlRss4

Positioning for maximum airflow: Think of an athlete who just ran the 100-yard dash or all the way downfield for a score. They might be sitting or standing bent over with their hands on their knees. Their back is not hunched but extended to open the chest. As they blow out, their shoulders fall back to their low resting position so they may fully empty their upper lungs. The athlete knows that this is a good way to get the most breath. This position works for COPD as well. Be careful to allow the back to extend on inhale and the shoulders to lower fully on exhale.

...Exercise and Cancer

This is a difficult topic. Each cancer is different. Each treatment regimen is different. Each case is different. Still, for most types and cases of even advanced cancer, the benefits of exercise outweigh the risks, and exercise is recommended.

Talk to your oncologist and radiation oncologist about exercise. Tell them what you want to do and your goals as clearly as you can. They may have specific recommendations or precautions and may refer you to a cancer-specialized physical therapist.

There is information on the Web, but there are too many types and presentations of cancer to give specific websites here. Type your specific diagnosis or treatment and "exercise" into your browser, and you should find several resources discussing specific issues. The American Cancer Society's Web page on exercise gives more-general guidelines that we found helpful: http://www.cancer.org/treatment/survivorshipduringandaftertreatment/stayingactive/physical-activity-and-the-cancer-patient.

The sections below discuss some symptoms and presentations that persist with many of the different types and stages of cancers and treatments.

Cancer-related Fatigue

For fatigue, shorter amounts of moderate-level cardiovascular exercise helps. You might consider the "rest day" described in the Basic Exercise Program listed earlier in this chapter. You may try walking 10–15 minutes (or even 2–3 minutes) at a time and at a level where you could still carry on a conversation without panting (the talk test). This can be done several times each day.

Keep an awareness of the overall amount of activity in a day. Expect good days and not-so-good days, and allow for a relative rest day or two following a big day. Try to keep the activity of the rest days within 30 percent of that of the big days, and the big days' activity level not more than double plus half that of the rest days. In other words, still get up and move on the rest days, and don't try to conquer the world on the good days. For more on fatigue, see Fatigue in Chapter 18, Managing Discomforts.

Blood work is usually closely monitored during cancer treatment and with advanced cancer. If the red-cell count (**hematocrit) is low**, expect fatigue, but in this case you may not want to exercise through it. Ask your doctor. If **platelets are low,** you may bruise easily or bleed excessively if cut. Be extra careful with bumps, pinches, or sharp things. This is also true if you are on blood thinners such as Coumadin. If your **white cell count is low,** you may be more prone to infection; consider avoiding the sweaty public gym and public pool. For more on this, see Infections and Compromised Immune Systems in Chapter 18, Managing Discomforts. If you have been vomiting a lot or have had severe diarrhea, you may have an **electrolyte imbalance**. This will also show up in the blood work and the doctors will make recommendations to correct it. Exercise should be avoided until it is corrected. You most likely won't really want to anyway.

Metastasis

Cancer *metastasis* (when cancer has spread from the original site to other places in the body) may weaken the bones. This is most common in the spine, ribs, and pelvis. If this is the case, the radiation oncologist probably took a bone scan or other images that clearly show it. It's nice to know just where it is and how much is there, so you can protect those bones. If there is just a little bone weakness, you can probably go about your normal exercise business with little worry. If it is more extensive, you should avoid loading much weight through any bone that is affected. Most often this is the spine.

Take care so you do not fall down. Any balance exercises should be done with guarding. Walking is usually still OK, as is everything in the Basic Exercise Program except the rowing exercises. A weight machine on which the trunk is supported on a bench allows you to work the arms or legs with little load through the spine. If the bony weakness is very severe, and if there are already fractures, the spine may need to be supported with a brace. We had such a brace, and with it and some creativity, Karen was still able to exercise her arms and legs. Your PT may be able to help here.

Other Concerns

During **radiation treatment**, the skin may be red and irritable. Avoid chlorinated or brominated pools and tubs. Pools and tubs should also be avoided with **external catheters, ports, or feeding tubes,** to minimize risk of infections. **Edema** is another common cancer problem, especially after radiation. Exercise is still possible, even recommended with some allowances. For more on this, see Edema earlier in this chapter. We also need to say here that **uncontrolled pain, nausea and vomiting, and diarrhea** are all good reasons to suspend any exercise program. This probably just makes sense.

...Exercise and Infections

Exercising with an active infection is not as forbidden as we used to think. The key is moderation. First, the infection needs to be well under control by the body. Any fever should below 100°F (37.8°C). The resting heart rate should be no more than 10 beats per minute above normal, and you should feel OK, well enough to exercise a little. If you are on antibiotics, you should be at least three days into the course.

At this point, a little *moderate* exercise can do the body good and help it fight the infection. This means gentle movements like the warmup and a little cardiovascular exercise in the Basic Exercise Program earlier in this chapter: about 30–50 percent of normal in both intensity and duration—for example, an easy walk. This should be enough to aerate the lungs, help with blood flow and fluid exchange in the body, help with sleep and rest, and help the immune system. It should not be enough to stress the body, which would tax the energy systems or immune system.

Avoid strength training until the infection is nearly clear, with no fever and a normal resting heart rate. At that point, you may try 1–2 sets with light weights, 10–15 reps, with a target of "I can feel my muscles work a little." Take extra time to relax and celebrate the workout afterward. Keep an eye on the fever and other signs of the infection over the next 24 hours.

...Exercise and Multiple Sclerosis (MS)

Every case of MS is different, depending on where and when the lesions develop in the brain. For most people near the point of needing caregiving assistance, the Basic Exercise Program listed earlier in this chapter will help them regain function and strength. It often helps to focus on functional core muscles (the muscles that help you sit up straight)—remember not to neglect the weaker side. There are a few other considerations as well.

Many people develop problems with **muscle tightness** and spasticity in the legs, especially in the calves, hamstrings, and quadriceps. When exercising, stretch the tight or spasticity-affected muscles first. It often helps to stretch five times each day to keep the tightness down and give the muscle more control. See more on spasticity at the National Multiple Sclerosis Society Website: http://www.nationalmssociety.org/Symptoms-Diagnosis/MS-Symptoms/Spasticity

Fatigue can also be a major issue. There may be days when you just don't feel like exercising. Try the warmups in the Basic Exercise Program for 5 minutes before you just call it in. You might feel better and keep going. If not, give yourself permission to skip a day or two, but try not to skip more than three. For more on pacing and managing fatigue, see Fatigue in Chapter 18, Managing Discomforts.

Avoid strenuous exercise, but moderate exercise works well, as well as strength training in the range of 2–4 sets, 8–15 reps per set, and only 4–8 total exercises for a session. Also consider strenuous activities (which make you breathe hard or sweat) as part of your exercise day. People often experience neural fatigue before muscle fatigue, where the nerve runs out of juice before the muscle. The strength often drops off sharply, often without muscle burn. Usually it recovers quickly, but stop there.

If key **walking muscles fatigue**, such as the muscles that lift up the toes (*dorsiflexors*) and the muscles in the hips that keep the body from leaning sideways when you step (*gluteus medius*), you may find it more difficult to walk later. It may help to train these, but if you find after a few weeks of training that those muscle are not getting any stronger, you may be better off by focusing on walking smoothly instead.

Giving the walking muscles a little assistance often helps. For **tipping sideways** (*trendelenburg*), a cane in the opposite hand as the tipping direction helps. For a little **dorsiflexion assist**, look at a Foot-Up: http://www.ossur.com/injury-solutions/products/foot-and-ankle/ankle-foot-orthosis/foot-up This simple device works with a laced shoe to give a little support just for lifting toes up. If you are at risk for **turning an ankle**, there are many other braces that may provide medial-lateral support.

Exercise typically raises your body temperature (that's why you sweat), and people with MS often experience increased symptoms, weakness, or fatigue when their **body gets too warm**. Keeping cool helps. Many people can exercise if they stay in a cool room, by a fan, or in cool water. Cooling vests and wrist wraps can help. You may find many different products by simply typing "MS cooling vests" into your browser. For more information, the Multiple Sclerosis Association of America (MYMSAA) can help people obtain these products: http://www.mymsaa.org/msaa-help/cooling/. In addition, the National Multiple Sclerosis Society http://www.nationalmssociety.org/ has a wealth of information of living with MS, including tips on diet, exercise, cognitive health, and emotional wellbeing. http://www.nationalmssociety.org/Living-Well-With-MS

...Exercise and Stroke and Hemiparesis

If you are reading this, you probably already know that most strokes affect one side of the body (*hemiparesis*). You also probably have read through the Basic Exercise Program earlier in this chapter thinking, "No, that one won't work, and not that either…" Well, you're probably right. If you are recovering from a stroke, you face special challenges. The involved body part is ignored or just doesn't work well, so the body and brain choose to do the task with the uninvolved side, further ignoring the involved side. Normal tasks and activities of everyday life are difficult and feel impossible.

Your world is full of Catch-22s: "How can I exercise? Won't that cause another stroke?" "How can I walk for exercise? Walking is so difficult or even impossible." It can take more than twice as much energy as it does for someone with a normal walk. Far too often, the person just does less, even to the point of staying in bed. Without movement and activity, the body gets weaker yet, making everything just that much harder. Without purpose and socialization, withdrawal and depression can creep in.

Yet exercise is still important—so important that it remains the cornerstone of most stroke rehabilitation programs. But it does need to address the special needs of someone who has had a stroke.

Medical Stability

The first need is medical stability. Stroke can be considered a symptom of a broader cardiovascular disease process. The risk factors need to be mitigated medically. The data clearly show that exercise after a stroke is quite safe once the major risk factors are addressed. Once the green light is given, exercise—particularly endurance exercise—can begin to reduce and even reverse some of the cardiovascular disease.

More so, cardiovascular exercise seems to be associated with increased brain-derived neurotrophic factor (BDNF) https://en.wikipedia.org/wiki/Brain-derived_neurotrophic_factor, which seems to be important for memory, learning, and brain recovery. It also helps with the depression that is so common after stroke.

Be sure to specifically **clear any squats** or other large leg-trunk exercises with your doctor. Those exercises tend to bump up the blood pressure while you're doing them. Mini-squats should still be OK. Usually doing squats with weight should be avoided.

Shoulder, Arm, and Hand

You must be especially careful with the **affected shoulder** after you've had a stroke. The shoulder joint is naturally lax, and its proper alignment is very dependent on the symphony of activation of the muscles around it, especially those supporting the shoulder blade and the rotator cuff. Poor alignment of the joint, spasticity, and muscle knots in those muscles can also be a source of pain. Pain just makes it more difficult to use the arm.

Look to the rehabilitation professionals early on in dealing with the **shoulder, arm, and hand**. Have the rehab team teach you what to do and continue to update the program as your condition evolves. The usual evolution is from limp and flaccid to some contraction, to spasticity, to improved active control. Shoulder pain sometimes develops two weeks to three months after the stroke. Gentle stretching and movement is good, but aggressive stretching, as with pulleys, usually makes it worse. Arm rests and pillows to support the elbow usually help. A short time in a sling or strapping system may help in the early stages, but long-term use of a sling doesn't help and instead contributes to many problems, including your never using the arm. Therapies that help the muscles of the shoulder become active again, help the muscle knots (such as massage), and help pain and inflammation all seem to help.

You may notice the arm and/or leg gets tight and draws into a **particular pattern of tightness.** As you begin to contract the muscles of a limb again, it may be very difficult to control how much contraction you give, the pattern of contraction, and shutting off that contraction. The muscles usually contract in a pattern that draws the limb up and in (*flexion synergy pattern*) or pushes the limb down and out (*extension synergy pattern*). To help control this excessive tone, rehab professionals use a number of techniques. They may be able to teach your caregiver some of the techniques they are using with you.

One of the simplest and most universal techniques is to gently help the limb move in the opposite synergy—that is, if it is pulling up and in, roll it down and out. Usually this occurs at each segment of the limb, and bringing one segment the other way can affect all the other segments. In other words, if your hand is pulling up and across your chest, have your caregiver use their relaxed flat palm to gently but firmly help your shoulder blade down and back to help your whole arm relax. If you try this, your helper should be gentle and smooth and not cause pain. Pain or jerkiness will cause more muscle contraction, not less. Your rehabilitation team has probably developed a pretty good strategy that works for you for both the pain and the **spasticity**. With this little help to control alignment and spasticity you should use your arm whenever possible. Every time you use it, it gets a little stronger.

Attend to your involved side too. A helper can stand toward your involved side, cuing you to look at them and acknowledge them there. Reach across your midline. Use your involved hand and both hands together as much as is reasonable. Move your chest and shoulder blade with your arm movement, chest "proud" for reaching up or out. Begin with gentle shoulder shrugs and circles, and shrug back as you lift your hand. Position things to add a rotational component to reaching movements, rotating palm-down for reaching in front, palm-up for reaching out to the side. Your caregiver may help guide your movement with their hand, but they should not fully lift for you and never push if there is pain in your shoulder. A mild pulling sensation or a sensation of muscular tiredness is OK, but any sharp pain or deep ache is not, and pain at the crown of the shoulder is usually not good either.

Aphasia

What do you do if you're in pain, and how do you communicate that, if you cannot talk? After some types of strokes, usually those that affect the right side of the body, you may have difficulty choosing words, forming words, understanding spoken language, reading, or writing. It's important to appreciate that in the brain these are all separate functions. One function may be affected, but another may be intact. You may be able to understand and write, but not speak.

The speech language pathologist (SLP) on your rehab team can help explain the details of your particular difficulties and help you with strategies to communicate. They may have signboards or picture boards or other special tricks and tools. There is a picture board for pain scale with faces on it to help communicate pain. It can be found online and in Chapter 17, Pain Management. SLPs also may have things they want you to practice. Darn, more exercise.

Beyond all that, consider that nonverbal communication usually remains universal. You can use grimacing, turning away, and the usual signs to let your caregiver know if something hurts. Your caregiver also can use nonverbal cues to communicate, but it is usually helpful if they continue speaking too. Speaking in their normal voice at their normal rate is usually the best idea. Remember, your brain is in the process of rewiring and your caregiver's voice will help you connect the sounds you hear to the actions you both do.

New Treatment Concepts

There are two fairly new treatment concepts for stroke and the hemiparetic arm.
Botox: Yes, the same botulinum toxin that politicians use to relax the wrinkles around their eyes can help temporarily shut down a spastic muscle, making it easier for you to use your arm after a stroke. This is a fairly new treatment idea that has many pros and cons. It's worth asking your rehabilitation professionals about it.

Constraint-induced movement therapy: This fairly new treatment concept addresses the Catch-22 formerly called "learned nonuse" ("It's difficult to use my involved arm, so I will just use the good side"). Lightly or not so lightly impeding the use of the good side forces your brain to develop movement strategies with the involved side. It's done in combination with intensive therapy to help you develop new strategies and control tone. Early on, it was called "oven-mitt therapy" for the oven-mitt device placed on the good hand.

Stroke-Specific Exercises

So if exercises given earlier in this chapter won't work, what will? Here are two programs from the National Stroke Association (NSA) for people with less severe and more severe involvement http://www.stroke.org/sites/default/files/resources/HOPE_Guide_2007_chap4.pdf. These exercises are geared more toward movement and skill. They are prescribed to be done 10 times each day. They also show how to get up off the floor.

The American Heart Association and NSA also recommend 3–7 days of cardiovascular exercise per week. As you look through the NSA recovery guide exercises, also consider stationary bicycling, or better, arm and leg machines like the Nu-Step http://www.nustep.com/our-products. Consider ways to add more or less resistance as necessary to make the exercises possible yet challenging. They recommend 40–70 percent VO2 max, just like we do. The activity helps mood, sleep, and appetite, helping with depression. Activity helps with socialization and so on. All the benefits are there.

Initially you may be able to exercise with only the uninvolved side. Early on, you may need to use your good side to help your involved side, but you should try using both sides at every opportunity. If you can exercise using both sides of the body, it will continue helping with the one-sided neglect and help to rewire the nervous system to use the affected side. Strong-effort exercise, especially **resisting an eccentric load**, helps drive the nervous system to recruit more nerve fibers and more muscle fibers.

Look again at the Basic Exercise Program. Depending on the nature and severity of the stroke, many of the exercises in this program will work if you are creative. Can a caregiver's hand gently guide your shoulder blade though the warmup exercises even if your arm can't raise? Can your helper assist, and even resist, your foot a little as you make circles with your toe? Can you move your knee instead of your toe? Neurologically it's halfway there. If you can walk, try the resisted walking. It might improve how you walk. Can your caregiver help hold your hand on a wall and support your shoulder for push-ups against the wall?

For all the exercises that won't work for you, what can you do instead? Can you ride a stationary bike or use Nu-Step instead of walking? Dance instead of walk? If you are continent, can you walk in a pool? Can you do the arm and shoulder exercises in water?

Take this list, the Basic Exercise Program, or any list you think might be close to what will work and honors the basic principles in this chapter, to your rehabilitation team. They can help you modify it to fit your needs. Ask them how to advance it as you advance. Things will change. Expect whatever you're given to need to be advanced in a couple weeks in a fairly new case and a month or two if the stroke was more than six months ago. The neurological system is our most adaptable organ.

For more on stroke, simply type "stroke" into your browser. There is a tremendous amount of information out there. Here is one fairly concise publication from the NSA that covers most bases http://www.stroke.org/sites/default/files/resources/HOPE_Guide_2007_chap1.pdf.

...Exercise and Dementia

There is a growing mountain of evidence and medical literature finding that exercise is one of the better medicines. Long-term regular exercise, especially 20–30 minutes or more of moderate endurance exercise, seems to be protective of the brain and nervous system against many of the mechanisms of dementia. It helps protect against small-vessel disease and cerebrovascular disease and helps with *neuroplasticity* (our neurons' abilities connect and to add and change function, allowing our nervous system to be resilient). It also seems to be protective against *proteinopathies* such as Alzheimer's Disease.

Exercisers typically showed more gray matter and larger *hippocampal* areas (where long-term memories are created) and scored better on cognition and dementia-screening tests. These direct benefits are in addition to the many other benefits. Stronger muscles and bones, more-flexible joints, and better motor skill means people stay more agile, more active, and more independent, and fall less—and get hurt less if they do fall. Physical activity helps mood, sleep, and appetite and is a terrific vehicle for social connection. People with profound dementia who were taken for regular walks tended to wander less and be less agitated.

In the **early stages** of dementia, make an effort to stay as physically active as possible. Connect exercise to social groups and to functional activities. Look up groups in your area. Consider offerings at local gyms such as the Silver Sneaker Programs and YMCA. Consider pool aerobics programs and swim clubs. Look into a tai chi or qigong class. Consider other local groups such as senior centers, church-based exercise programs, mall-walk clubs, and exercise groups at adult day-care facilities. All this not only helps keep you fit and active with a healthy brain, it also helps build new social connections and exercise habits. At this point, learning something new and making new friends might be a good idea. It also helps to develop the exercise and activity routines you can keep into the middle and later stages.

In **middle and later stages**, considering what you have done in the past for exercise and activity becomes more important. How can these activities be modified so you may do them safely now? If it involves a social or led group, you may need help to attend these at your regular time. Allow yourself to make errors. Allow yourself to slow down a bit. Keep it fun. Try to keep it to things you can do so you don't become frustrated. Music you like really helps. Oftentimes people with dementia can sing better than they can talk and can dance better than they can walk.

If equipment (weights, bands, exercise balls) needs to be set up, lay it out in the order you will be using things and put away things you are not going to be using. This helps you sequence and make choices. Limit distractions; turn off the TV—that's bad for the brain anyway. Close out bright lights and turn off loud noises; softer lights and music help, but glare and blare don't. If you become agitated and your behavior inappropriate, you may need to leave the situation to a quieter place for a little while.

Helping a Loved One with Dementia Exercise

If you are a caregiver who is exercising or doing activities one-on-one with your loved one, here are some tips that might help you communicate and guide them:

- **Let them see you before you start talking.** Approach them from the front. Make eye contact.
- **Let them know what you are doing** or talking about before you get into details.
- **Keep your directions short and concrete.** *Eliminate* all those *extra words* that we usually stuff into each rambling sentence we utter in our normal conversations. If I were to try to communicate this preceding sentence to someone with memory and processing problems, I would say, "No extra words." Abstraction and metaphor usually don't help either. Keep it concrete and direct.
- **Speak clearly, in a voice loud enough for them to hear you,** but at your normal pace and tone. Talking too slowly doesn't seem to help.
- **Give them time to respond** to you before repeating yourself. Consider that their processing may be slow. If you do repeat yourself, use the same words, the same way. Paraphrasing yourself will only cause confusion.
- **Use gentle touch** to bring them back from distraction and to guide them. Placing your hand gently on their hand works well.
- **Use modeling;** let them mirror your movements.
- **Allow them to make errors.** Don't sweat the small stuff; that only causes frustration.
- **Give them rest breaks** as they need. Often the nervous system gets tired before the muscles or heart. You may see a decline in their ability and an increase in movement errors and how frequently they get distracted. They may simply stop. Allow them to rest for a minute or two before continuing.
- **Try using distraction** for getting them unstuck from an idea. Don't argue. Don't try to reason it out. Try asking them about something they know, usually an older memory like their prior work or the garden they kept.
- **Walking is good exercise.** For more exercises, see Late-Stage Exercise later in this chapter.

If they must learn something new, consider that even though their implicit memory processing may be very poor, their procedural memory may still work. This means that they can learn to *do* something even if they cannot remember how they know it. To help teach this way, do the task the same way each time. Use the same setup, the same words and touch cues, even the same time of day if possible. Give good feedback when they do it right, but avoid excessive feedback. Have patience with their learning. It may take up to 40 times before they have learned it as well as they can.

By the way, all these tips may be helpful for communication and activity in general. You may find more tips on managing agitation in Delirium: The Hard Road in Chapter 18, Managing Discomforts, and in Chapter 19, Dementia.

...Exercise and Parkinson's Disease

Parkinson's is primarily considered a disease of movement. This may make exercising seem pointless, but as with anything, movement gets better with practice. In fact, exercise—strong, vigorous, challenging exercise—has proven to be one of the most important parts of treatment. At the time of this writing, we haven't pegged out what type of exercise works best, but it seems that in the early stages, more is better. It seems to help the dopamine we have, and the cells that produce it, work better. Exercise should start as soon as possible, the day of diagnosis or sooner, and continue through late stage. Include cardiovascular (endurance) exercise and skill exercise. For more on exercise and Parkinson's Disease, including a terrific specific program for middle and later stages, look into the program and book *PWR!Moves* by Becky Farley, PT http://www.pwr4life.org/product/pwr-moves-book/.

By the time you are reading this book, you are probably beyond the early stages. You may have a pronounced tremor. You may have trouble initiating movement, controlling it, and stopping it again once its purpose is done. You may have many problems, but listing them here won't help. Let's focus on exercise. Here are some tips that will help.

If you are **becoming stiff**, especially in the trunk, begin with gentle rhythmic motions and gradually work into stretching. The warmup described in Day 1 in the Basic Exercise Program earlier in this chapter works well if you begin with easy, rhythmic partial motions. Your caregiver may guide your movement with their hands or do it with you, allowing you to mirror them.

Rhythm helps with **movement initiation** too. We sometimes use a metronome set to a slow beat, 30–60 beats per minute, but I like music, and if it's a song you love, all the better. Practice reaching across your body; your caregiver can resist your push and pull for a resistance workout and to challenge your balance and weight shifting. Having a visual target and time to work out the coordination helps with the shuffling movement (*fenestration*). This could be reaching toward your helper's hand or, if you're walking, it could be a visual line to step over. Dancing with your caregiver is terrific. You're nice and close, so it's easy for your helper to give movement cues and support. It helps you weight shift and move in all directions without having to think about it so much too. Most importantly it's intimate and fun. Singing is also wonderful for working on **breathing, voice control, and speech**. What songs do you love? Try a duet with your caregiver.

You may have trouble with **balance orientation**. Most often you feel as if you are falling forward while you are actually leaning way back. Before you attempt to stand, take time to just sit to help get reoriented from lying down. Focus on other senses, such as the pressure from your caregiver's hand as they hold you up, or look to the side to find visual cues such as a vertical door frame, might help you reorient. Stretching the calves helps too.

Sometime, when your systems that plan and sort movement become a bit overwhelmed, you will just **freeze**. If this happens while you are walking or standing without support, it may cause you to fall. This can happen in visually busy situations like crowds or in tight places like doorways. It's important for you not to fight the freeze. If you feel it coming on, purposefully stop trying to force the movement and hold on to something solid. To unfreeze, take a moment to straighten up. Take a deep, relaxing breath and begin to shift your weight from foot to foot. You may do this until you are ready to take big, complete steps again. For more on fall prevention, see Home Safety and Fall Prevention in Chapter 16, Basic Mobility and Transfers.

Also consider that late-stage Parkinson's can affect your perception and processing of visual edges. Caregivers can augment important edges, like the edges of stairs, with contrasting or bright tape to help you see them earlier. In late-stage Parkinson's Disease, much of the brain will be affected. Some of the tips offered in Exercise and Dementia above may prove helpful.

...Late-Stage Exercise

I originally came across this program in an article published through the National Institute of Health (NIH) by the Mayo Clinic regarding dementia, but it is very similar to things we PTs commonly employ in rehab and nursing homes all over the country. This is a good functional exercise program you can use for many different situations:

- **When sitting at the edge of the bed,** side scoot toward the foot of the bed and back again to the middle. This helps exercise the muscles needed for standing up from a bed or chair.
- **Balance in a standing position.** You can hold on to a solid support if you need, to or hover your hands above the support for increased challenge. This exercise helps with balance and posture.
- **Sit unsupported for 1–10 minutes each day.** This exercise helps to strengthen the stomach and back muscles used to support posture. This activity should always be carried out with someone else present if there is a risk of falling.
- **Lie as flat as possible on the bed** for 20–30 minutes each day, trying to reduce the gap between the curve of the back and the mattress. This allows for a good stretch, strengthens abdominal muscles, and gives the neck muscles a chance to relax. Consider lying on the tummy, also known as *proning*, for more stretch. For more on this see, Positioning for Comfort in Chapter 15, Basic Mobility and Transfers.
- **Stand up and move about regularly.** Moving regularly helps to keep leg muscles strong and maintain good balance. Consider repetitive functional activity such as sweeping.

The most important gift in all this exercise is the close, intimate time you spend doing, dancing, singing, and sharing together with your caregiver. I saw this again just last week at a transitional-care facility where I was doing some PT work. This lovely woman who was just struggling made more progress in the two days her family was there than she had made in the prior two weeks. We all had to rewrite our prognosis and plans. When her husband, impressed with her progress, thanked us, I said, "No, we should thank you. It's the power of your love that's making her better."

Chapter 14.
Sleep

Sleep is the other side of the stress-rest cycle, and it is just as important to our health and sense of well-being. As a caregiver you know this. You also hopefully have read Sleep in Sleepless Times in Chapter 4, Dancing in the Rain: Healthy Habits for Caregivers. Many of the tips there can also help your loved one, and you may recognize some of those tips here in this chapter too. Your loved one's issues are not the same as yours, however, so some of the strategies here are different. First, let's talk about sleep so you can help choose strategies that make the most sense for them.

The Normal Sleep Cycle

There are two basic parts of sleep: rapid-eye movement (*REM) sleep*, or dreaming, and non-REM sleep, or *restorative sleep*. We usually cycle through restorative sleep, stages I through IV, three to five times a night, with REM sleep usually following stage IV; then we have a period of light stage-I sleep when we move around a little to readjust our position before heading back in for another round. We usually go into REM sleep longest and deepest in the very early morning (like 4:00 a.m.) and wake up from there to the morning sun and our next lovely day.

Some Sleep Problems

Problems can occur with this normal sleep cycle. A person may have trouble falling asleep (*sleep onset*) or staying asleep (*sleep maintenance*) or have poor-quality sleep (not enough or too much deep restorative sleep or REM sleep), *parasomnia* (sleepwalking, night eating, talking in one's sleep, etc.), and/or changes in the normal day-night rhythm (*sleep-wake syndrome*). People with a sleep disorder may be irritable, depressed or anxious and/or have difficulty concentrating or remembering. They often have more difficulty with inflammation, healing, and maintaining body weight and lean muscle mass. You may see these signs directly, such as night waking or sleepwalking, or you might not, such as poor-quality sleep. A lot can be answered with the simple questions "Do you sleep well?" and "Do you feel rested in the morning?"

If you suspect your loved one has a sleep disorder, take it seriously and discuss it with your loved one's health-care team. Try to record when and what occurs. A **sleep disorder assessment** includes a physical examination, health history, and sleep history and may include a polysomnogram https://en.wikipedia.org/wiki/Polysomnography.

Sleep Hygiene

This section describes a series of suggestions we call sleep hygiene that are somewhat universal. They are addressed to your loved one rather than to you, the caregiver, but if they aren't able to implement these suggestions themselves, you can help them with their sleep hygiene. Some suggestions address more than one sleep problem at once; some are for one problem only. As you read through these two lists, see if you can figure out which aspect of sleep each suggestion addresses.

...Universal Suggestions for Better Sleep

1. **Appoint a worry time** during the day. Write your worries down. When you write, try to have the writing reach some resolution. If there is more to do, appoint a time to do it. If you're not working with it at the moment, put it on the shelf and don't worry about it until you are ready to work on it more. This is to avoid ruminating and taking your worries to bed.
2. **Exercise regularly 5–6 hours before bed**, but not less than 3. (There's that darn exercise again)
3. **Eat a bit of protein 2 hours before bed,** which helps with sleep.
4. **Take a bath 1–2 hours before bed.** The cooling of the body afterward signals sleep.
5. **Enjoy a glass of warm milk or chamomile tea 1 hour before bed.**
6. **Eat a turkey sandwich** with your milk or tea; the tryptophan in turkey is a natural sleep aid.
7. **Eat some carbohydrates 1 hour before bed**, but don't eat a lot—it's good for sleep, but not so good for the waistline.
8. **Have a presleep routine**: Brush teeth, stretch, do a relaxation breathing exercise or meditation, say your prayers … Your routine before sleeping helps signal your body that it is time to go to sleep.
9. **Go to bed and get up at the same time every day**, even if you slept poorly.
10. **Make your bed environment as comfortable as can be.** The room should be as dark as is safe. The bed should have clean, dry sheets without wrinkles. Have enough blankets to be warm in bed, but the room should be cool. Use pillows to support neutral positions and sore knees, shoulder, or whatever else (see Positioning for Comfort in Chapter 15, Basic Mobility and Transfers). Eliminate disturbances from your sleep environment: noise, light, pets, that annoying partner … anything that wakes you up.
11. **Drink water and fluids in the day, but not before bed** if you have trouble with having to get up to pee.
12. **Use the toilet before bed** to minimize having to get up in the middle of the night. If you must get up, light the way with red lights to minimize the light disturbing your sleep cycle.
13. **Use sleep medications sparingly** and only as needed; be extra careful with using sleep medications for someone with Alzheimer's or another dementia.
14. **Review all your medications** if you are having trouble sleeping. Some meds may be contributing to poor sleep. Some chemotherapies, corticosteroids, antidepressants, anticonvulsants, hormone therapies, and sedatives all can cause sleep problems. Do not go off medications, especially sleep medications, abruptly without your health-care provider's supervision. That could lead to more sleep problems—or worse.
15. **Get exposure to daylight** in the morning to signal to your brain that it is time to wake up and get up. If daylight is not available (for instance, if you live in Seattle in the winter), consider using a blue light. Look up seasonal affect disorder (SAD) for more information.
16. **Have a purpose in the day.**

...Things to Avoid

1. **Don't nap late in the day;** a short 30- to 45-minute nap at lunch is good for the energy level, but a 3-hour nap in the afternoon will make for difficult sleep that night. Avoid day sleep after 4:00 p.m. no matter how tired you are, especially if you suffer from depression.
2. **Don't let pesky caregivers wake you up at all hours of the night.** Sometimes they need to, to provide medication or monitoring, but sometimes they can be better about minimizing it. If you have been having trouble sleeping, ask that they adjust their care plan to minimize the disturbances. Put a sign on your door to help them stick to it.
3. **Don't eat a high-fat diet.** Excessive fat in the diet causes more breathing problems, less REM sleep, and more unrest during the sleep cycle.
4. **Don't spend excessive time in bed.** Don't lie awake in bed. If you can't sleep, get up and do something. Go to another room. When you're sleepy, go back to bed.
5. **Don't sleep excessively during the day.** Many times people who are ill or injured require more sleep, but until near the end of life, they shouldn't sleep all day; it puts them at risk of offsetting their normal day-night rhythm. This is especially true with Alzheimer's and other dementias, in which it is known as sundowning. This is also often associated with delirium.
6. **Don't look at television, computers, and other blue-screen devices 2 hours before bedtime.** If you must use them, wear amber glasses to cut the blue light. For more on amber glasses, see https://www.lowbluelights.com.
7. **Don't do things in bed other than sleep and sex,** such as reading or watching TV, especially things that stimulate your brain's visual centers (visual imagination). This helps you to associate the bed and the bedroom with sleep.
8. **Don't take stimulants, especially 3–4 hours before bed.** This includes coffee, black or green tea, chocolate, nicotine, and many soft drinks. Read the labels.

Special Sleep Problems

The general suggestions in the section above will help most people get a better night's sleep, but they are not universal for every sleep problem or the special needs of someone with a specific illness. This section discusses some of the trickiest sleep problems, which revolve around poor-quality sleep.

...Sleep Apnea

In sleep apnea, a person may repeatedly stop breathing for 10 seconds or more. The most common type, **obstructive sleep apnea**, is often associated with sleeping on one's back and with snoring. Often the sleeper is unaware of the problem because they never fully wake up, but they often report not feeling rested and may have trouble with irritability, depression, anxiety, poor memory, and obesity. Obesity results because the growth hormone that helps one stay lean is produced mostly in stage III and IV sleep. The catch-22 is that obesity often causes snoring and obstructive sleep apnea. The partner of someone with sleep apnea knows full well the problem. They have heard it.

Often the cure is simple: prevent or disrupt the snoring. If the partner can gently cue the sleeper to stop snoring, that might be enough. Karen said I snored, and she would pinch my nose, making me take "guppy breaths." Crude but effective. I would stop snoring and breathe normally. Sewing a small irritant into the back of the nightshirt, such as a tennis ball or a rolled towel, might cue someone not to sleep on their back. Little stick-on strips are available to help open the nose, which helps some people. The most common are called Breathe Right strips. Special dental appliances, which must be fitted by your dentist, hold the jaw forward to prevent snoring.

Using a CPAP or VPAP (continuous or variable positive air pressure) machine is the most effective—but also the most invasive—treatment. The sleeper wears a mask that is hooked to a machine, which pumps warm, moist air into the sleeper's nose and possibly their mouth. The positive pressure of the air holds the throat open, preventing apnea. For more information, see http://www.sleepapnea.org/treat/treatment-options.html. I've read that up to two-thirds of stroke survivors have sleep disorders related to breathing, with apnea being the most common problem.

...Restless Legs

Restless legs often rob older people of a good night's rest by both not letting them get to sleep and disturbing their sleep cycles. Generally it's an uncontrollable urge to move the legs during rest and is often associated with aching or burning. We don't know exactly why it occurs, but it may be associated with multiple sclerosis, Parkinson's Disease, diabetes, kidney problems, neuropathies, and just being over 65. It also may be aggravated by certain medications and alcohol.

Addressing the problems directly works best, so better controlling these diseases and a review of medications are good ideas. Mild exercise during the day, massage and stretching before bed, relaxation techniques like relaxation breathing or meditation, and counterirritant creams like Ben Gay may help enough to let them sleep. There are medications that may help as well. For more information, see http://www.ninds.nih.gov/disorders/restless_legs/detail_restless_legs.htm .

...Sleep Jerking

Periodic leg movement during sleep (PLMS) or periodic leg movement disorder (PLMD) occur during sleep, before REM, while restless legs happens mostly while a person is trying to get to sleep. These terms are all closely related, so for the purpose of this discussion I will talk about them as one. Classically with PLMS, the great toe pulls up. This may be followed by the ankle, knee, and/or hip drawing the foot up. It can occur in the arms as well, but this is rare. As with apnea, the sleeper may not know they have it, but their sleep is disturbed (and their partner usually knows all too well). Mostly it robs the sleeper of deep restorative and REM sleep, so they experience all the problems listed with apnea.

Many people who have restless legs also have sleep jerking, but they are not the same thing and the correlation does not fit the other way around. Some of the same things that cause restless legs can cause sleep jerking, and many of the things that help restless legs may help PLMS. A sleep disorder assessment is recommended. For more information, see https://www.sleepassociation.org/patients-general-public/periodic-leg-movements-during-sleep-plms/about-periodic-leg-movements-during-sleep/.

...Nighttime Heartburn

Nighttime heartburn or gastroesophageal reflux disease (GERD), also called gastric reflux, is when acids from the stomach backflow into the esophagus. This happens most easily when people lie down, and it can make it quite difficult to get to sleep and/

or stay asleep, or it can disturb the normal sleep cycle. It tends to run in families but also may be aggravated by obesity, smoking, alcohol use, fatty or acidic diets, or any foods that can make heartburn worse. It's much more common as people age as well.

If you suspect this problem, do alert your loved one's health-care team, as it can be made worse by certain medications, and it can cause a number of other problems. There are also a number of changes in diet and habits that can help. As it relates to sleep, avoid eating large meals, especially before lying down. Chewing gum may help, as saliva may help soothe the esophagus. Eating while relaxed, and being relaxed before bed, helps. Avoid anything associated with heartburn, including:

- **eating acidic foods** like citrus and tomatoes
- **smoking**
- **drinking caffeinated drinks and eating chocolate**
- **eating spicy foods** like garlic, onions, and peppers
- **eating fatty foods**

If all these measures aren't enough, try having your loved one sleep on their left side or elevating the head of the bed a few degrees. A hospital bed makes this easy, but this can also be done with a shallow, wedge-shaped pillow. You may also tilt the whole bed up slightly with 4- to 6-inch blocks under the feet of the bed frame at the head end of the bed.

...Insomnia

Having trouble falling asleep or getting back to sleep once one is awakened is insomnia. Sleep hygiene suggestions 1–10, 14, and 20–24 earlier in this chapter are all geared toward helping someone fall asleep. If someone has had insomnia long enough, they often have reached the point of associating going to bed with another anxious night lying awake. The suggestions listed above help, but if sleep anxiety has crept in, those suggestions may not be enough.

We often look to some types of cognitive behavioral therapy techniques to help the person change these destructive associations. These are in the realm of sleep psychology. The focus here is often changing the anxiety of "why can't I sleep, I need to sleep, I'll feel terrible tomorrow if I don't sleep" to "just relax a while, this feels great." Methods include reassigning sleep associations (sleep hygiene suggestions 8 and 9 touch on this), sleep restriction (sleep hygiene suggestions 9, 17, and 21), and relaxation therapies such as meditation, imagery, and self-hypnosis. Consider talking with your loved one's medical team about a referral to a sleep psychologist.

...Pain and Sleep

Pain can rob sleep. Control pain early and as effectively as can be. For more on this, see Chapter 17, Pain Management. If your loved one is waking up in pain, report this to their medical team to consider longer-acting pain medications. Also look again at sleep hygiene suggestion 10 as well as Positioning for Comfort in Chapter 15, Basic Mobility and Transfers. If pain is keeping them from sleeping, consider more seriously using all those gentle massage and light touch tricks. Sometimes a gentle back rub will work miracles. Karen would relax and fall asleep well with a gentle head scratch or gentle foot rub. After a good night's sleep, you may be surprised at how much better their pain is.

Disease- and Condition-Specific Approaches
This next section addresses some of the conditions that usually cause sleep problems and may have more-unique approaches to addressing them. We refer to the sleep hygiene suggestions listed earlier in this chapter by number and also reference other places in the book to help you. Following this we discuss medications for sleep problems.

...Sleep and Depression and/or Anxiety
Both insomnia and early and excessive REM sleep are associated with depression and anxiety. Often a depressed person is sleepy and lethargic, so simply getting more sleep doesn't really help. Resetting their sleep pattern is what works here. Purposefully retard their sleep by not letting them sleep late, nap, or go to bed early for a night or two. Get them up, into the morning sunshine, and as active as they can be, with lots of physical and psychological stimulation in the day. Then try to reset their normal sleep cycle with normal bed and wake-up times. Sleep hygiene suggestions 2 and 16 are aimed at this.

The brain center called the suprachiasmatic nucleus (SCM) in the hypothalamus may be affected by the brain changes with depression. It is associated with our normal sleep-wake cycle. It can be reset by morning light (blue light) and may be disturbed by blue light in the evening. Sleep hygiene suggestions 9, 15, and 22 address this problem.

Depressed people and people suffering with anxiety often spend too much time in bed and/or with computers and television. Look again at sleep hygiene suggestions 17 and 20–23. If they have trouble falling asleep (insomnia), look at sleep hygiene suggestions 3–6, 8, and 19—and especially suggestion 1 for rumination and "monkey mind."

Selective serotonin reuptake inhibitors (SSRIs) can help restore a more normal sleep cycle, but be careful with serotonin norepinephrine reuptake inhibitors (SNRIs), as they may make it worse. Diet is often a problem in depression. For more on this, see Eating and Depression in Chapter 12, Food and Nutrition. Sleep apnea is often associated with depression, but we don't know which is the chicken and which is the egg here. Either way, see Sleep Apnea earlier in this chapter and consider that it may be a part of the problem. You may read more about depression in Chapter 5, A Brief About Grief.

...Sleep and Aging
Aging itself is not a disease, but it definitely brings changes in sleep patterns and some difficulties. As we age, we tend to go to bed a little earlier and wake up a little earlier. We take longer to get to sleep, have longer periods of light sleep, and wake up more often and more fully. This makes it seem as though we need less sleep or more sleep, depending on whom you ask, but in fact the total optimal sleep time remains pretty much the same throughout our adult lives.

These sleep changes with aging are normal, but this new sleep pattern tends to be more fragile, and we tend to collect more health problems and medications as we reach older age. All this adds up to more than 40 percent of older people reporting insomnia at least a few nights per week and having problems with daytime sleepiness. Now that you know what is normal, you may tease out the individual problems and treat each one accordingly.

Some of the most common problems for older folks include some pain, GERD, the need to urinate frequently at night (*nocturia*), restless legs and sleep jerking, apnea (especially if they are overweight), depression and anxiety, and mild to severe dementia (Alzheimer's and Parkinson's are discussed later in this section). If they are retired, they may not have a normal structure to their stress-rest and/or sleep-wake cycles. Sleep hygiene suggestions 9, 15–17, and 20–23 are especially important. Naps are OK, but sleeping longer than 3 hours, or later than 3:00 in the afternoon should be avoided. Sleep hygiene suggestions 11 and 12 help with the nocturia.

A good medication review is important too (sleep hygiene suggestion 14), especially if they are taking heart medications, steroids, or asthma or allergy medications. Gentle stretching, hot packs to arthritic joints, and good positioning (see Positioning for Comfort in Chapter 15, Basic Mobility and Transfers) may help with arthritis and muscle tightness aches and pains.

Many older people like a drink in the evening and more still smoke. Unfortunately, the nicotine is a stimulant even though "it relaxes me," and the alcohol—though it may help them fall asleep—will tend to make sleep lighter and will add to their need to pee. I mention these two topics last as they may be the hardest habits to change. Choose your battles wisely; you may want to read Dignity: Practical Considerations and Respect in the Introduction: Advanced Basics.

...Sleep and Lung or Breathing Problems

People with COPD, emphysema, and other breathing problems may awaken with a drop in their blood oxygen level when they are asleep. A breathing treatment an hour or two before bed may cure this problem. Supplemental oxygen often helps too. They also may be affected by frequent urination; see sleep hygiene suggestions 11 and 12, and consider the red-light lighting system discussed in suggestion 12.

...Sleep and Cancer

It's estimated that over 50 percent of cancer patients also suffer from sleep disorders. Pain is the first most-obvious problem (see Pain and Sleep earlier in this chapter). For most people, having cancer is just plain stressful, and one night spent worrying often leads to more long nights.

Karen and I did many things to help with the stress. Sleep hygiene suggestion 1 may help. You may also find suggestions that work for your loved one in Sleep in Sleepless Times in Chapter 4, Dancing in the Rain: Healthy Habits for Caregivers. Counseling may also help, especially sleep psychology.

Karen and my mom both slept well in the hospital, but many people don't. Bringing their own pillow helps, as does bringing other familiar things from their bedroom. Minimizing intrusion from the health-care team helped a lot too (sleep hygiene suggestion 18). The drugs used to treat cancer can also cause problems. If your loved one is having trouble sleeping, discuss it with their health-care team.

Before accepting a sleep-aid medication, review their current medication list. Also review all their signs and symptoms. The progress of the disease itself can cause a rapid heart rate, night sweats, anxiety, stomach and/or bowel problems, bladder problems, and breathing problems. Look at the sleep hygiene list again to see what suggestions might apply, and look to the sections in this book that address each one of these symptoms separately.

Some things you just cannot control with medications or techniques. At one stage in the journey, Karen would just wake up at 4:00 a.m. She didn't fight it by lying in bed. She got up and enjoyed the quiet private hours of early morning. She could make up the sleep time with a siesta, being careful to wake up before 3:00 p.m. so as not to make it hard to fall asleep that next night.

...Sleep and Multiple Sclerosis

MS lesions may cause such a broad array of symptoms that can affect sleep that it is difficult to discuss all the possibilities here. The medications used to treat the disease and address its symptoms may further complicate the picture. It's not surprising that more than half of people with MS describe sleep problems. You may already be identifying problems and possible solutions as you've read through this chapter so far. Insomnia, pain, depression, and anxiety are all discussed above, as are restless legs and sleep jerking.

Look to Exercise and Multiple Sclerosis (MS) in Chapter 13, Exercise, and to Fatigue and Anxiety in Chapter 18, Managing Discomforts, to help make exercise more feasible and anxiety more manageable. Sleep hygiene suggestions 11 and 12 may help with frequently needing to get up to pee. Stretching, specifically two-stage slow stretching (classic stretching) done frequently in the day and before bed, may help with the spasticity. Relaxation techniques such as relaxation breathing and meditation can help here too.

Obstructive apnea is a problem in MS, but so are other types of more nervous-system-related apneas. Again, a sleep disorder assessment is recommended. All that said, getting enough sleep may still be a problem. Consider catnaps and meditation for ways to augment sleep. A fuller discussion and instructions for this are in Sleep in Sleepless Times in Chapter 4, Dancing in the Rain: Healthy Habits for Caregivers. For more information on sleep and MS, see the National Multiple Sclerosis Society's website: http://www.nationalmssociety.org/Living-Well-With-MS/Diet-Exercise-Healthy-Behaviors/Sleep

...Sleep and Parkinson's Disease

Parkinson's comes with its own list of possible sleep problems. In many cases, insomnia seems to precede Parkinson's by several years. One unique problem that has to do with the dopamine system is called REM behavior disorder (RBD). The normal mechanism that keeps us from physically acting out our dreams breaks down somewhat. People may grind their teeth, kick, yell out; they may even have pretty violent behaviors, attacking their caregivers. Dopamine-related drugs like clonazepam may help. Stimulants in the day may help. Often we just have to protect the patient and their sleep partner by separating them. A baby monitor or video monitor helps a caregiver keep tabs on a patient. We also pad the floor and/or put the bed close to the floor to minimize injuries from falling out of bed.

Someone with Parkinson's may wake up in the middle of the night, often at the same time every night. This may be caused directly by the changes in the brain with the disease process. Again, drugs like clonazepam might help. It may be related to position and comfort. They may get increased muscle stiffness or tremors and rigidity. Gently rocking them, as well as stretching and moving an hour before bed, may help (see Exercise and Parkinson's Disease in Chapter 13, Exercise). They may be unable to roll in bed. Rolling and repositioning may help (see Positioning for Comfort in Chapter 15, Basic Mobility and Transfers).

Frequent urination is another problem they face. For this see sleep hygiene suggestions 11 and 12. You might also have a bedside commode or urinal. Red-light night lighting may allow them to see but not wake them up fully with blue light.

...Sleep and Alzheimer's Disease

With Alzheimer's, sleep may change directly from the disease's effects on the brain or can be affected by any of the secondary problems people experience. Anxiety, depression, restless legs, and apnea are common contributors to sleep problems. If you suspect any of these problems, look to the sections earlier in this chapter that address these individually.

People who can't sleep usually cannot lie still, making it that much more difficult on caregivers. They often fidget, pulling out catheters and other lines, yell out, or even wander, putting them at very high risk of falling down. Treating the sundowning is first (sleep hygiene suggestions 15, 17, 18, and 21). Reviewing their medications is second. Helping them fall asleep (sleep hygiene suggestions 2–8 and 10) and stay asleep (sleep hygiene suggestions 10–12 and 18) is important too. There are medications that may help, but again, sleep medications must be used with caution. If they are used, begin with a low dosage and go slow when increasing dosage. Monitor for increased confusion. For more information, see http://www.alz.org/alzheimers_disease_10429.asp .

...Sleep and Stroke

It's common for a person to require more sleep and to have periods of being quite sleepy in the day when recovering from a stroke or brain injury. Sleep helps the brain recover. The cruel irony is that sleep is often compromised. Obstructive sleep apnea is the most common problem after a stroke, but it may be hard to tell if this is a problem if they're sleepy anyway. Do they snore strongly? Do they stop breathing or have repeating cycles of altered breathing? Look again at Sleep Apnea earlier in this chapter. Try the simple suggestions first. These might work well for up to two-thirds of the cases. Other sleep breathing problems—and other sleep problems in general—can occur, especially if the stroke occurred deeper in the brain. A sleep study might be warranted.

Insomnia and depression are sometimes a problem as well. Look to Insomnia and Sleep and Depression and/or Anxiety earlier in this chapter for help. Give special attention to sleep hygiene suggestion 14, medication review. Discuss the risks and benefits with your loved one's doctor, as some blood pressure medications can cause sleeplessness. If they are sleeping in the day and unable to sleep at night, they may have an alteration in the normal day-night cycle; sleep hygiene suggestion 15 is most important here. Sleep hygiene suggestions 2, 4, 8, 16, 17, and 20–23 also play a role and can be helpful.

If shoulder pain is keeping them awake, supporting the arm and shoulder blade often helps. A pillow under the arm and a little under their shoulder blade can support the arm in a neutral position. For this and more ideas on making the bed comfortable, see Positioning for Comfort in Chapter 15, Basic Mobility and Transfers. Feel the shoulder to make sure the top of the arm fits into the shoulder with much the same shape of the other shoulder. If the bone feels too far forward or down, it may be partially dislocated (*subluxed*). If it's only a little out, sometimes very gently pushing it back into normal position is all it takes. If it's more than a little out, contact their doctor right away. It may be dislocated. You should still support the arm as described above, but usually it's a bit of a trick to reduce (put back) the shoulder, and that trick is done at some risk to the cartilage ring around the joint.

...Sleep and Brain Injury

People with a brain injury can have all the same problems as someone with a stroke. Because brain injuries can be more diffuse and often affect deeper centers in the brain, people with a brain injury can have a host of other sleep problems as well. Parasomnias are often the most confusing of the sleep disorders. They can range from grinding the teeth, kicking, or yelling out to full-on sleepwalking and other REM behavior disorders (RBDs). Though obstructive sleep apnea can be a problem, some breathing disorders arise from the brain rather than the throat. Listen to their breathing when they're asleep. If they don't snore or their breath doesn't seem to get stuck in their throat, yet they still stop breathing for periods or change rhythm a lot, the suggestions for obstructive sleep apnea may not help much.

Relaxation techniques before bed such as relaxation breathing, a gentle stretching routine, and meditation can help with sleep disordered breathing and RBDs and may also help with sleep jerking too. A night guard can help protect the teeth from teeth grinding. If they are experiencing these problems more than just a little, a sleep study may be warranted.

...Sleep and Other Conditions

As you've read through this chapter, you may have noticed problems your loved one has that are described under another diagnosis's heading. Don't panic. This doesn't mean that your loved one now has MS or cancer. We've made efforts here to discuss problems that are more usual to certain diagnoses, but individuals are, well, individual. You may use the suggestions found in any section to address a problem you see. You may also find more and often-useful information by typing the name of the diagnosis and "sleep" into your search engine.

Sleep Medications

By Seth Fadar D.O.

This section reviews the most common classes of medications used to help treat insomnia. These medications will either work on helping people fall asleep (sleep onset) or stay asleep (sleep maintenance).

Sleep medicines have the potential for side effects, and care must be taken when combining them with other medications. Working with your loved one's physician to tailor medication therapy to fit their needs is essential to maximize the benefit of restful sleep.

...Benzodiazepines

Benzodiazepines are a potent class of medications often used to treat anxiety. They bind to gamma-aminobutyric (GABA) type-A receptors in the brain, which increases the potency of these inhibitory neurotransmitters. Activating these receptors reduces anxiety and causes sedation. These medications also cause muscle relaxation, amnesia, and can cause both respiratory and cardiovascular depression. Benzos speed the onset of sleep and prolong the duration of sleep so they are often used as a strong sleep aid. They also may be used to help treat anxiety and, with their anticonvulsant effect, used to treat seizures.

Benzos come in several strengths and duration of effect, ranging from short- to intermediate- to long-acting. As a general rule, it's best to use short- to intermediate-acting medications to avoid or limit excessive daytime sedation. All benzodiazpines can accumulate in fat tissue, so regular use of higher doses can build up a reservoir of medicine, triggering side effects, especially in obese patients. Caution should be taken when using these medications in the elderly, and long-acting benzos should be avoided for sleep. See Delirium: The Hard Road in Chapter 18, Managing Discomforts.

Alprazolam (Xanax): This very short-acting benzo (11 hours) can cause sedation even in low doses, so it can be used as a sleep aid when appropriate. This medication comes in an extended-release form that can reduce rebound side effects and is likely less habit forming.

Diazepam (Valium): This is very long-acting benzo (30–60 hours) is a well-known medication used to treat anxiety, alcohol withdrawal, muscle spasm, and seizure. It should be avoided for the treatment of insomnia, since daily use can cause a buildup of the active form in the body, causing prolonged side effects. It's also famous for being addictive.

Lorazepam (Ativan): This is a common short-acting benzo (12 hours), though it's slightly longer-acting than alprazolam. It is effective for panic attacks, acute anxiety, and even nausea. It is a very common first-choice medication to try in this class. Starting dose is 0.5 mg daily to twice daily.

Temazpam (Restoril): This benzo can be very effective for sleep and often is well tolerated by elderly patients. Side effects include sedation, memory loss, delirium, confusion, loss of balance and coordination, and respiratory and cardiac depression.

Triazolam (Halcion): This is a short-acting benzo that is more commonly used for insomnia, both sleep onset and sleep maintenance. There are several drugs, including opioids, which may interact so be sure all prescribing doctors know if this medication is being used. Common side effects include headache, tingling or prickly sensations in the skin, dizziness and loss of coordination, which can increase the risk of falling. Like the other benzos, it can be addictive. It also should not be taken by pregnant women or anyone under 18.

...Nonbenzodiazepines

Nonbenzodiazepines are a class of medications that have more focused action on the GABA type-A receptors, causing sedation but not reducing anxiety or seizure activity. Like benzodiazepines, they come in different durations of actions: Short-acting forms should be used when the person mainly has trouble falling asleep. Longer-acting forms are a better choice when someone is having trouble staying asleep. The most common side effects with this class of medication are headache, somnolence (sleepy feeling in the morning), and dizziness, which increases the risk of a fall. They can also cause diarrhea or constipation and increase risk of sinusitis.

Eszopiclone (Lunesta): The longest-acting medication in this class is used for both sleep onset and sleep maintenance. Women metabolize these medications much more slowly and should avoid higher doses. It can give an unpleasant metallic taste.

Zaleplon (Sonata): This medication has a short duration of action and would be great choice for someone who needs help with sleep onset but may not work for people who wake up frequently. This medication is metabolized by the body quickly, and so it is less likely to cause side effects the next day, such as a "hangover" feeling.

Zolpidem (Ambien): This is the most commonly used medication in this class; it now comes in short-, intermediate-, and long-acting forms. Intermediate-acting forms come in a dissolvable pill or oral spray; this would be good choice for someone who cannot swallow a pill or who wakes up in the middle of the night. The standard form of this medication, which is more intermediate-acting and longer-acting compared to zaleplon, is indicated for short-term use for insomnia. The extended-release form (**Ambien CR**) releases a second dose of medication during the night, which helps people who often wake up during the night; it is indicated for chronic insomnia. The extended-release form is also considered a better choice for long-term use, because it seems to cause fewer side effects. Women should avoid higher dosing since they do not metabolize this medication as fast as men; also use the lowest possible dose with men.

...Melatonin Agonists

Melatonin agonists bind very strongly to melatonin receptors in the brain and stimulate these areas for a much longer period of time, which can help some people fall asleep and stay asleep longer. These medications are metabolized by the liver and should be used with caution by people with impaired liver function or who abuse alcohol. Avoid using them if the person is currently taking the antidepressant fluvoxamine, which can prolong the effect of these medications. Melatonin agonists tend to have fewer side effects than benzos and nonbenzodiazepines, the most common being drowsiness.

Ramelteon (Rozerem): This medication works better to treat sleep onset and is not the best choice for people who fall asleep but then wake up during the night (sleep maintenance).

Tasimelteon (Hetlioz): The newest medication in this class, this is currently approved for treating a condition called non-24-hour sleep-wake disorder, which affects people suffering from blindness.

...Orexin Receptor Antagonists

Orexin receptor antagonists are a new class of medications recently approved for the treatment of insomnia. Orexin A and B are neuropeptides produced in the hypothalamus in the brain that regulate the sleep-wake cycle and help maintain alertness. **Suvorexant (Belsomra)** blocks the orexin receptors, causing sedation. This medication can impair alertness the following day, cause rebound insomnia when stopped, and be habit forming.

...Antidepressants

Certain forms of antidepressants can be used for the treatment of insomnia. The reason these antidepressants promote sleep is their anticholinergic and antihistamine effects (blocking acetylcholine and histamine) cause sedation. For more details on these medications, see Pain Medication in Chapter 17, Pain Management.

Amitriptyline (Elavil): This antidepressant, like **trazodone,** can be used for someone with both insomnia and depression, but neither is currently FDA approved for the treatment of insomnia. It's unclear as to the long-term benefit..

Doxepin: This has been approved by the Food and Drug Administration (FDA) at low doses for the treatment of insomnia. This medication would be a good first choice for older people.

Mirtazapine (Remeron) is an antidepressant to consider for people with insomnia and depression associated with weight loss or decreased appetite, since it can stimulate appetite and promote weight gain. Sedation tends to occur at the lower dose of 15 mg at bedtime; sedation tends to improve with a higher dose up to 45 mg daily.

...Other Medications

Muscle relaxants are a class of medications used to reduce muscle spasm; most are centrally acting, directly affecting the brain and spinal cord. We still do not completely understand the mechanism of action of these medications other than a general understanding of certain receptors stimulated and the effect of muscle relaxation and often sedation. Medications such as **tizanidine (Zanaflex)** inhibit motor neurons by stimulating alpha-2 receptors, which can reduce spasticity and can assist in sleep, such as for someone with significant musculoskeletal pain with muscle spasm.

The **anti-seizure** medication **gabapentin (Neurontin)** can be used as a sleep aid for those with painful neuropathy or restless leg syndrome. It is commonly used since it is both effective and generic. There is a long list of more common side effects to be aware of including trouble with balance and coordination, nystagmus (jerking of the eyes), depression, irritability and other mood changes, and fever. If your loved one experiences these, contact the prescribing physician right away.

...Over-the-Counter Substances

Diphenhydramine (Benadryl) is a potent **antihistamine** frequently found in over-the-counter sleep medicines. This medication is not recommended for insomnia, aside from very brief and infrequent use, and has several side effects such as a "hangover" effect, dry mouth, blurred vision, urinary retention, and constipation and can increase eye pressure.

There are also several **herbal products** marketed for insomnia such as **valerian** and **chamomile**. Not a lot of research has been done on herbal products and these are no exception. There is some literature saying that valerian can cause side effects when compared to placebos, and there is concern about irritation to the liver. Karen found some help with these herbs in tea before bed.

Melatonin is a natural hormone produced by the pineal gland in the brain, and it promotes sleep; it is a well-known over-the-counter supplement. People with low melatonin levels or a delayed sleep-wake condition (changes to the normal sleep-wake pattern) may benefit from taking melatonin. The medical literature finds that this condition is not common, but the medication seems to help sleep anyway. Perhaps placebo is also powerful medicine. Melatonin does appear to be safe to try when used for short periods of time.

Alcohol consumption, unfortunately, is also commonly used as a sleep aid because it can shorten sleep onset, but it can have a negative impact on the normal sleep cycle and usually causes restless sleep and increases sleep apnea. It is not typically recommended for the treatment of insomnia.

Chapter 15.
Basic Mobility and Transfers

At the start of this chapter, I must at least mention the most important factor in helping your loved one keep or get back safe, happy, optimum mobility: Simply enough, help them stay as healthy as can be. Exercise, nutrition, sleep, and pain management all help with this. Though in this moment you may need to focus on this chapter to help your loved one move, don't forget the other chapters in Part 3, Caregiving Skills and Advice from the Field. You may do more to help their mobility by helping them exercise and get a good night's sleep than by getting them the best wheelchair.

Fall Recovery: How to Get Back Up

Let's hope that this is not why you are now looking at this chapter. If it is, you need this now, so let's get right into it.

Before they move, are they conscious? breathing ok? Do they have a pulse? Is it regular enough? If the answer to any of the last three are no, consider their advance directives or POLST, call 9-1-1 and start CPR if that is their wish. Are they hurt? in pain? Is a limb or their neck in an awkward position? Does their hip hurt? Can they feel and move their fingers and toes? Again, consider calling 9-1-1. If you're trained in first aid you may be able to safely log roll with the limb or spine supported so they may be in a more comfortable position. You may give them pillows and blankets to help make them more comfortable and keep them warm. Generally, don't move an unconscious person unless their position is dangerous and you know their spine and bones are ok.

If they can move, even with some help, you have options:

The standard way is to roll to their side, then up on hands and knees, crawl to some furniture like a couch or heavy chair, then up to kneeling and up to the chair. Caregiverstrianingvideos.com has a nice video of how to do this without help. https://www.youtube.com/watch?v=99GnNHk71Qw This video from Cure PSP demonstrates how to assist with this. https://www.youtube.com/watch?v=10jR0zjI19Y

There are other options. Homeability.com Gives many ways to get back up independently or how to get to a place to call for help. Many of these ways can be assisted too. https://www.youtube.com/watch?v=4ETgQD8QhZs

If they are **safe to move, but can't help much**, there are several methods to move or lift someone depending on how fragile they are, how strong you are, and how much help you have. CERT has produced several excellent videos for their citizen first responders. Here is the one on the **log roll and blanket lift and carry**. https://www.youtube.com/watch?v=66qCkgqVhaI We used this method with Karen with only two people who were each strong enough to gently carry half her weight. You get the blanket under them using the same method we use for rolling and to change the bed with the patient still in it. When you roll them to their side be careful to keep their head and neck supported. When you lift them, have a hand on each side be in line with the top of their neck and another hand with their knees so as to provide a supportive hammock.

If it is just you, consider again if you really need to move them. You might not be able to lift them if they cannot help, but if you must move them you can use the blanket to drag them. This is a lovely demonstration from Pocket Tools Training

NCOSFM https://www.youtube.com/watch?v=ZHzXFgKYii0 .For many people lifting their arm all the way up is difficult. When you roll them you may also support their head and neck with a pillow or a rolled towel.

Like with all mobility skills, it is best to practice these skills before you need them. It also best to prevent a fall in the first place.

Fall Prevention

How do you know if your loved one is at risk of falling? How do you know if they need someone close by or even holding on to catch them if they lose their balance? The truth is that we don't really know. Everyone standing up is at some risk of falling down.

That said, having a recent history of falling while doing something normal is probably the clearest indicator of high risk. If they have suddenly gotten much weaker, have a newly increased difficulty with moving, or have a new balance problem, they also might have a new increased level of risk of falling. As their condition improves again, the risk may indeed go back down. How do you know when it's OK to let them walk on their own again?

...Fall-Risk Assessments

Physical therapists can help assess the risk of falling with a number of different assessment tools. The reason there are different tools is because some tools are better at looking at certain problems than others, so I cannot recommend one test over another here, but I can give you the basics to help you make a good educated guess of your loved one's risk of falling:

- **To balance on two moving feet,** a person needs to have an awareness of upright balance.
- **To not trip,** a person needs to clear the floor with their feet when they walk.
- **To catch themselves if they do take a misstep,** they need to have the strength, speed, and accuracy of movement to get a strong foot out to catch themselves.

Different medical situations challenge each of these different aspects of not falling. If you know they have challenges in one or more of these areas, then you know they have some increased risk. They also need to make good choices and be appropriately cautious in considering their abilities and difficulties.

Two of the most commonly used risk-assessment tools are the **Tinetti Gait and Balance Assessment** and the **Berg Balance Scale**. Typing either of these names into your search engine will lead you to the tests, scoring systems, and even videos. Let's look at how your loved one moves and some of the tests within these tools to help you make a good choice:

- **Can they sit up unsupported? Can they stand? Can they do these without wavering?** Good, they have some basic balance. If they cannot stand or sit unsupported, they definitely need assistance and guarding.
- **What happens if you challenge their basic balance a little? Can they stand with their eyes closed? Can they stand while looking over their shoulder? Can they turn around?** If they cannot do these things and aren't trustworthy with a cane or walker, they are probably at high risk of falling and need guarding. Difficulty with these indicates that they may rely heavily on vision

for their balance. They might seem fine in most circumstances but will have much more difficulty in the dark or in a visually busy place like a busy street or market where things are moving around them. Using night-lights in the dark and walking sticks may help a lot.

- **Can they stand with their feet together? Can they stand with one in front of the other? Can they stand on one foot?** Each of these is an increased level of challenge to their balance. If these are a problem, add them in with other things you see.
- **Do their feet clear the floor when they walk? Is their stride strong and even? Can they walk quickly? If they step up onto a stair, does their foot clear?** All these indicate a higher likelihood that they may catch a foot and have more difficulty getting the other foot out to catch themselves.
- **Can they get up quickly with steadiness? Can they sit back down without using their hands?** These are good functional indicators of balance and strength. If they have problems with more than two or three of the tasks on these last two bullets and aren't trustworthy with their walker or cane, they may need assistance or guarding.

Note: The last piece of this puzzle—judgment to know their limitations and make accommodations—is probably the most important. **Are they forgetful, impulsive, or just too damn stubborn to use a cane or walker?** If so, and if they have trouble with the things above, they may need supervision and/or changes in their home and the places where they go.

In this chapter you can learn about modifying their environment to make it less likely to trip them up, some of the assistive devices out there, and how to physically help them move around safely.

...Home Safety

The most obvious thing to do to make getting around the home easier and safer is to clean out the clutter. Imagine their usual walkway paths inside the home. Now consider removing the newspapers, boxes, plants, and so on to make this pathway clear and smooth. **Walkways should be at least 3 feet wide, smooth-surfaced, uniformly well lit, and not too busy visually.**

Remove things that will make your loved one trip or slip. Area rugs can be taped down with two-sided carpet tape or just rolled up and put away. Electric cords should stay tight to the wall and not cross pathways. While you're doing this, check for loose or uneven floor surfaces and threshold transitions. Oftentimes people don't pick up their feet the way they used to, so remove or secure things that could grab a sliding foot.

People will use furniture as a handrail. It should be sturdy enough to lean on and its edges free from clutter or that menagerie of dustables people tend to collect as they travel through life. Be aware of sharp edges on furniture and countertops. If these are next to a doorway, a turn in their pathway, or another place where someone is more likely to fall, sharp edges are kind of like a punji spike waiting for them. Padding or removing sharp edges can help prevent a more serious injury.

Stairs should be well lit, and it's best if there is a light switch at both the top and bottom of the stairway. Check the handrail to make sure it is smooth and secure. A handrail on both sides is best. If vision is a problem, apply some bright or color-contrasting tape on the steps to help them see the edges. If the stairs could get slippery, apply some nonskid tape.

It's a good idea to help them **live on one floor**. It's best if they don't need to go down rickety stairs to the basement. You might negotiate bringing up those things that they need to the main floor while moving the clutter items down. You might help them do some of those basement tasks so you can help them get upstairs, or simply assign those tasks to someone else. Of course all this goes for the attic too.

Most people eventually make a **bedroom on the main floor,** eliminating the need to travel the stairs to go to bed. For us this worked well. We had a futon sofa that Karen liked to sleep on. It was comfortable, low, and quite adaptable for positioning like a hospital bed. Most importantly for us, it kept her in the heart of the home and engaged with all the activity there. If you don't have a "command center" sofa, there are several options for hospital-type beds that can help. They are discussed in Mobility Aids and Adaptive Equipment later in this chapter.

In the **kitchen**, try to keep the things they use most in easy-to-reach places. Placing things at a height between the knees and shoulders works best. This concept is true all over the house. Where are the towels, the bedding, their clothes, the stuff they use and will reach for? If they must use a step stool, one with a handle at waist height helps. If someone tends to get fatigued, a chair and table or a stable stool at the countertop allows them to sit while preparing food or working on things.

In the **bathroom,** simply cleaning the soap buildup on the shower or tub helps make it less slippery. Nonslip strips can help more. Secure the bath mat with two-sided tape or use a nonslip bath mat. Mount grab bars in the tub or shower and consider a bath chair and handheld showerhead. A grab bar or set of toilet bars can also help them get on and off the toilet more easily and safely. If the towel rack is in a place they are likely to try to use as a handle, replace it with a grab bar that won't break off. We also discuss grab bars and bathroom accessories in Mobility Aids and Adaptive Equipment later in this chapter.

Outside, keep walkways clear and well-lit just like inside. Think of the path from the car to the door and from the door to their favorite outside space. If they love the garden, consider paths there too. Install lights in entryways and walkways. Repair holes and uneven sidewalk joints. Secure any broken handrails on stairs, or perhaps install one. Consider installing one on both sides. Consider whether you may eventually need a ramp. Salt or sand sprinkled on walkways in cold weather will keep the ice clear. For people with memory or cognitive issues, we discuss more safety modifications in Chapter 19, Dementia.

Now that I've discussed all this stuff to change, I beg you to choose your battles wisely. Changing a person's home is disruptive. In college I lived in a house with an interior designer. She would routinely rearrange the furniture, and we found ourselves constantly running into end tables and tripping over this or that. If your loved one is older, frail, or just more set in their ways, it can be downright disorienting.

Also, this is *their* home. Most people don't want their things moved or removed. Adding a little light is an easy change. Taping down throw rugs, stabilizing wobbly furniture, and taping cords out of the way are also changes that are pretty well accepted. Removing some clutter may be just a bit harder. It might be clutter to you, but to them, it's their stuff. Getting rid of stuff wholesale, especially mementos, and moving furniture may be the hardest change of all. Doing a little at a time may work better than trying to get 'er done all at once.

...Medical Alert Systems
"I've fallen and I can't get up!"

Most of us are familiar with this advertisement tag line from Life Alert. They offer a wearable emergency button (pendant or wristwatch style) that communicates with an in-home monitor, which then links to a call center. For many people, this gives them peace of mind and enough protection against the catastrophe of a fall and injury or other emergency to allow them to continue to live independently. The Life Alert ad, though we all make fun of it, has worked and they are the second-largest provider of these services, behind Phillips Lifeline.

There are other companies too, and there are pros and cons to each. For an excellent breakdown of these services, check out http://medicalalertsystemshq.com/compare-medical-alert-systems. We encourage you to read the small print, especially of a longer-term contract.

More and more people routinely carry a cell phone and are familiar enough with it to call 9-1-1, even in difficult times. This, perhaps coupled with a carbon monoxide detector, may be another option for similar security.

Mobility Aids and Adaptive Equipment
"Mobility aids" or "mobility devices" or the more general term "assistive devices" refers to all manner of canes, crutches, walkers, and wheelchairs. It's any device that helps someone get around. There are lots of options. A physical therapist or occupational therapist may be the best at making good recommendations for your loved one's particular needs. One thing to keep in mind is that anything you use doesn't need to feel stuffy or medical. It can be as individual as you are.

The first mobility aid Karen had was a cane I fashioned for her from a stick of driftwood. My great-grandmother had such a walking stick: gnarled, polished with love, and full of character. With a belt sander, I shaped the handle to fit the curves of Karen's right hand. We cut its length so it came to the top of her hip for support and finished its foot with a rubber crutch tip. This lovely custom walking stick eased the idea of using a cane. It was as interesting and beautiful as Karen. She could lean on it a bit and with it walk with more ease without the encumbrance of a "medical device." Later, when she needed two canes, we were blessed with her best friend's trekking poles. And later still, we pimped out her wheelchair with red handles and handlebar tassels and all kinds of decorations.

This section provides you with some basics about the various types of mobility aids. Each basic type is outlined below, along with some of the options and features, pros and cons, and how it might be used. Much more information on each type can be found online by typing into your browser the name of the device you are interested in.

...Canes
Canes can be used for support or for balance. The size for each is a little different, as is the technique for using them. For **support**, the person will generally use it on the opposite side from the weaker leg. We fit it about hip high (top of the upper leg bone,

or great trochanter) to give a slight bend to the person's elbow when they're using it. This allows them to rest their hand against their hip to stabilize the handle as they put their weight on the stick. The stick moves along with the weaker leg, parallel to the leg, as they walk.

For **balance**, the cane is a bit longer, about the height of the fleshy bit between the top of the leg bone and the crest of the pelvis. This allows them to comfortably place it a foot or so in front of them without having to bend over. The person often uses it in their dominant hand, forming a strong tripod with both legs for balance. In walking, the stick can move separately from each leg, like a separate third leg (three-point gait) or with the opposite leg (two-point gait). Three-point is more stable, two-point tends to be faster and smoother. Here is a video we made for you: https://youtu.be/pTJVaoYTnXw

Canes and walking sticks are inexpensive at drug stores and medical supply stores. Wooden ones can be cut to fit, aluminum ones are often adjustable. A wide selection of trekking poles can be found at hiking and mountaineering stores like REI.

There are canes with three or four points on the bottom (fig. 1), allowing the cane to stand up on its own and making it more stable to put weight on. We usually use these with one-sided weakness such as from a stroke. Walking with one of these is a bit slower, as the cane doesn't roll and tilt with the normal walking cycle. These are usually available only by the recommendation of a physical therapist.

Figure 1. Four-point cane

...Crutches

Crutches are used to supply more weight-bearing support than a cane provides. One might need this with an injured leg that can't bear any or only a little weight. Crutches take much more upper-body strength and control and usually aren't useful for people who need caregiving. There are two basic types:

Axillary (armpit) crutches (fig. 2) are the standard. Fit the handle at wrist height, like you do a cane for support, and the pad so you have two fingers of space between the top of the pad and the armpit. Be careful not to put weight on the armpits, as there's a bundle of nerves and blood vessels in there you don't want to squish. There's a bit of technique to using them, too much to list here. I found this website and video fairly complete and helpful http://www.physiotherapy-treatment.com/walking-crutches.html.

Figure 2. Axillary (armpit) crutches

Forearm (Lofstrand or Canadian) crutches are the ones that have a cuff around the forearm instead of an armpit pad. These are better for longer distances and higher-level mobility. Some people feel much more stable on them, but some people feel more stable with the pad under their arms. I used the Lofstrand in my times on crutches.

Good features of the Lofstrand crutch are, there is no weight bearing or chafing near the armpits, and they allow

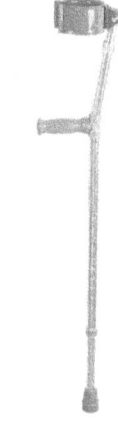

Figure 3. Forearm (Lofstrand or Canadian) crutches

the arms to move fully at the elbow, which means the person can move faster and easier up- and downstairs or over obstacles.

A feature that is not so good is that more of the weight is on the hands. This can be hard on the wrists and takes more upper-body strength and control.

Other crutchlike devices include various types of scooters or platforms that support the lower leg for an isolated foot injury. **Leg scooters** (fig. 4) allow weight bearing through the injured side, but are sometimes more difficult to use and cannot be used if the knee, hip or upper leg is involved. This would be something to ask the doctor or PT about.

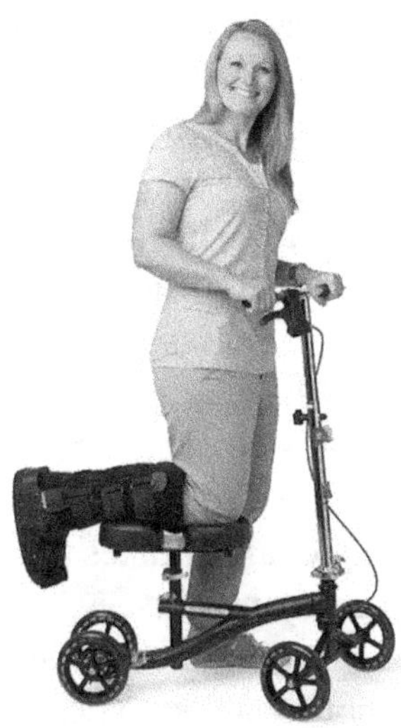

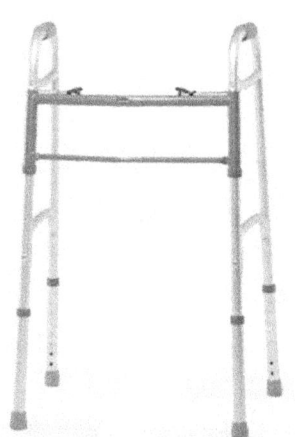

Figure 4. Leg scooter

There are **platform crutches**(fig. 5) that bear weight on the forearm if the person's hand is unable to bear much weight. The forearm platform is much like the one on the platform walker shown Figure 10 in the Walkers section below.

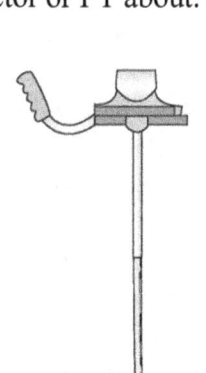

Figure 5. Platform crutch

...Walkers

Walkers are much more stable than a cane or crutches, and like a cane, can be used for support of an injured leg or for balance. The handle height should fit just like a cane for support with a small bend in the elbow, or slightly taller for balance. The standard **four-point walker** (fig. 6) is lightweight, easy to use, and stable. It's especially useful when someone needs to put a lot of weight on it, such as after a hip or knee replacement or fracture. These walkers fold up so they are easy to fit in your car or to carry upstairs, but they don't work so well to help a person get upstairs. These can be found for less than $50 and are available at medical supply houses, Walgreens and other pharmacies, and online.

Figure 6. Four-point walker

Front-wheeled walkers (fig. 7) can be used for balance and/or weight bearing. Among their **good features** are that they can roll on a smooth, clean surface, like a hospital floor. They're also almost as good for stability as a four-point walker; if a person puts weight on them, the back points keep the wheels from rolling out from under them, and they are better for balance, as one doesn't have to pick it up to move it. We like to put tennis balls or other types of skids on the back feet so they slide quietly. They're not so good outside or on varying surfaces.

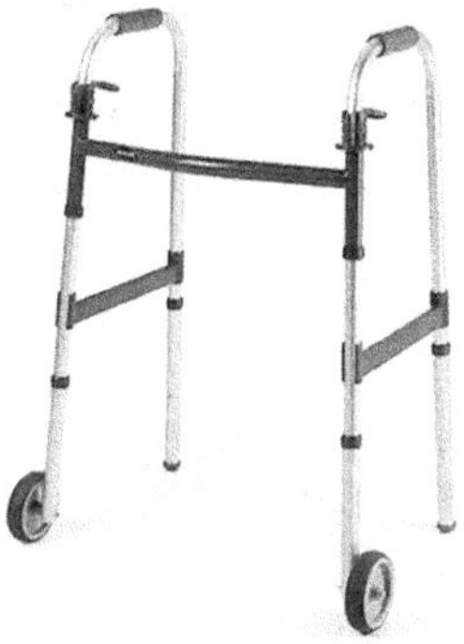

Figure 7. Front-wheeled walker

Here are two videos to help with fit and use. http://www.hugoanywhere.com/video-instruction-for-how-to-properly-use-your-walker/ and http://monkeysee.com/how-to-use-a-walker-to-prevent-falls/

Four-wheeled walkers (fig. 8) are good for balance help inside and outside and over rougher surfaces. One of their **good features** is that they usually have larger, softer tires that roll smoothly, even outside. They are heavier and more stable for balance, and some have a seat to rest on. They have lockable brakes and can even have storage and carrying bins.

Among their **not-so-good features** are, they are not so stable to bear weight on and they are a bit heavier and more awkward to transport. They

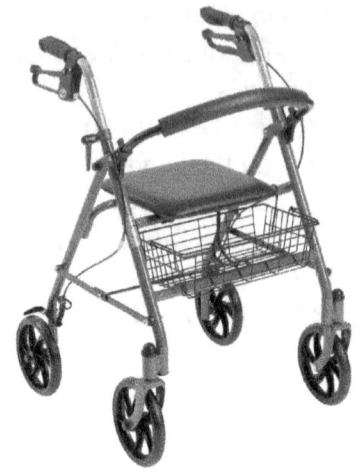

Figure 8. Four-wheeled walker

also are more expensive ($100–$300) than a four-point or front-wheel walker. They can be purchased or rented at medical supply houses and online. Here are a couple videos to help your loved one learn to use a walker.

Hemi walkers and other special options are available for stroke or other one-sided weakness. A **hemi walker** (fig. 9) is a walker meant to be used in one hand. It is kind of like a wider, more stable four-point cane. Physical therapist Kim doesn't recommend these, as they tend to lead to a poor walking pattern, which makes rehabilitation more difficult.

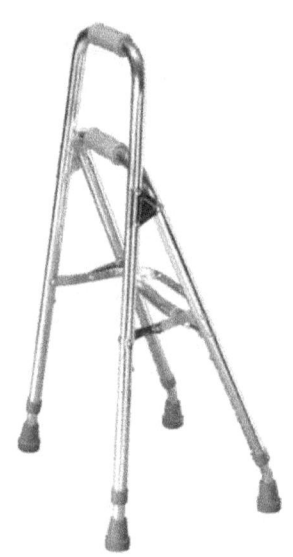

Figure 9. Hemi walker

A **platform walker** (fig. 10) can have one or two arms. These are useful if there is a hand or wrist injury and a walker is needed. A tabletop platform on the walker may also be used. It can have wheels, allowing the person to fully lean on the walker and roll the walker forward. These are usually intended for use in the realm of the rehabilitation gym and not for home use. In fact,

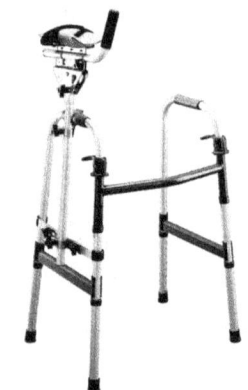

Figure 10. Platform walker

there are many different clever adaptations of walkers for most every special need. Your physical therapist can help you here.

...Wheelchairs

Wheelchairs can be very specialized. The basic one pictured in Figure 11 has large rear wheels with a handrail, allowing the user to propel it with their hands. If the seat is low enough, they may also pull it along with their feet. It has handles in back so a friend

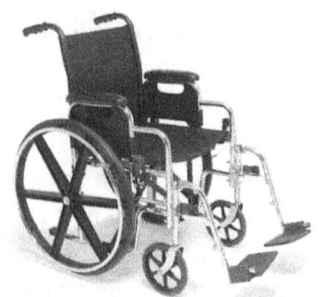

Figure 11. Wheelchair

can push it or the user can use it as a wheeled walker for balance. Careful with this, however; it will tip back and roll out if they put much weight on it. There are tilt bars low in the back to make it easy for a helper to lift the front wheels to clear a curb or obstacle. The brakes should be set before the person gets in or out of the wheelchair. It may also have removable footrests that swing out of the way and lift off. Most wheelchairs are foldable for transport and storage.

Usually when someone needs a wheelchair, a physical therapist will be called in to train them and their caregivers in the specific skills they will need. You can find several videos online that will also help. https://www.youtube.com/watch?v=EZestPFcvP0 by Medifecta provides good general information on helping someone who might need a wheelchair or walker. The series by Craig Hospital on curbs and stairs is brief, clear, and well done. Charlie Croteau has produced a comprehensive handbook and video mostly geared for para and quadriplegic wheelchair users. Still, many of the techniques will help most anyone in a chair. http://www.wheelchairmobility.org/mobility_video.html. https://www.youtube.com/watch?v=b2mWfFPbTkA is the most friendly and practical video I've seen, probably because it was made by regular people like you and your loved one. For more on how to assist someone get in and out of a wheelchair, see Physically Helping Your Loved One Move later in this chapter.

Features and Options

Tilt back: This allows the wheelchair's back to recline, which is good for people with severe blood pressure problems, like quadriplegics. This option does add weight and complexity to a wheelchair.

Elevating footrests: These are good for someone with a knee or foot problem and are helpful with edema. They also may be used in combination with a tilt back to help with blood pressure. Downsides to them are that they are a little heavy, more expensive, and more cumbersome.

Reclining or tilt in space chairs: The whole seat tilts back, footrests and all. This can help with blood pressure problems as a tilt back does. This kind of chair also relieves pressure on the seat and allows the user's legs to come up higher and more comfortably than with elevating footrests. This can be much better for edema problems. It is also good for people who tend to squirm out of the chair because it makes it more difficult for them to fall out.

Removable armrests: These are helpful if the person will be sliding in and out of the wheelchair from the side; it is a standard feature on many chairs.

Small rear wheels: These "transport chairs" don't allow the person to self-propel with their hands or set their own brakes. These wheelchairs are lighter weight and less expensive, though, and quite a bit easier for the caregiver to fold up and put in a car.

Special seat padding: Usually a special seat cushion can be placed in any wheelchair. These are great at relieving pressure and decreasing the chance of the user getting a pressure sore. Generally they are foam, air, or gel. There are advantages and disadvantages to each type. Deeper, softer seats may be better at relieving pressure but may make transfers more difficult. A PT can make the best recommendation for each case.

Various widths and sizes: Wheelchairs come in different widths and seat-pan heights. When the user is sitting in it, there should be just a little room on the sides of each thigh. If there is too much room, it is difficult for the user to reach the wheels and brakes, and the chair is more cumbersome in tight spaces; if the fit is too tight, there may be a risk for skin breakdown on their hips and thighs. If the person will be pulling the wheelchair along with their feet, the top of the seat pan should come to the crease in the back of their knees if they were standing, to allow their feet to reach the floor. Otherwise, a little extra seat height is no problem. A higher seat or a cushion in the seat can make getting up easier, as they are starting from a little higher position.

Special seating and positioning options: The length of the seat pan, tilt, and the position of the backrest work together to support the person in their best posture. Having a good fit to begin with helps. The seat pan should be long enough that you can place at least two fingers behind their knee without touching the pan. The tilt should support the pelvis and back in as neutral a position as possible (see Positioning for Comfort later in this chapter) so the curves of their back are supported and they don't slump or slouch. Most of these fitting techniques just make sense, and you may do quite a bit with pillows and pads in the backrest and the seat to accommodate their special needs.

Padding: The user should be protected from any sharp edges in the wheelchair that may bruise or cut them with repeated contact. We often use pipe insulation, a tube-shaped piece of foam you can get at a hardware store, to pad any edges. Special bolsters and padding or other modifications can be made to the wheelchair to support a person and protect them from any pressure points. This is especially important with spasticity and certain deformities. Fitting someone with special seating needs is an art, something a specialized physical therapist will help with.

Lightweight and sport chairs: There are many options here, too many to discuss in any detail. These are not usually something that someone in a caregiver situation is concerned about, though. If this is something you are considering, a simple internet browser search for "sport wheelchair" will get you started.

...Power Wheelchairs and Scooters

I mention these devices together because Medicare, and thus many other payers, will pay for one or the other of these but not both, and they are expensive. Be careful choosing one of these, as Medicare generally won't consider paying for a second chair for five years, and they may require the one you have to be repaired rather than replaced. If you suspect your loved one's needs will change and they may need the support and operation of a power wheelchair, do not let Medicare pay for a scooter.

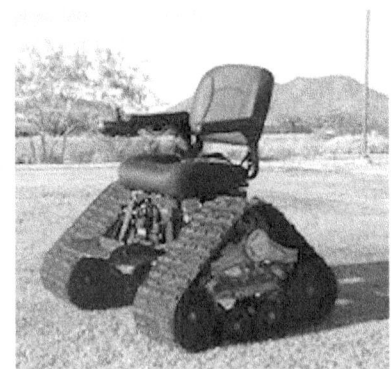

Figure 12. Not your typical Scooter

Power wheelchairs come in many shapes and sizes. They are often controlled with a joystick but can have different options to utilize nearly any movement the person has to control the chair (fig. 12). They also have a wide variety of changeable seating options, which allow the person to be supported and secure and allow them to tilt back with their legs supported (fig. 13). The range of features and options is huge, but this is not something you will be buying on your own. The rehabilitation team you are working with will work with your loved one on the purchase, and on how to use it. Proper fitting, use, and selection of options is a bit of an art.

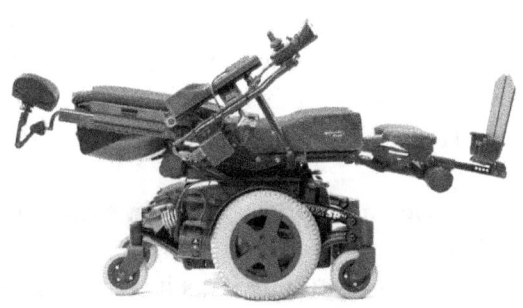
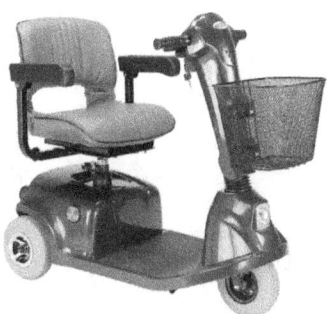

Figure 13. Power wheelchair in tilt back position

Figure 14. Power scooter

Power scooters give a longer travel range than most motorized wheelchairs and are thus better for community mobility (mobility outside the home). Many of them can be easily disassembled to put it in a regular car, whereas power wheelchairs will need a special carrying rack or a roll-in van. Most city buses in the United States have boarding methods for either scooters or wheelchairs. Scooters usually do not have much in the way of seating options and require handlebar control.

...Access Ramp

If your loved one has entry stairs for getting into the house and they are using a wheeled device, they may need an access ramp built or installed. The Americans with Disabilities Act (ADA) requires that a ramp be at least 3 feet wide, give no more than 1 inch of height for every 12 inches in length, allow at least 5 feet by 5 feet of flat landing at each end, and have handrails between 34 inches and 38 inches high. At the time of this writing, Massachusetts and California required 48 inches in width. Premade ramps are commercially available. Most contractors can build one as well.

...Slide Board

A slide board acts as a bridge across the gap between a chair, bed, or such, to allow the person to scoot over rather than standing up. This is often useful if they have good upper-limb strength and very poor lower-limb strength. This device is one to ask the PT or nurse about whether it might be helpful. If they're using the slide board bare bottomed, don't forget the baby powder.

...Lifts

A **sling lift or Hoyer lift** is a small hydraulic crane that allows one person to safely lift and transfer someone who is mostly unable to help with the lift. The device uses a sling that can be placed under the person (Your health care team or the vendor of the lift will show you this). The sling hooks to the lifting arm of the crane, the caregiver gives a few pumps of the handle or presses the button, and voila, the person is suspended above their bed. The lift has wheels so it can be moved over a chair, gurney, or anything else and then the person is lowered again onto the new location. For more on Hoyer lifts and other total-assist lifts, see http://en.wikipedia.org/wiki/Patient_lift.

...Grab Bars and Poles

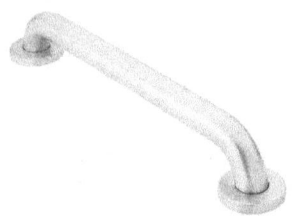

Figure 15. Grab bar

Sometimes just having a handle in the right place can make getting around much safer and easier. Grab bars are inexpensive, relatively easy to install, and available at many hardware stores. In fact, the picture in Figure 15 is from the Home Depot of one of the many grab bars they stock.

There are two basic types: **screw-in grab bars,** which should be secured to the studs of the house (check the stud spacing before you buy it, as it will need to be screwed to a stud on each end), and **suction-type grab bars**, which need a smooth surface such as tile.

Generally grab bars are placed on the wall of the bathtub or shower surround and maybe next to the toilet. If the towel rack is in a place that makes a good handle, it might be a good idea to replace it with a grab bar, which won't break if someone puts weight on it.

A pole can serve as a strong handle and doesn't need to be near a wall. The **Superpole** by Healthcraft (fig. 16, 17, and 18) offers easy installation in most locations, and it can have attachments such as a horizontal bar (fig. 17) or a trapeze—a handle over the bed (fig. 18). The pole is especially useful for one-sided weakness such as a person might get with a stroke.

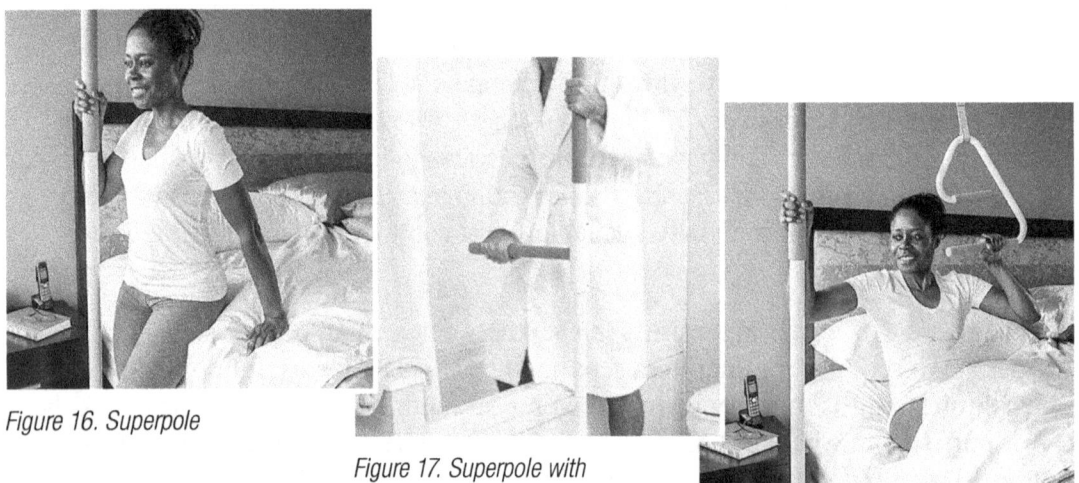

Figure 16. Superpole

Figure 17. Superpole with side handle

Figure 18 Superpole with trapeze

There are also inexpensive **bed rails** that secure with a piece under the mattress to provide someone with a handle to use to get up from bed. There are many different types; PT Kim recommends the Freedom Grip Economy Bed Rail by Mobility Transfer Systems. Careful with bed rails with anyone who is not cognitively alert and intact. There are people who have gotten an arm stuck which can be disastrous. Bed rails should help mobility, not prevent it. They should never be used to keep someone in bed. That's just a small soft prison.

Having handles on either side of the toilet can help someone get up and down safely and easily. Figure 19 shows a handle frame that is commercially available. For Karen, we were able to place her walker backward over the toilet so that its grips served as handles.

...Bathroom Aids

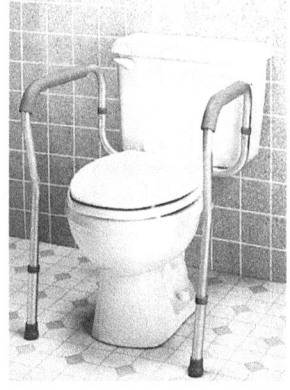

Figure 19. Handles for the toilet

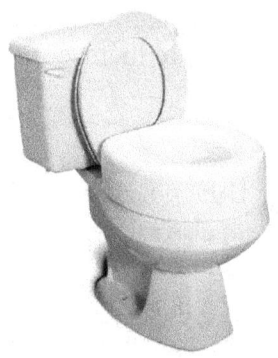

Figure 20. Raised toilet seat

While we're in the bathroom, we may as well discuss a **raised toilet seat** (fig. 20). This simple device fits on top of the toilet, making the seat higher. This enables a person to not have to squat down so low, which is especially important after hip replacement surgery or some fracture repairs.

A **bath chair** (fig. 21) and handheld showerhead can allow someone to shower sitting down at normal chair height. A wide version can straddle the side of a standard tub, allowing the person to slide across the chair to get out of the tub. Don't forget to keep gloves in the bathroom because you'll probably use them there.

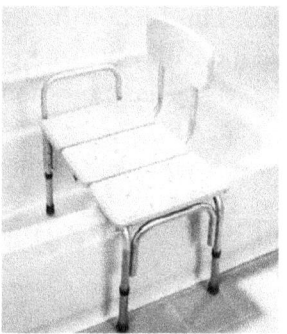

Figure 21. Bath chair

When the bathroom is just too far for your loved one to get to, a **bedside commode** (fig. 22) can be placed just about anywhere. This is used like a regular toilet, but it is designed to be a bit higher than a toilet so it doesn't need a raised toilet seat, and it comes with its own handles. For instruction for bathing and toileting, and the bedside commode, see Chapter 16, Hygiene, Bathing, and Toileting.

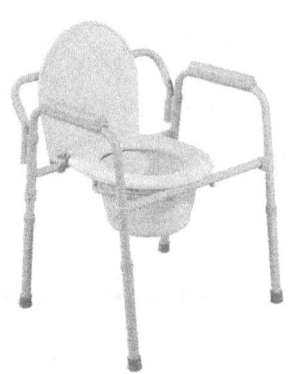

Figure 22. Bedside commode

...Hospital Beds

There may come a time when you want a hospital-type bed. This can be in their bedroom, another room, or on the main floor in the center of the home. Hospital beds are usually narrow enough that you can reach your loved one from either side, making it easier for providing care and for them getting out of bed. Hospital beds may also have removable rails on either side to make getting in or out easier and to prevent falling out of bed.

These beds **can be raised at the head or foot**, making positioning easier too. Be careful not to have the bed head up too much. It's good for eating, reading, etc., but this position puts more pressure on the buttock, especially the tailbone, and can make pressure sores. Having the knee bent all the time can make their knees stiffen in this position (knee contracture). For more on this, see Positioning for Comfort later in this chapter.

Often the mattress is waterproof, which has its advantages for hygiene. However, **waterproof mattresses** don't breathe as well, so they may be less comfortable and make someone a little more prone to skin breakdown. There are **special mattresses designed to prevent pressure ulcers**. These used to be quite expensive and needed to be prescribed specifically for people who could not move in bed themselves (making them high-risk patients) or who already had advanced bedsores that weren't healing. These rather complex mattresses and mattress tops float the person on a pillow of air that can change pressure from side to side as well as top to bottom, changing where the person bears weight. It may be more difficult for the person to move themselves, sit up, or stand up from one of these mattresses.

Assistive Devices

"Assistive devices" refers to all those clever items that can help with the kinds of simple tasks we do every day, such as getting dressed and preparing a meal, also known as **"activities of daily living" (ADLs)**. There are thousands of such devices, many developed by people like you and me and the ones we care for to help with our specific need. This section discusses some of the most universally useful ones, but keep in mind that there may be a more specific solution out there for your loved one. Your occupational therapist is the professional master here and your best resource for techniques and devices to help. Also, typing "assistive devices for (fill in your specific need here)" into your browser will yield pictures and descriptions of some more of what's out there.

...For Grasping Things

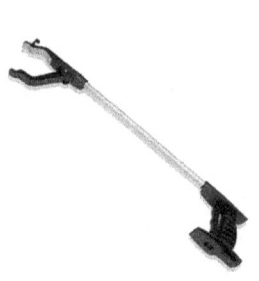

Figure 23. Reacher

The **reacher** (fig. 23) is probably the most universally handy item. These are cheap, usually under $30, come in different lengths, and can have a side pull or an open jaw type grip. Normal length is about 2 feet. Longer is more cumbersome but gives more reach, and both grip styles are popular and useful, so which one to choose depends on tasks and tastes.

Around the house, **doorknob grippers or handles** can help the arthritic hand open the door, and **key holders** allow a troubled hand to operate a key. There are also **special knobs** for light switches and **handles** for electric plugs.

...For Getting Dressed

If tying shoes is a problem, **elastic shoelaces** allow someone to pull a laced shoe on without having to untie and retie laces. A **shoehorn** helps with all types of slip-on shoes, and a **long-handled shoehorn** helps if someone also has difficulty reaching their feet with their hands. A **sock aid** (fig. 24) holds open the stocking, allowing the person to push their foot into it without having to be able to reach their feet.

A word about socks: Socks are something we generally don't think much about unless you happen to be long-distance hiker, but there are a few considerations here.

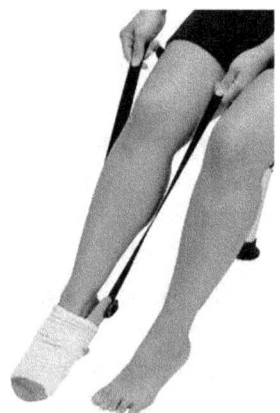

Figure 24. Sock aid

For anyone with poor sensation in the bottoms of their feet, such as diabetics with foot neuropathy, we strongly recommend white socks. This allows anyone to easily spot blood or fluid stains and alerts us to any wound. This little tip may just save a foot. For someone with edema, be careful the sock does not roll down or form a restrictive ring around the ankle. Socks with tight tops should be avoided here as well.

Zipper pulls are simply a string looped through the zipper pull and knotted, which is easier to grasp than the zipper pull itself. (We also use these loops in our outdoor gear so we can work a zipper without taking our gloves off.) A **button aid** is a clever looped hook that allows someone to pull a button through the buttonhole with one hand.

...For Cooking and Eating

Most assistive **cooking and eating equipment** focuses on use with only one hand or being easier to grasp and hold. A spike in the cutting board holds your vegetables so you may cut them with one hand. A sticky pad can keep the cutting board or plate from sliding. Cooking and eating utensils can have wide or curved handles, or grips which allow the utensil to strap or hook onto the hand. A bowl or plate can have a steep rim or scooped side on one side to allow a person to more easily scoop food onto a spoon. Plates can have separators like picnic paper plates and can be brightly colored to make foods easier to see and manage. There are hundreds of different designs and products to meet specific needs. Elderstore.com http://www.elderstore.com/kitchen-and-dining_51.aspx is one vendor, and their site is easy to navigate and loaded with pictures of creative products. Chapter 12, Food and Nutrition discusses a little more about helpful plates and utensils and Physically Helping Your Loved One Eat.

...For Viewing and Listening

There are **headphones and earpieces** that connect to the telephone, television, or radio. Some **hearing aids** come with features that allow this as well. There are also **large-text voice-recognition screens** to help someone who is profoundly hard of hearing communicate by telephone, but as with most of our current voice-recognition devices, it sometimes gets it wrong, which may prove frustrating or really funny, depending on your outlook. Again, here is a link to Elderstore.com http://www.elderstore.com/auditory-visual_21.aspx

Obtaining and Paying for Mobility and Assistive Devices

In the United States, Medicare is the chief driver of the policies regarding paying for **durable medical equipment (DME).** There has been a lot—think billions of dollars—of abuse over the years getting Medicare to pay for expensive medical equipment, so entities like Medicare and Medicaid have responded with ever more difficult and complicated rules aimed at preventing abuse. The rules change year by year, so what's written here today may be somewhat different by time you read it. Private insurance, military insurance, and workman's compensation insurance all have their own rules but tend to follow Medicare. They all have their own vendors by region, so any discussion on this topic for Seattle wouldn't work for Portland, let alone London. That said, there are some terms and basic concepts that will help you navigate this ever-changing terrain.

Are They Medically Necessary?

Basically Medicare and all the other payers want to be as sure as they can that they are buying something for your loved one that will make them more independent, prevent further health problems, and save them money on medical care in the longer run. When you think about it, what they want is really quite reasonable. To help them be sure, they want anything they're paying for to be a **medically specific device and be medically necessary**. This means the doctor needs to prescribe the equipment and the doctor's and rehabilitation specialists' (PTs, OTs, and SLPs) notes need to support the need for the equipment. This also means payers aren't buying something that, though it might help the patient, could be for general use, like an air conditioner or stationary bicycle. There is specific language that Medicare reviewers want to see; the language isn't 100 percent necessary, but it does make it clearer for reviewers. That's rehab's job, not yours, but you might hear everyone talking in these funny terms or see them on your Medicare statements, and that's somewhat the reason why.

Assistive devices should allow the person to be able to complete their **activities of daily living (ADLs),** such as getting dressed, making a meal, eating, bathing, toileting, etc., when they otherwise couldn't. Rehabilitation professionals will be working toward the **least-restrictive device** to help someone get around safely in their home, improving their **mobility** with things like getting out of bed and getting around in the home without falling down. It's much less likely that someone will fall from a wheelchair than with using a cane, but being confined to a chair is pretty restrictive. **Community mobility**—getting around outside—is considered different from **in-home mobility**. Medicare is primarily concerned with mobility in the home.

One more thing. Durable medical equipment must be in fact, durable. DME cannot be supplies that are used up or disposable like gloves or Band-Aids. Medicare won't cover modifications to the home like ramps or grab bars, or things that could be considered for convenience like a stairway elevator.

Who Orders and Pays for Them?

Getting things ordered and paid for is most often something done by the health-care facility staff. This often falls to the PT's, OT's or social workers, but may be part of the rehab team's responsibility. Any **ordering** they're doing should start early, as it may take a while from order to confirmation of benefit to delivery, and the order can be cancelled if it is later determined that it's not needed.

Hospice has access to most of the medical equipment you'll need. This may be coordinated through the nurse or social worker on your health-care team, and things are usually supplied immediately with no fuss. These are loaned for use during the hospice period, whereas Medicare pays for your purchase of DME.

To get things on your own, some **private insurance** plans do allow for reimbursement. Read the policy for the details. Knowing the above-listed terms will help. There also may be **charitable organizations** in your area that help people with medical equipment. Senior centers, church organizations, community organizations such as Shriners and Rotary, and disease-specific organizations such as local chapters of the Arthritis Foundation are full of people giving of themselves to help in this difficult time. The social work department and community resource center of your local hospital may be able to help with more information on local resources.

For smaller, less expensive items, such as walkers and special dishes, if you're not connected to a care facility you might find it easier to just **pay for them yourself**. There are a huge number of online vendors and usually a few local vendors in each community. Of all the professionals I spoke with, none had a recommended website, but simply typing the name of the device you're interested in or just "mobility aids" or "adaptive equipment for …" into your browser will lead you to a plethora of sites with pictures, prices, and lots of options.

Sammons Preston (Now Patterson Medical) is one of the largest suppliers for professional organizations. They have one of the most complete, somewhat overwhelming catalogs, but they do have pretty much everything and can help you get an idea of what's out there. Colonial Medical Supplies also has a fairly friendly site to help you see what's out there. Elderstore.com also has a fairly friendly site with good pictures and prices listed.

If you have time and little money, you might look at the local thrift shop for something used and cheap. People often donate equipment when it's no longer needed. If you need it *now* or need something specific, this isn't the best option. The professionals at any hospital or rehabilitation facility you are in contact with may also be able to steer you to a local source for **used equipment.**

Physically Helping Your Loved One Move

One of the most intimate yet frightening aspects of caregiving comes as the person you care for begins to need physical help getting around safely. People often have an image of their loved one falling and of having to catch their full weight in some awkward way. They wonder if they'll have the strength or if their back can take the load. This mental image is paralyzing to potential caregivers and often leads to people being placed in a facility when they don't have to be.

Long before physical therapy school, I volunteered at the Flagstaff Medical Center PT department. There I met a most talented and powerful therapist who, to be generous, stood all of 5 feet 3 inches tall. She was also quite pregnant at the time. Still, in her care, profoundly disabled people who were easily twice her weight seemed to move effortlessly about the gym and hospital floors. She began to show me how she performed her daily mobility miracles. "The basic principles are easy," she would say:

- **Set up the area** to help them with their success as much as is reasonable.
- **Allow the person to do as much for themselves as possible.**
- **Use their strength and your leverage** to help them.
- **Consider what is weak or fragile** to give support and protection.
- **Keep them and yourself safe.**
- **Respect their dignity and independence** as much as possible.

These principles are woven into all the techniques we teach to all caregivers, professional or otherwise. They will help you make getting around safer, more comfortable, and easier for your loved one and for everyone involved.

...Standby Assist and Contact Guard Assist

The gentlest form of assistance you can give is to simply be there, helping make things easier and safer for them. They may need help with setting up the area, getting assistive devices like a cane or walker within reach, and being cued to use them properly. They might need help opening doors or knowing where they are going. They need someone close by in case they lose their balance or footing, but aren't so unsteady that you need to be holding on to them. We call this kind of assistance **standby assist (SBA).**

Contact guard assist (CGA) is the point where they do need someone holding onto them. You're not lifting them, but you are physically holding onto them to steady them *and should be in position* to catch a fall. Here are some tips:

- It is standard care to **wrap a gait belt** around their waist and snug it so that you can slide two fingers under it fairly easily. A gait belt is simply a wide belt with a secure clasp. It gives you a handle but is not intended to be a harness with which to lift them. *If they have a wound or tube or some other reason not to put the belt around their waist, you can wrap it around their chest.* I like the buckle a little to the side so it doesn't pinch them when they bend and tails of the belt tucked back into the buckle to keep them out of the way and to make it easier to take the belt off again. When you remove the belt, don't pull it out as though you're spinning a top. Use your hand and arm between them and the belt to protect their fragile skin as you gently pull it from the side.
- **Use as light a hand as possible**, giving only the balance or position correction they need. Try to be smooth and steady rather than abrupt or sharp.
- **If you are using any kind of belt,** you may hold it gently palm up so if they do fall, they fall into your hand. This allows you to relax your hand and arm.
- **If you are catching a fall,** use your body as a chair or a wall, using your strong hips and legs rather than your back or arms. You will see what I mean in the videos.

Here are three basic videos on SBA to CGA:

Contact Guard or Catching a Fall:
https://youtu.be/KziiwT8VVCM

Guarding Someone on the Stairs [Farmington Valley]:
http://www.youtube.com/watch?v=XeY4YbmTxro

Car Transfer with Minimal Assist:
http://www.youtube.com/watch?v=9FPo7dyCWag

...Minimal, Moderate, and Maximal Assist

This section discusses when you begin to physically help them move. **Minimal assist** means they are doing better than 75 percent of the effort, with you providing the rest. This is usually light assistance, providing them support and perhaps giving them a little lift under the shoulder to help them stand. **Moderate assist** refers to them giving up to 50 percent of the effort, perhaps blocking their knees with your knees to assist their strength and keep their knees from buckling as you help lift them. And **maximal**

assist is you providing up to 75 percent of the effort. The techniques for these three categories are somewhat similar, whether you are helping them with a **stand-pivot transfer** or a **sit-to-stand transfer.** Here are some training videos from Farmington Valley Visiting Nurse Association:

Assisted Stand-Pivot Transfer [Farmington Valley]:
http://www.youtube.com/watch?v=71WzN6oO6s4

Slide-Board Transfer [Farmington Valley]:
http://www.youtube.com/watch?v=oIT9mJmLsR8

Car Transfer Minimal to Maximal Assist:
http://www.youtube.com/watch?v=BYXNusXA_q4

This next clip gets into more-advanced techniques, more specific to hemiplegia (one-sided weakness) that one usually sees as a result of a stroke or other one-sided brain injury. The techniques shown here are not for everybody. For example, there is no way Karen, with her fragile spine, could have used this method for getting off the floor. Still, the skills shown are wonderful, and the practitioner is very good at demonstrating the basic principles:

Patricia Neal Mobility Video: http://www.youtube.com/watch?v=I_NftgBc2tY

Practice the Techniques

Begin practicing the basic techniques with your friends and family, especially with the other caregivers on your team and, if possible, with professional caregivers. PTs are best here ... or is that just some professional snobbery on my part? Take turns being the patient so you can also feel what it is like to be assisted. As the patient, try helping a lot, a little, and not at all; you will find that it is difficult to not help. Give each other feedback and be willing to laugh through the awkwardness; the times we did this in our house, it was a giggle fest. Have fun with it. You won't be perfect at first, but I saw excellent lifts (better than the YouTube training videos) from software engineers and photographers. As you practice, keep the basic principles in mind.

Look at the setup. Before you begin to move, clear the path. Remove any clutter, especially on the floor, even if it's an end table or a slippery throw rug. The path should be wide enough and smooth enough for everyone. Make sure there is enough light for your loved one to see. This may be more light than *you* need. If you can, try to decrease the total distance your loved one needs to travel. Position the chairs, cars, car doors, etc., so that everything is as easy to reach as possible.

If they have a strong side and a weak side, set up so they move toward their strong side; it's easier to shift weight toward the strong leg. Place pillows behind them to catch a backwards fall; you may also use pillows to cover hard edges or corners. Both you and your loved one may use natural "handrails" like countertops and doorknobs (if the door is braced) to help steady and support them. You may try to design the path so these are within reach.

Be sure to **secure all the brakes** on wheeled walkers, wheelchairs, and hospital beds, and hold the walker so it can't tip. Help them don any shoes (don't try to walk in slippery socks), braces, or anything else. Secure any lines, like IVs or oxygen hoses, to allow for travel.

Communicate:

Use simple verbal commands, gestures, modeling (giving them an example by doing what you want them to do), and tactile cues (guidance through touch) to communicate. The more your loved one knows what to do, the easier it is for them to anticipate you and help.

Be loud enough for them to hear and understand, but soft enough to support calm confidence. Consider whether they are hard of hearing on one side. When possible, communicate at eye level. Think of where they are and where they are facing. If your gestures aren't in their field of vision, then they didn't see you. The "one, two, three" count is pretty universal; most people know it's time to go on three.

A little encouragement is good, but lots of "atta-boys" and "good jobs" can get annoying. Your loved one is not a Labrador. I'm not really joking here; just ask anyone who has spent too much time in the hospital.

Use the body's handles to better communicate and help to move or lift your loved one. That therapist from Flagstaff Medical Center knew the body's handles. These are usually bony prominences such as the brim of the pelvis or the tops of the leg bones. Let's try a little exercise to help you and your care team practice with these.

Face your partner and reach out above their shoulder to the back of the shoulder. Feel the **shoulder blade**. If you allow your hand to palm against its contours and gently but firmly pull it toward you, you will find their whole body follows you. You have found the first handle. You can find it again from under the arm, this time bringing the rib cage along with you. This is another handle. Slide your hand down their **forearm** to find where it widens at the elbow. This is a handle as well, but it is not as direct as the shoulder blade.

On the pelvis and hips, find the **bony prominence on the outside of the hip**, about a palm's distance below the belt line. This is the greater trochanter of the femur (upper leg bone), and it makes an excellent handle for scooting, rolling, or lifting. Now go back to the belt line to find the **crest of the pelvis**. This is great for scooting and rolling. Now hook your palm on the **fleshy bit just behind and above the knee**. This handle works well for lifting or bending the knee.

For more support, try cradling the base of their head in your hand, allowing your forearm to support the spine. Your other hand can spread across the top of the chest to the shoulder. **Cradling** like this allows a very supportive way to roll someone forward and back. When you are helping someone roll or move, think of them as a tree or log, so that the pelvis moves in sync with the shoulders, avoiding putting excessive twisting in the spine. Practice finding the comfortable places on these handles. Practice moving your partner around with them. We created a short video to help you practice this and to show you more about the body's handles. Patient Transfers like a Pro: The Body's Handles https://youtu.be/VXey98ydF6o

Remember that you can **use your whole body to help**, not just your hands. Your knees can meet their knees. Your feet can help secure or guide their feet. If you are behind them, your thigh can become a bench or your hip a wall. Consider positioning yourself so you can fill any holes in their environment. If you are against the edge of the bed, you become a bed rail. If they might fall backward, you might be behind them to catch them; this is especially an option with two caregivers. Don't be afraid to kneel to be a support or handrail for them.

Try not to tower over the person or put them in a compromised position. You should not need to manhandle them. We try to keep the patient in as natural a position as possible. If it all feels easy, you are probably doing it right.

Move Safely

As you practice both as the patient and the caregiver, try to **feel in balance with your partner**. If you know how to partner dance, consider what it feels like to lead. That is essentially what you are doing here. You may use the same skills to help weight shifting so they may step. You may use a partner-dance approach in your contact with them: firm enough to communicate, without being tense. Allow your weight to counterbalance theirs.

Allow your back to be in a neutral position. I've used this term before. It is generally the natural curve in your back that you have when you stand or sit upright. This is the form that weight lifters use because it is the strongest and safest position for the spine. Bend at your hips and knees. You might feel most stable with your feet shoulder-width apart or a bit wider and maybe staggered, with one in front of the other. Generally it works best to have the foot you are turning toward in the back. This keeps you from getting your feet tied up as you pivot. For more on this, see our video link Neutral Spine: Back Safety in Patient Transfers https://youtu.be/05Wfb7llZl8.

Our Videos

Consider again the **special needs and strengths of the one you are caring for**. Do you need to modify the basic transfers to make them useful? Karen had a very fragile spine, but she had been a gymnast, a figure skater, and a mountain climber. She knew how to challenge her body safely and was usually aware of her limits. She had strong arms and, most of the time, good balance. She was patient with herself and with us and could communicate what she needed and usually follow directions. We could not use a gait belt, but her back brace also gave us a handle, so we didn't need the gait belt. There was pressure on her spinal cord, so her leg might suddenly weaken or have spasms. Usually how she moved gave us some warnings before this happened.

Below are some short training videos that we produced to help train our caregiving team. Please take a moment with them. Appreciate the standard techniques and what we did that was unique to Karen. You may notice how we were especially careful about positioning and protecting her back. You may also notice how we used the bathroom door, first as a handle and then as a wall to protect against a forward fall, as well as to give her privacy.

You may notice how, even though she was quite sick, she could do a great deal for herself. This was brought home to us when, a week before she died, she took us to one of her favorite places, the Chihuly Museum of Glass. It was wonderful for all of us. Your patience, skill, and confidence can open a lot more than the bathroom door. It can hold open the door to the world so you all may continue to embrace life together.

You can also produce your own videos that are specific to you, your loved one, and your home. It's not difficult, it's fun to do, and it will end up being very helpful for others on your care team. For more on this, see Producing and Publishing Training Videos in Chapter 1, Building a Caregiving Team.

    Karen's Training Video 1 of 6 Back Brace https://youtu.be/1Fv2RIRVHIQ
    Karen's training video 2 of 6 Contact Guard Assist https://youtu.be/PCDbXj5DgEk
    Karen's training video 3 of 6 Wheelchair https://youtu.be/Q6vpPg98gp8
    Karen's training video 5 of 6 Snuggle https://youtu.be/L8EfoaOqMYg
    Karen's training video 6 of 6 Transfers https://youtu.be/v1tc1nZf01A
    Karen Bathroom Transfer https://www.youtube.com/watch?v=gaSTuy8qyU0&t=93s

...Total Assist

There may come a time when the person you're caring for can help very little (less than 25 percent) and needs help with basic mobility such as rolling in bed. You are now beginning **total assistance,** where some of the techniques change but the basic principles remain.

Why They Need to Move

Have you ever seen fast-motion video of people sleeping? They kind of dance around, they move so much while asleep. When someone is very sick and cannot move so well, you need to perform this dance for them. If they have been lying on any part of their body for a while, blood either pools there or is squished out. Either way, their circulation is compromised. Movement is life, and they need to move to keep the blood flowing and the tissue, especially the skin over the bony bits, alive and healthy. Did you ever sit through *Gone With the Wind*? Did your butt get sore? Even if your loved one doesn't seem to want to move, they need to move about every two to three hours.

Positioning for Comfort

So they need to move, but where to? What positions are best, and how do we get them there? **Most comfortable positions are near "neutral" for each joint.** Imagine relaxing in warm water, floating tummy down, your arms and legs hanging loosely in front of you. Your knees and elbows will be slightly bent, your legs slightly bent and a little apart. Your spine will maintain its natural curves, a little in at the neck, out at the ribs, and in again in the low back. This is all near "neutral."

    Now turn that position over into a **"race car seat" or "beach chair" position.** It's still near neutral. Now imagine where the pillows go to support this. You're probably thinking, "under the knees, perhaps a little between, under the seat to form the bucket seat and keep them from sliding down, a small pillow to support the low back and prevent slouch. Perhaps the knee pillow should also take the pressure off the heels." Don't forget that the sheets shouldn't pull the feet hard into the down position. They might get stiff that way, making it very hard for them to stand up again. You might even support the arms and elbows and the crook of the neck. This probably sounds a lot like an easy chair—that's probably why easy chairs are so easy.

To help your loved one be **more upright in bed**, you may use a firm cushion behind them, still making the shape of the curves of the spine. This will be easier than trying to get them scooted back farther to lean against the headboard, as you or I might do. You also might consider having a hospital bed brought in. It can raise and lower, taking the place of the pillows to prop them up or elevate the knees.

OK, so you've done all that work to get them positioned just perfectly, but now it's been three hours: time to move them again. Even the best position isn't good all day.

Now think of that same body position, only with them **lying down on their side.** Now where do the pillows go? You're right: between the knees, under the head and neck, but not the down-facing shoulder, maybe under the upper shoulder and arm. You may need to make the knee pillow keep the ankle bones from resting on each other. If they have hip pain, you may pad above and below the sore bony point of the hip, or simply don't rest them on that side. You may consider supporting them from in front or behind with pillows. A squished pillow behind them allows them to lie a little toward the back without just rolling back onto their back. A pillow in front allows them to lie more toward the tummy, in what we call **three-quarter prone.**

Proning, or lying on the stomach, is hard to do if their neck doesn't turn well or their shoulders won't allow their arms to come up and out enough. This said, it is an excellent position for stretching and straightening out the hips and knees and getting off the backside for a while. It also is good for letting the back aspect of the lungs drain and giving the gut a different position, helping it move. Usually people don't stay prone for long, perhaps 20 minutes. It really helped with Karen's breathing and blood pooling on the back side of her body. If they cannot tolerate proning, three-quarter proning with the lower leg straight works pretty well. We give you a how to for rolling and proning next.

...Maximum Assist Bed Mobility

How can you help them move when they can hardly help and/or are very fragile? There are, of course, a few tricks, but all the same principles still apply. The main difference is that now you may need to do more of the moving for them. Still, set it all up for success before you start. Communicate, even if you think they don't hear you or won't understand. Allow them to do as much for themselves as possible. Use the body's handles, and use your back-neutral biomechanics to help them move easily and to keep yourself strong and healthy as you help them. Consider their special strengths and needs.

Scooting Them Up, Down, or Sideways Using a Draw Sheet

The **draw sheet** is simply another sheet laid out on top of the bed's bottom sheet—but the draw sheet is not tucked in. You can set it up when you make up the bed. It has many uses, from helping your loved one to move, to changing the bed with them in it. Using the draw sheet is the easiest of all the bed mobility techniques, as you simply clear the area enough to move the person and pull the draw sheet they are resting on. You are basically sliding the "ground" underneath them and they move with it.

Use two hands, one near each corner of the draw sheet, as wide apart as you can to get a comfortable straight pull. If you're moving them up, pull on the top two corners; if you're pulling them down, use the bottom two corners; if you're moving them from one side of the bed to another, pull on two side corners. You can easily slide them up, down, or sideways in bed with a draw sheet. If you have a hospital bed you might flatten the bed so you are not trying to scoot them uphill. Be sure to straighten the wrinkles out of the sheet when you're done.

Sitting Up Straight Using the Draw Sheet

To sit straight up in bed, they will probably not be able to do a sit-up. You may help them from in front of them using the draw sheet, pulling it up and forward to lift and cradle their upper body. It might work best to pull from their low chest level. It's probably not so good to lift them from the shoulder from behind, as this places a lot of flexion torque on the trunk, squishing them into a slump. You can use the sheet to temporarily support their trunk as they sit. You may then build a false backrest out of firm cushions as described in Positioning for Comfort earlier in this chapter. Again, have everything in arm's reach before you lift, and have them help as much as they can.

Rolling Them onto Their Side

Let's consider helping the one you're caring for to roll to the right. Do they have, and will you have, enough room? Remove the dishes and magazines and such, clearing the area of anything that will be in the way of where they will be going or where you need to be. You may need to use the draw sheet to scoot them away from the direction of the roll so they don't roll right out of bed. They should be lying pretty flat on their back before you roll them and have a flat, smooth area of the bed to roll onto. Adjust the pillows to be close to the position they will be in at the end of the roll.

To roll them to the right, bend their left knee or both knees up. Bring their right arm into the position they will want to lie on it, usually out about 70 degrees. Ask them to reach toward you with their left hand; you may want to give them a target, like your hand, to reach toward. As they reach, have them push with their left foot. You can assist at the pelvis and at the left shoulder blade, either from above or below the arm. Presto, they are now lying on their side.

Going from Supine to Sitting at the Edge of the Bed

To move them from *supine* (on their back) to sitting at the edge of the bed, begin with rolling them onto their side (see the section above). They may position their down-facing elbow against the bed in front of them and the up-side hand also on the bed, usually close to the elbow. Sliding their feet over the edge of the bed allows them to use the weight of their legs as a counterbalance for their torso. It may help to have them cross their legs at the ankles for this. As their legs slide off the bed into your hand, they push with their hands, propping themselves up. You may also help this movement with your arm supporting their head and your forearm and hand helping to lift their torso as they come up. Be patient and communicate well so they may do as much as they can to help. This video from UNMC gives a pretty good demonstration and discussion. https://www.youtube.com/watch?v=eR8H_JvrQXM

Going from Sitting at the Edge of the Bed to Transferring to a Wheelchair or Commode

If someone does not have enough leg strength to stand up, even with your assistance, you may still transfer them using a squat pivot technique. This works very much the same as the stand pivot, only they do not stand up fully. We kind of just lift their bottom and swing them over. How much they can help will determine a lot of your technique. You may need to clear the path for the swing by removing any armrests. It helps to have the surface you are moving to level or a little lower than where they are moving from. This is usually done quickly so it might help to have their hands on you to keep them out of their own way. I like to use a pillow to pad their knees as I cradle them in mine. Scooting with a draw sheet, rolling to the side, sitting up, and the dependent "squat pivot" transfer are all demonstrated in our video Patient Transfers Like a Pro using the Body's Handles https://youtu.be/VXey98ydF6o Farmington Valley also has a good demonstration of this independent Stand Pivot Transfer. http://www.youtube.com/watch?v=fXXXUnpM-Ss

Changing the Sheets with the Person Still in the Bed

If you can help them roll onto their side in bed then you can bring a sheet under them without their having to get up. Begin by rolling them to the side. Lay the bedding out with the first third to half that is toward you laid out as if it was under them already. Accordion-fold or roll the rest up, leaving the top edge exposed. Tuck this under them tightly along the length of their body where their body meets the bed. Now roll them to their other side, over the rolled-up sheet. You may now pull the part of the sheet that you accordioned or rolled up out from under them. We use a similar technique for giving a bed bath in Chapter 16 Hygiene. You will find a good video there as well.

Using a Mechanical Lift

If your loved one needs a mechanical lift (Hoyer Lift) you should definitely receive training from the rehab team and probably from any vendor supplying the lift, so I won't give you instructions here. There are some tips that can help.

- Make sure you have plenty of room to roll the lift around. Try moving the lift through the area you will need before you lift your loved one to make sure.
- You can approach bringing the sling under them from the top down, having them sit up, or from the side in, having them roll much like changing the bed with the patient still in it (above section).
- If they will be using a commode or bathing you cannot use the draw sheet to sit them up and may need to remove the sling once they are in their new place. If the head of the bed elevates this helps tremendously with sitting them up.
- Double check all your attachments and bring the feet of the lift into the wide position before you make the lift. Everyone makes errors. It's easy to double check.

Rolling to Prone

To move them to prone, begin with rolling them to lying on their side (see the section above). Remember that you will need more room to roll them at the start, so you might want to slide them over farther before you begin the roll. Once they are in side-lying position, they may position the down-facing arm either tucked deeply downward and tight against the body or up all the way so their forearm is under their head and the pillow. Bring the pillow back to about their ear so that when the roll is completed, their face will be free from the pillow but their head will still be supported and their neck not turned so sharply. Straighten the down-facing leg and continue having them reach out with the up-facing arm. They will then roll toward their tummy.

Once they are completely on their tummy, their down-facing arm is free to come out from below their torso or out from under their head. For three-quarter prone, both arms may stay in front of them. They might like a pillow under the ankles, slightly bending the knees and letting the feet hang without being pressed into pointing down.

We used this as an opportunity to give a little back rub. It surely made the effort worth it for Karen.

Chapter 16.
Hygiene, Bathing, and Toileting

Helping someone bathe or go to the toilet is intimate, loving, and, well, technically challenging as far as mobility and caregiving go. Intimacy is two ways. As your loved one needs help, reach into your heart to be as gentle and loving with each other as can be. As we begin to explore this topic, you may want to recall Dignity: Practical Considerations, Respect, and Exercise Your Compassion in the Introduction: Advanced Basics. See how you can apply those lessons now. Each person, and each situation, is different. The skills you use here bring together many of the mobility skills discussed thus far in Chapter 15, Basic Mobility and Transfers: setup, transfer, adaptive equipment, and peri-care. Oh, we haven't discussed peri-care yet. We will here, toward the end of this chapter.

Bathing

Karen loved to take a tub bath. Typically, we physical therapists consider that most people with difficult mobility will use a shower chair or bench and handheld shower. For Karen and me, she was small enough and I was strong enough to cradle her in a towel and gently help lower her into the tub. In this way I could help her in and out of a lovely warm bubble bath. Again, every situation is different.

...Adaptive Equipment

Consider what your loved one will need. Can they stand? How much support do they need? Can they stand with one hand free? Two? Can they lift each foot high enough to clear the shower or tub threshold? Can they bend to reach all body parts? Can they sit without support?

Now consider the space you have. If they need a wheelchair, can you get it into the bathroom close enough to the shower chair? Take a look again at Mobility Aids and Adaptive Equipment in Chapter 15, Basic Mobility and Transfers. Here are suggested aids for various levels of ability and need for support:

- **If they are not so sure of foot:** grab bars and nonslip strips in and near shower
- **If they don't stand well:** shower bench or chair; handheld showerhead; shower door removed and replaced with shower curtain
- **If they can't walk to the shower:** wheelchair or 4 wheeled walker that will fit close enough to the shower bench so they may do the type of transfer they can do—stand-pivot, step-pivot, scoot, slide ...
- **If they can't reach all body parts:** long-handled scrubby; basket or other secure place within reach to keep soap and bath products
- **If they use primarily one hand:** pump tops on bath products

...Setting Up and Gathering Supplies

Towels: you need one for your loved one and probably one for the shower and bench. You will also need any **dressing materials for wound care** if you are changing dressings. **Bath products:** skin-care products, lotions, and potions. **Clothes** for after the bath. And, of course, **gloves for yourself.** I like the large, long kitchen utility gloves for this job. I also like to have a **warm rice bag** or other microwavable hot pack nearby for after the shower. If they get cold, this feels great. Wrap it in a towel: you can't wash it. Rubber ducky? Got it—OK, we're ready.

...The Sequence

Some people can wear a robe and nonslip slippers to get to the bathroom, but some might want to stay dressed and keep shoes or nonslip socks on until they are securely in the bath. This means they will be getting in and out of the shower or tub dressed. So the sequence would look something like this:

1. **Prepare:** Set up the bathroom, assemble what you need, etc.
2. **Transport:** Help them get to the bathroom.
3. **Transfer:** If they are in a wheelchair or wheeled walker, help them transfer to the shower chair.
4. **Undress.**
5. **Bathe.**
6. **Pat dry.**
7. **Apply lotions and potions.**
8. **Change dressings,** etc.
9. **Get dressed.**
10. **Transfer.**
11. **Transport.**
12. **Celebrate.**

Oh, I almost forgot: if they are going to get dressed sitting on the shower bench, the lovely game of picking clothes is now part of the "prepare" step before getting to the shower. Try to plan out the sequence you will need before you start.

...A Few Tips

Here's a few more tips: **Check the water temperature** on yourself first. The back of your hand or wrist is a nice sensitive area. Don't check the water temperature on an area on them that has poor sensation, such as their involved side after a stroke.

If you are using a shower chair and a shower curtain with a liner curtain, you can help **keep water from getting all over the bathroom and yourself.** Simply cut two vertical slits in the liner curtain in line with the edges of the shower chair. Then, if you tuck the middle section into the slit in the shower chair, you can get your arms around that section of curtain to help your loved one. It protects you and the whole bathroom. It also gives your loved one just a little more privacy.

If they are going to dress in the shower, dry the chair before they put their pants on.

Here is a nice video by the Family Caregiver Alliance on bathing and dressing: https://www.youtube.com/watch?v=lvQtjY3-bcE.

If you need to **keep a wound, picc line, port, or something else on the body dry,** you can cover it with Tegaderm or Aquaguard. These medical products are effective but expensive. If adhesives are not such a problem, you can use sport tape or nylon tape to secure Saran Wrap or Glad Press n Seal over the area. If the sensitive area is on a limb, you may **cover the whole limb**. Place a large trash bag over the limb and tape the top shut, taping on the plastic, not their skin. You can then wrap another bag or more plastic wrap around the top so it acts like a shingle, and this time tape the edge onto the skin: now the limb should stay quite dry. Please follow any special care instructions for wounds or lines that you received from the doctor or on the hospital discharge instructions.

The question I asked when first approaching this subject was, **How do you wash the parts they are sitting on?** This touches on the topic of *peri-care*. The simplest answer is to have them stand up. If this is not your answer, can they lean over to one side, then the other? If this is still not an answer for you, there are commode-type shower chairs that allow access from below. Another possibility is a bidet toilet seat, if they can use a toilet. There are inexpensive ones and very interesting and quite luxurious Japanese models. Try typing "bidet toilet seat" into your search engine. The first time we traveled in Japan, giggles bubbled from the bath as each person in our party played with the buttons.

...Giving a Bed Bath and Changing the Bed with the Patient in It

Now that you can help your loved one roll in bed (see rolling them onto their side in bed and change the sheets with the person still in the bed Chapter 15 Mobility) you can give them a bath while they are still in bed. As with any time you are helping them move, get everything set to go and within reach first.

Bed Bath and Bed Changing Supplies

For the bed bath, you will probably want these:

- latex gloves; I like to double-glove if there's a mess or use long kitchen cleaning gloves
- several washcloths
- baby wipes
- bucket of warm, clean soapy water
- bucket of warm rinse water (for rinsing the patient, not the washcloths)
- dirty dump bucket or trash can with a plastic liner for dirty linens
- lotions and powders and any other skin-care or dressing-changing supplies
- fresh clothes

For changing the bed, you will probably want these:

- sheets and bedding material
- clean chuck pads (absorbent pads, usually about 3 feet square, usually with a moistureproof backing, kind of like a cross between a diaper and a sheet; they go under the patient's pelvis to catch leaks)
- a bucket or bag-lined trash bin if the bedding is soiled (you can use the dirty dump bucket we mention for the bed bath).
- An extra blanket to put over them to help them keep warm and protect their modesty while you are changing the linens

The Sequence

The Bed Bath: Begin by **cleaning all you easily can with the patient on their back**. Start with their face and eyes. For their eyes, no soap please, and wipe from in to out (near the nose to near the temple); use a clean and separate side of the washcloth for each eye. Encourage and help them do as much as they can for themselves. Gently wash their arms and torso. You can keep them covered where you are not currently bathing to help them stay modest and warm. If you're going to be using a lot of water, you might place a towel under a limb or near their trunk to keep too much water from getting in the bed. With them still on their back, you can wash their legs and around their pelvis. This is also a good time to **inspect their skin**, especially the around the pelvis, the nether regions, and the bony spots for redness or skin breakdown (see Wound or Ulcers in Chapter 18, Managing Discomforts). Consider sliding the patient toward you a little to allow room for them to roll, then **roll them onto their side** and wash their back and bottom, all those parts that you could not reach with them on their back.

Changing the Bed and finishing the bath:

1. **Roll the dirty bedding** up toward the patient's back and tuck it tight into where their body line meets the bed. If the bedding is soiled, you may want to put a towel over the soiled bedding and the patient to protect the clean sheets as you lay them out.
2. **Next, lay out the clean bedding,** with the half that is toward you just as you want it on the bed and the other half up and onto the patient. Try to keep the clean bedding as straight and wrinkle free as you can. Wrinkles in the bedding catch the cracker crumbs and other unwanted foreign material and create pressure points that may lead to skin breakdown. Consider chuck pads first, then the bottom sheet, then the draw sheet, or maybe another layer of chuck padding. It might help to start with the draw sheet a little low as patients usually slide down in bed.
3. **Now scrunch or fold like an accordion the half of the clean bedding** that is on top of the patient and tuck that under them next to the rolled-up dirty bedding, with the leading edge of the clean bedding on top and tucked as far as you comfortably can under the patient.
4. **Next, roll the patient onto their clean side, on top of the clean bedding.** Finish washing any areas you couldn't reach, then roll the soiled bedding out of the way and into the bucket.
5. **Now pull out the clean bedding,** perhaps rolling the patient just a little farther, smooth out all the wrinkles, and **finish making that half of the bed.**
6. **Finish positioning them with the draw sheet** now to help them be just where they want and as comfortable as can be (see Positioning for Comfort in Chapter 15, Basic Mobility and Transfers). Apply any lotions and dressings and, if appropriate, help them dress.

Here is a lovely video out of Singapore that gives a nice demonstration. In this, the caregiver also helps with dressing, oral care, and grooming: https://www.youtube.com/watch?v=P0N5KXDT_iE .

Oral Care

By Sue Vetter DDS

Dental disease has a great impact on the general health of patients. Poor oral hygiene and dental disease may be more prevalent in patients with chronic illness or disabilities due to the effects of their condition and medication on the oral environment. Problems of the teeth and mouth affect patients' ability to eat and communicate. This section provides caregivers with information and knowledge to prevent oral disease such as gum disease or tooth decay and to treat and maintain good oral care for loved ones with special needs.

It is important to establish a relationship with a dentist prior to the start of any cancer treatment or before the patient becomes immunocompromised. This will help your loved one maintain regular dental visits during the course of medical treatment as well as having an established dental provider to go to in case of a dental emergency.

...Assess Their Ability for Oral Self-Care

First, determine if your loved one has the ability to provide dental self-care. Can they brush and floss on their own? Do they require partial or total oral care by a caregiver? Make an assessment to see if your loved one has the adequate range of motion and grip strength to perform daily oral home care. Observe them and make any modifications necessary to enable them, and you as the caregiver, to be successful.

Range of Motion

If your loved one can't reach their mouth, you may be able to extend the toothbrush or floss holder by attaching it to a wooden stick or ruler. If they can't fully bend or extend their wrist or elbow, try using a toothbrush that has a compact or smaller brush head as well as toothbrushes that have bristles surrounding the surfaces of the teeth, such as the Surround toothbrush www.specializedcare.com or the Dent Trust three-sided toothbrush www.kleenteeth.com.

Grip Strength

If your loved one has **weakened grip strength or difficulty holding a narrow toothbrush handle**, modifying the size of the handle will make it easier to hold. The brush handle can be bulked up with a foam toothbrush holder, or you can wrap a washcloth around the handle or stick the base of the toothbrush into an easy-to-grip ball. Power toothbrushes also have a bulkier base and are easier to hold.

...Daily Oral Care Routine

The bathroom is not the only place that daily home oral care can be performed. A sink is not necessary if your loved one can spit into a bowl or cup. They can recline in a chair, couch, or bed or can sit in a wheelchair or on the floor. Use pillows or props to brace or stabilize their head. Position yourself to have the most optimal visibility into their mouth. Make sure to protect their airway to avoid their aspirating water or toothpaste.

Use a regular **toothbrush** with soft or extrasoft rounded nylon bristles or a power toothbrush like Sonicare, Oral B, or Spin Brush. Replace the toothbrush every three months. **Toothpaste** is not necessary, but if it is used, a small pea-sized amount of toothpaste with fluoride is sufficient. If your loved one has difficulty spitting, use a nonfoaming toothpaste or none at all. Here's the sequence:

1. **Brush the front, back, and top of each tooth.** Gently brush back and forth and in a circular motion.
2. **Gently brush the tongue** after you brush the teeth.
3. **Help the person rinse with plain water.** If they can't rinse, give them a drink of water or consider sweeping the mouth with a finger wrapped in gauze or thin washcloth or one of the sponge-on-a-stick devices (you may ask your nurse about these).

Flossing removes plaque and debris between the teeth where a toothbrush can't reach. **String floss** comes waxed or unwaxed, and either one will work. Here's the sequence:

1. **Use a string of floss about 18 inches long.** Wrap that piece around the middle finger of each hand, leaving a couple of inches in between to floss with.
2. **Hold the floss between the thumb and index finger** of each hand.
3. **Pass the floss through the contact points between the teeth,** curving or wrapping the floss in a "C" shape around each tooth and flossing down below the gum line; make sure not to force the floss, which can injure the gums. Floss gently up and down between the teeth one side at a time on both sides of every tooth.

Floss picks or floss holders are an option that allow you to floss with one hand, but they are not as effective as string floss due to more-limited control of the floss. **Oral irrigators** such as Water Pik or Air Floss are helpful when manual flossing is not an option. The oral irrigators use pulsating or a stream of water to rinse food particles and plaque from in between the teeth.

Fluoride- and xylitol-containing gels or rinses can be beneficial to decrease the patient's risk for tooth decay. Use daily after brushing and flossing.

...Dentures or Partial Dentures

If your loved one wears dentures or partial dentures, remove and clean them after every meal. Use a soft toothbrush or thin washcloth or gauze to wipe the soft tissues and bony ridges in your loved one's mouth. Wipe gently with a massaging motion to stimulate circulation. Remove dentures at night during sleeping hours and soak them overnight in a denture solution. Also disinfect them once or twice a week.

...Oral Complications with Cancer Treatment or Other Drug Interactions

Problems such as dry mouth (*xerostomia*), dry lips, painful tissue inflammation and ulceration (*mucositis*), oral fungal infection (*candidiasis*), oral viral infection, oral bacterial infection, or canker sores (apthous ulcers) are common. Check with your loved one to see if there are any areas of concern. Perform a visual check during your daily home oral-care routine to see if there are any dental or soft-tissue concerns such as loose or broken teeth or restorations, mouth sores, redness and moderate to heavy bleeding, or white coating of the tissues.

Managing Oral Complications

Besides the specific suggestions that follow, avoid dry, spicy, or acidic foods.

Dry mouth: Encourage them to consume freshwater by sucking on ice cubes or ice chips, saliva stimulators like xylitol or sugar-free lozenges www.oracoat.com, or saliva-substitute products www.biotene.com.

Dry lips: Have them use lip balm or lubricant.

Pain: Try using systemic over-the-counter or prescription pain medications, topical lidocaine, and/or soothing oral rinses.

Mouth Rinses

Saline mouth rinse: A saltwater mouth rinse throughout the day can be used to clean the mouth and remove food debris. Use 1 teaspoon of salt to 2 cups of freshwater. Make sure to follow a saltwater rinse with a plain freshwater rinse.

Milk of magnesia (Maalox) and diphenhydramine (Benadryl) rinse: Mix these over-the-counter meds in equal amounts and have them rinse with 1–2 teaspoons of the mix every 2 hours, especially before meals, and then expectorate. Refrigerate the unused mix.

Lidocaine HCL (Xylocaine) viscous solution 2%: This local anesthetic solution requires a prescription. Follow the instructions as prescribed.

Treating Oral Infections

Prescriptions for bacterial, fungal, or viral infections also must be made by their dentist or physician:

Bacterial: Antibiotics can be prescribed for oral bacterial infections.

Fungal: Antifungal rinses such as Nystatin can be prescribed for oral fungal infections.

Viral: Acyclovir ointments or tablets can be prescribed for oral viral infections.

Contact your loved one's dentist if there are issues beyond your scope of care. It is important to know when professional dental help is needed.

Toileting

If someone needs help with standing and walking, they will most likely need help in the bathroom as well. This is where caregivers begin to get squeamish, but in most cases, all you will be doing is walking them to the bathroom, helping them get ready to sit down, and leaving them alone. You may preserve their dignity while protecting them from a fall by creating a safer independent environment and giving them as much privacy as possible.

Consider ways you might create a temporary barrier that can **keep them from falling off the toilet.** Our bathroom was configured so the door swung in front of the toilet. By blocking it with a foot and or hand to keep it from moving, the caregiver could be on the other side of it, out of sight. Once Karen was settled, we could shut the door and stand outside listening for when she might be ready to get up again.

If your loved one needs **help wiping up**, cleanup can be performed with them standing. Sometimes its easiest for everyone for you to help steady them while they wipe up themselves. If they need **help getting their clothes back in order**, this can also be done with them standing, or you can close the toilet lid and have them sit down again. Sometimes Karen needed some help with her pants. Instead of trying to pull them up for her, we steadied her so she could pull them up and fasten them herself. Even though she usually used a wheelchair at that point, I kept a walker in the bathroom that could be placed in front of her so she could use its handles for support. We also could place it over the toilet for grab handles on either side. When we needed to remove the bathroom door for a wider opening to accommodate a wheelchair, we could position the chair in front of the toilet, also to act as a wall to prevent her falling.

Transfers in toileting work the same as the minimal assist, stand-pivot, and sit-to-stand transfers and other transfers in Chapter 15, Basic Mobility and Transfers.

Every situation is different. Your bathroom may be bigger or smaller and configured differently than ours. You may have grab bars already. You may have a raised toilet seat to make getting up easier. If you have questions or helping them use the bathroom does not seem so easy, a home safety evaluation may be prescribed by your love one's attending doctor or as part of hospice. They may help you with **bathroom aids** (see Chapter 15) and also with technique training specific to your needs.

Keep **supplies**—gloves, hand sanitizer, hand soap, hand lotion—within arm's reach in the bathroom. If you are going to be helping them with anything more than sitting and standing you will want gloves. You may also keep a few pairs of those thick household cleaning gloves handy too.

...Bedside Commode

For times when the bathroom is just too far away, you may keep a **bedside commode** in your loved one's room. The commode (see Bathroom Aids in Chapter 15, Basic Mobility and Transfers) looks like an overgrown walker with a toilet seat and a bucket beneath, but somehow it can be inconspicuous in the corner of the room and pulled out if needed.

Keeping about 1–2 inches of water in the bucket makes it function more like a regular toilet and makes **cleaning it out** *much* easier. This is one place where the thick household cleaning gloves are handy. Most commodes come with a lid that can be placed tightly over the bucket. Generally this lid stays off when the bucket is clean, but it is good to have a little later when you are transporting the bucket. Oh, yes, bring the bucket low and close to the toilet when you empty it—no splashing, please. Once it's empty, you can use the laundry sink or bath faucet to rinse and then wash the bucket with soapy water, then 10 percent bleach water.

...Urinal

A **urinal bottle** is usually a wide-mouth plastic bottle with the top bent toward the front a bit. Men might use this to urinate without getting up to the toilet. It is somewhat intuitive to use for most men. Raising the head of the bed about 45–60 degrees and having them open their legs a bit helps. Sometimes they might need help to get into position. If this is the case, you will want gloves and probably a warm wet washcloth or baby wipe for any cleanup needed afterward. Use a towel or dry washcloth to dry the area after cleanup. Often you can just give them the washcloths and wipes.
Clean the urinal as for the bedside commode, above.

There are urinals of various designs for women. These aren't yet common and there is no standard design or method yet. Typing "female bed urinal" into your browser will give you images, discussion, and instructions. For women, remember to wipe from front to back.

...Bedpan

A bedpan is useful when a person just cannot get out of bed to the toilet. When you help them use the bedpan, they can either lift their hips or turn (or you can roll them) onto one side, then slide the bedpan under their buttock, have them turn back onto their back, then adjust their hips and thighs so **the person is centered on the bedpan**. Elevate the head of the bed so the person is in as much of a sitting position as possible, which makes it easier to use the bedpan. Allow privacy and plenty of time—often it takes people longer to go on a bedpan, especially if they are not used to it.

When the person is done, lower the head of the bed and hold the bedpan straight while they lift their hips or turn onto their side so you can **remove it without spills**. You can hold it with one hand while you help them move their hips to the side with your other hand.

If they had a bowel movement, you may want to wear a double pair of gloves so that if your gloves get soiled, you can remove the top pair and your hands are still protected by the pair underneath. If they need assistance to wipe, be sure to wipe from front to back in order to prevent infections. If there is a lot to clean up, you may need to come back to do that after you empty the full bedpan. Empty and **clean the bedpan** as for the bedside commode, above.

A couple more tips: If it's a metal bedpan, running warm water over it before use will help with the cold shock for the person using it. A little baby powder on the rim will help it slide under better too. Here is a simple video https://www.youtube.com/watch?v=ld5ivhqkgSw.

Incontinence and Peri-care

Let's start this section by saying that those flimsy blue-backed disposable chuck pads that hospice brought over were psychological protection only. If a real accident happened, they just wouldn't hold. The plastic-lined fabric ones do actually work.

This is a messy topic that, for ample reasons, scares many caregivers. We had an agreement with our team of friends that if Karen became routinely incontinent, we would have full-time CNA help. This understanding put everyone at ease, but when accidents did happen, people took it in stride, heroed up, and, without being asked, performed excellent nursing care.

...Cleanup

Get things clean and dry immediately. This is not only much nicer for everybody, it helps prevent skin breakdown and infections where no one wants to have one. **Glove up.** I preferred to double-glove in case one tore. My nurse friends kind of laughed at me a bit for this. For big messes, though, we all used the big latex cleaning gloves as they are much more durable and go up the arm a ways. If you suspect splashing might occur, a pair of glasses is also recommended.

...Cleanup Supplies

Get all your materials in place before you begin. For a small mess, your cleaning supplies may be only some baby wipes and the bag-protected waste bucket. For anything larger, you may need:

- several washcloths
- baby wipes and/or toilet paper
- a bucket of clean soapy water
- a bucket of rinse water for rinsing the patient, not the washcloths
- a dump bucket for used washcloths and dirty clothes and bedding
- clean bedding, with new chuck pads and a draw sheet
- lotions and powders
- fresh briefs if your loved one uses them
- fresh clothes
- I like a little air freshener too.

I also like to have a warm rice bag hot pack to help them stay warm or to warm up again fast after the cleanup. Wrap the rice bag in a towel because you cannot wash it. If this looks a lot like the list for the bed bath it is because it is nearly the same list.

...The Sequence

For cleaning someone in bed, we use the same technique as the bed bath earlier in this chapter.

Begin by **cleaning all you can easily with the patient still on their back.** Helping them lift and spread their legs a little will make things easier to reach. Don't be afraid to do a little spelunking to clean all foreign material from any nooks or crevices. Washcloths work fine here, but once dirty they are done. Don't rinse and reuse as that spreads germs around. Baby wipes (don't flush these) or toilet paper are good here and they are disposable. Wipe front to back to avoid bringing bacteria forward, which can cause a urinary tract or other infection. Work from the middle outward toward each side. You can use the washcloth after the wipes for better cleaning. Make sure that any place where the skin folds is clean and dry.

Protect any area that gets wet with a barrier lotion. You can ask your loved one's pharmacist for recommendations. Nurse Julia prefers types with zinc oxide. This is also a good time to inspect their skin, especially around the pelvis, the nether regions, and the bony spots, for redness or skin breakdown.

Roll your loved one onto their side and clean up as you need to. Again, wipe from front to back and from their middle outward. You can use washcloths for large areas and baby wipes for small messy spots. Roll the dirty bedding up toward your loved one's body and tuck it tight into where their body line meets the bed.

Put a towel over this and your loved one to protect the clean sheets as you lay them out. Now **lay out the clean bedding** with the half that is toward you just as you want it on the bed and the other half up and over the clean towel you just laid out. Try to keep the fresh bedding as straight and wrinkle-free as you can.

Now **scrunch or fold like an accordion that half of the clean bedding on the towel and patient**, and tuck that under them next to the rolled dirty bedding. Try to end up with the leading edge of the bedding on top and tucked under as far as you can comfortably so you can pull it out when you roll them back.

Then **roll your loved one to their clean side,** on top of the clean bedding. Finish cleanup and roll the soiled bedding out of the way and into the bucket. Now, perhaps rolling your loved one just a little farther, pull out the clean bedding, smooth all the wrinkles out, and finish making that half of the bed. If you are using briefs, you can wrap the upper leg in now.

You can **finish positioning with the draw sheet** to help them be just where they want and as comfortable as can be (see Positioning for Comfort in Chapter 15, Basic Mobility and Transfers). As you roll them back onto their back or even a little farther, you may pull the rest of the brief together and attach it around the other leg. There, that wasn't so hard, was it. This video shows in great detail a good sequence for cleaning the peri area and pericare. https://www.youtube.com/watch?v=Qp78x7NxUho

If the person is seated, you will need to stand them up (see Toileting earlier in this chapter). Otherwise, cleanup is the same as describe above. If they need more than a minimal assist to stay standing long enough for you to clean them up, this may be a two-person job. If you don't have someone else to help you, you may need to transfer the person onto chuck pads on the bed.

Managing Incontinence

If you can help your loved one be as regular as possible, you might have more of a **rhythm for toileting** or peri-care. The body forms habits. Often, bowel movements are linked to habitual actions. I wake up, get up, have breakfast with coffee, and go to the bathroom. If you can help them toilet in the same step in their rhythm of the day, it might help minimize accidents. If they take some type of bowel stimulant like senna at the same time every day, chances are that they will begin to have their bowel movement at the same time too. All this allows you to plan ahead to get them to the toilet in time. Look into Eating to Avoid Constipation and Eating After Having Diarrhea in Chapter 12, Food and Nutrition, and Constipation and Diarrhea in Chapter 18, Managing Discomforts, for excellent information about helping treat someone with constipation or diarrhea and keeping them regular.

Take them to the toilet frequently to help them keep their bladder empty and their bowels moving. This will help them decrease accidents. This is true even if they are using a bedpan or bottle-type urinal. Getting them up and moving, even if it's just the act of toileting, may help stimulate the bowel and help them go. For a good how-to, see Toileting earlier in this chapter.

For many people, an accident is more embarrassing and personal for them than it is for you, the caregiver. Toileting is a fact of life, but for most of our lives it is a very private fact. Try to **keep this in mind if any accidents do occur.** It's OK to be squeamish or a little embarrassed; it's natural. Keep it honest and respectful, while you keep them clean and dry. And don't forget to check their skin for redness or breakdown.

You can help minimize accident mess by having them use **incontinence products** such as briefs, adult diapers (Depends), or underwear pads. For small amounts of urinary leakage, a maxipad might do. If they don't move around much, these products can be worn loosely just to catch and contain anything but still allow ventilation. You can keep a **protective pad** (chuck pad) over their seat cushion in their chair, but just be careful about folds and wrinkles, as they create pressure spots.

In the bed, keep the chuck pads under their middle region. I like to have two pads overlapping like a shingle, with the head-end one on the bottom. If the mattress isn't waterproof, we do this both under the bottom sheet and under the patient. Under the patient, it can also serve as your draw sheet Again, be careful to smooth out the wrinkles. If they don't move around much, sometimes you can just wrap a chuck pad around them loosely like a swami.

There are **moisture-detecting alarms for urinary incontinence.** These save you and your loved one from frequent checking, allowing you both to get a better night's sleep. The best alarms for adults are pads that slip under the sheets and wirelessly alert the caregiver so cleanup can happen quickly. I found the best listing by typing in "moisture alarm for adult incontinence" into my browser.

Sometimes the doctor may order an indwelling **catheter**. This can help if voiding the bladder is a problem. It can also make life much easier for someone who just can't get up to use the toilet or a bedside commode. For men, a condom-style catheter works. The fit needs to be right, but they do come in different sizes. Any catheter can be a problem for the busy patient. If they fidget or move around a lot, they may pull it out or off. A catheter must be kept clean and dry and the urine bag emptied as needed. For people who get up and maybe walk a bit, a shorter tube and a leg bag might make moving around easier.

Here is a lovely video from a series by Caitlin Morgan and the Family Caregiver Alliance outlining incontinence-management strategies for the caregiver: https://www.youtube.com/watch?v=4DvYE12CM0c .

Sometimes **having a professional handle peri-care** may be more comfortable for both you and your loved one. If these words resonate with you, you might look into Chapter 2, Calling in the Pros.

Chapter 17.
Pain Management

Pain is a remarkably complex perception. It is more akin to an emotion than a sensation. In fact, emotional pain and physical pain share many of the same neural pathways. Many parts of the brain, the nervous system, and other tissues of the body are involved in and affected by the perception of pain. The neurons involved, like most neurons, act like weighted switches, requiring multiple excitatory inputs to reach their threshold for firing and carrying the signal forward, while also being affected by inhibitory inputs, bringing them further away from firing.

What inhibits pain: Many different neurons in the brain and spinal cord are inhibitory. Beta-endorphin, noradrenalin, and serotonin are all *inhibitory neurotransmitters* in key circuits involved in the perception of pain. Many of the medications we use to control pain act by mimicking these molecules. Firing inhibitory neurons is also quite effective in blocking pain. Having something else that is important to pay attention to, purposefully paying attention to other things, disassociating the sensations from the emotional weight of pain, or simply being distracted at the brain, spinal cord, or peripheral receptor (in the body) level all can inhibit pain.

What intensifies pain: On the other hand, fear, anxiety, or even the memory of something painful can key the system up, making pain more intense. This is so powerful that even imagining moving in a way that might be painful can be painful for some people. Emotional pain such as sadness, depression, frustration, and angst all add to the physical pain symphony, making pain worse.

Inflammation and pain: Several of the molecules associated with inflammation also excite neurons associated with pain. Another possible method for decreasing pain is to tone down the body's inflammation response in some way. One example of this is the common over-the-counter medicine ibuprofen. It is also called a *COX-2 inhibitor*, as it inhibits the cyclooxygenase (COX) enzyme, which results in the inhibition of the inflammatory hormones prostaglandins.

How the Body Adapts to Pain

The tissues of the body tend to adapt so they get better at doing whatever you're doing with them. If you lift weights regularly, your muscles get bigger, more efficient, and stronger. Your bones, connective tissues, blood vessels, and energy systems all adapt to the stress of weight lifting to get stronger as well. The nervous system holds some of the most adaptable tissues in the body. Every time a neuron fires, it gets a little closer to its last input, and that connection gets a little stronger. It grows new connections and stocks more receptors and more vesicles to produce the neurotransmitters.

If what you are doing is suffering from pain, those neurons, and many other tissues in the body, get very good at generating pain signals. In the spinal cord, long-term chronic pain can make the supporting cells there generate molecules that further sensitize the pain circuits. At the nerve endings, continually perceiving pain seems to cause inflammation in the surrounding tissue.

In the brain, the interaction of pain perceptions on the different centers and circuits is amazingly complex. The algorithm flow chart looks something like spaghetti. Most notable in this algorithm is that long-term suffering activates the centers in the *amygdala* (our attention-switching house) associated with anxiety. It also leans on area CG25, associated with sadness and depression, and shuts down the prefrontal cortex. Anxiety and depression only make the pain worse, and the cycle can be vicious.

Controlling Pain

However, if what you're doing is controlling pain, then the systems associated with control can also get stronger. It seems that the big difference between suppressing pain, keeping it in check, and suffering—pain that runs away with us—is a sense of control. Since the turn of the 21st century, the medical community in the United States has become more aware of this and is doing more to control pain early.

There are multiple options for pain medications, and patients are given more control of what and how much medicines they use. We are also getting better at maximizing other ways to control pain. When someone is very sick, most likely they will have pain, but they should not have suffering. You can help them in many ways to find the right combination at that given hour to keep their pain in control.

Measuring Pain

Pain is a subjective experience, but in order to help your loved one control their pain, you need to know how severe it is. We do find that we can get a somewhat reliable number rating on pain in several ways. Below are the most common ways to rate pain.

...A Pain Scale

Ask your loved one to rate their pain from 0 to 10, where 10 is screaming agony, the worst pain you can imagine, like giving birth or cutting your legs off slowly. A 5 rating would be the pain is so bad it makes you stop what you're doing; 1, you feel it; and 0, you don't notice any pain. For Karen, the number that meant we had to act to decrease pain was 4. For your loved one, it will be whatever it is. Be wary of people who calmly report 11. They may be a little too focused on their pain or be over-reporting.

...A Visual Analog Scale

Ask your loved one to make a mark on a line that is 10 centimeters long (such as the one below) indicating how bad their pain is. You can describe 0 centimeters, 5 centimeters, and 10 centimeters in the same way as the pain scale above. This visual analog scale is usually used on intake forms in the physician's office:

0cm	5cm	10cm
No Pain		Worst Pain

You then measure where their mark is in centimeters along the line. The number on your ruler is the rating.

...Pain Faces

This pain-rating tool is a sheet of paper with stick-figure faces ranging from smiling to agony. Ask your loved one which one shows how they feel. This rating system might be useful if words and numbers are difficult for your loved one to use. The original scale is known as Wong Baker Faces http://wongbakerfaces.org/

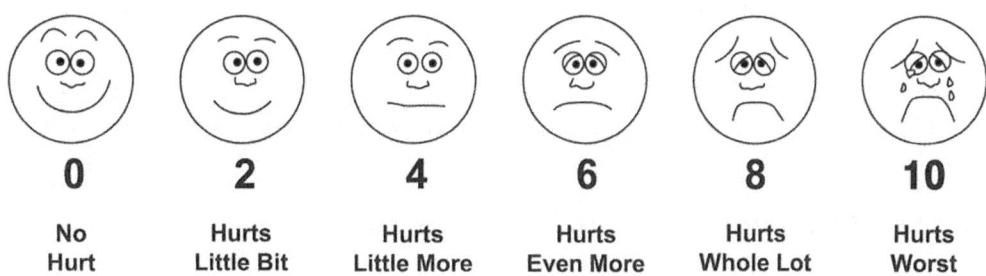

Pain Medications

The attitudes toward taking pain medications are as varied as the individuals taking them. My family has always been stupidly stoic, erring on the side of taking less medication. I remember Karen insisting that I take the pain prescriptions when we were trying to drive over the mountains while I had a tooth abscess; "sleeping Dave is better than screaming Dave," she would admonish as she handed me another pill. Others are just the opposite, reaching for the answer in pill form long before most would, and perhaps not looking into all the other nonpharmacological ways to manage pain.

The balance might be hard to find in general and harder to find minute by minute. As caregivers, we must balance our own attitudes against the attitude of our loved one. If you read the introduction to this chapter, you know that attitude is important in the perception of pain. You also know how important it is not to let your loved one suffer.

You, as caregiver, probably will not prescribe medications, but you are part of the health-care team because often you will be the one making decisions on how much and what to administer and when. Having a set pain-scale number to act on helps. Having information on what you're giving, how it works and interacts, and the signs of possible bad reactions will help too.

This section provides a brief description of the major classes of medications used to treat pain. You may also look into Drugs.com https://www.drugs.com/, which provides a drug index, side-effects listing, interaction checker, and reviews. You may also look up each medicine online or in the *Physician's Desk Reference* (PDR) and check the information sheet given to you by your loved one's pharmacist. Also, if you haven't done so already, look at Keeping a Medication Log and Using Basic Charting Techniques in Chapter 11, Medications.

...Acetaminophen

Acetaminophen (Tylenol) is the number-one over-the-counter (OTC) pain medication; it is often used for headaches, arthritic pain, and fever. We still do not know exactly how Tylenol reduces both pain and fever. This medication does not reduce inflammation and swelling.

Unfortunately, acetaminophen is the number-one cause of acute liver failure from overdose. The maximum short-term dose should not exceed 3.25 grams, and regular use should be no more than 2.5 grams daily.

It is a good choice for moderate pain and/or fever. When Tylenol is combined with short-acting narcotics as with Percocet, Ultram, and Vicodin, it can have a synergistic effect, which can reduce the dose of narcotic needed. When using it, take into account the person's age, liver function, and other medications being taken that are metabolized by the liver. Discuss long-term use with your loved one's physician and pharmacist to ensure no drug-to-drug interactions. By the way, it seems to act on emotional pain too.

...Nonsteroidal Anti-Inflammatory Drugs (NSAIDs)

Nonsteroidal anti-inflammatory drugs (NSAIDs), like aspirin, ibuprofen, and naproxen, are some of the most popular medications used worldwide for treating acute and chronic pain, inflammation, and fever. NSAIDs block cyclooxygenase (COX), an enzyme needed to form prostaglandins and other hormones involved in the inflammatory cascade. There are two forms of cyclooxygenase, called COX-1 and COX-2, which is important to know since some of these NSAIDs affect both forms (nonselective) while others, such as Celebrex, affect COX-2 only (selective). Selective and nonselective NSAIDs can further be categorized as short-acting (lasting less than 6 hours) or long-acting. NSAIDs also reduce inflammation by slowing down white blood cells' (*macrophages'*) ability to migrate to the source of injury, which reduces the release of inflammatory *granulocytes*. These medications also can help limit dilation of blood vessels, helping to control local swelling.

NSAIDs are metabolized in the liver and are transported in the blood tightly bound to serum protein, so patients with low *serum albumin* (blood protein), such as with liver disease or rheumatoid arthritis, will have higher concentrations of active medicine circulating and may require a lower dose. COX-2-specific inhibitors have a lower risk of causing gastrointestinal injury but may have a higher potential to cause a cardiovascular event or stroke. Since these block cyclooxygenase, this can cause restriction of blood flow to the kidneys. Exercising caution or avoiding use of these medications with patients who have poor kidney function is recommended. This effect on blood flow can also raise the concentration of other medications that are metabolized by the kidneys.

...Opioids (Narcotics)

B-endorphin is the most well-known pain-inhibiting *neuropeptide*. It is a very powerful inhibitory neurotransmitter that acts to suppress pain transmission in the brain and body. Deep within the brain, it also serves as one of our body's key reward or pleasure molecules. Its name literally comes from *endogenous* (the body's internal) *morphine*. The sap of the opium poppy from which morphine is derived contains a molecule that mimics B-endorphin in such a way that it can bind with and stimulate the same receptors in our bodies. The term *opioid* refers to all the synthetic and poppy-based drugs that do this. Opium, and later morphine, has been used for many centuries to treat pain and many other maladies. It and its derivatives also have one of the most infamous histories for addiction and all the troubles that come with that.

Currently, opioids like morphine sulfate, codeine, and Fentanyl, are the most commonly prescribed medication for moderate to severe pain. This medicine, traditionally used to treat cancer pain, over the past twenty years has seen a rise in treating *nociceptive* pain (pain from the damage detectors in the body) such as arthritis, orthopedic injuries, and back pain. Opioids are also used to treat *neuropathic* pain (pain from the nerves, like sciatica) if the first-line medicine is not adequate.

In addition to pain relief, opioids produce a wide range of brain and body responses, including sedation, decreased gastrointestinal (stomach and gut) activity and constipation, itching, respiratory depression, heart rate and blood pressure changes, nausea, euphoria or *dysphoria* (bad feelings or anxiety), mental clouding, delusions, and hallucinations. Wow, that's a lot. It works on three different receptors—mu, delta, and kappa; these different receptors have somewhat different effects, and different opioids may act on them differently. If one opioid medication is giving nasty side effects, another might be better. Also, the different drugs can become less effective at the different receptors by different mechanisms at different rates. This might result in someone needing more of the drug to control pain at the mu-1 receptor but still being sensitive to dysphoria and delusions at the delta receptor.

Over time, the body's endorphin receptors become less effective in the presence of the drug and most people do develop a tolerance. Dosage must be increased to gain the same effect. By January 2013, our little princess Karen was routinely taking 10 times more morphine in each dose than would probably kill me.

Abruptly stopping medicine will cause withdrawal. The nasty list of withdrawal symptoms include dysphoria, anxiety, mood swings, chills, stomach cramps, vomiting, diarrhea, elevated blood pressure, increased heart rate, sweating, restlessness, and pain. Patients should always plan ahead in acquiring refills to avoid running out, which would result in both a return of the pain and onset of withdrawal symptoms. Discontinuing opioids should be done slowly, tapering the dose by about 10 percent per week; some patients require inpatient detoxification. The medication suboxone is used to help patients with withdrawal symptoms come off narcotics. Addiction is both physical and psychological. Anticipate complete addiction recovery treatment when stopping morphine.

Because opioids decrease gut activity, one of the most common side effects is constipation. To avoid this unpleasant and potentially hazardous symptom, preventive therapy is recommended. Treatments include stool softeners, contact cathartics that stimulate the colon, and osmotic laxatives, which help maintain fluid in the stool. For more on this, please refer to Eating to Avoid Constipation in Chapter 12, Food and Nutrition, and Constipation in Chapter 18, Managing Discomforts.

Another common side effect is sedation. This often improves over time. Karen was even allowed to drive once her dose became more stable. We were all a little scared about this. If excessive sedation continues, consider a 25 percent reduction in the dose. If sedation symptoms persist, consider a different opioid. Some people require stimulants such as methylphenidate or modafinil to compensate for the sedation.

Over longer-term use, some people may also experience opioid-induced *hyperalgesia*, a condition of having increased sensitivity to painful stimuli, and *allodynia* (pain from typically nonpainful stimuli). I have seen this in several chronic-pain patients, including my brother. It was amazingly paradoxical that getting off the high doses of pain medication actually decreased his pain.

Initiation of opioid medication is done on an individual basis, taking into account the person's age, current and previous use, and other health conditions. As a general rule, we start a low dose of fast-acting medication. The medication dose can then be converted to long-acting form once a therapeutic level is achieved. Using long-acting preparations for chronic pain often reduces the amount of additional short-acting drugs needed for "breakthrough" symptoms.

Since opioids have such a high potential for addiction and abuse, patients should be evaluated for alcohol and drug abuse or any addiction problems prior to initiating therapy. It is now a Washington State law to inform patients of the risks and potential side effects of this medicine. Patients requiring regular use of this medicine are now required to sign a pain contract. This sets clear guidelines for using this medicine in an attempt to avoid people becoming addicted or overdosing. These guidelines include filling prescriptions at the same pharmacy, taking medication as prescribed, and regular office visits, including periodic drug screenings. The need to adopt such guidelines is due to the fact that from 1999 to 2007 the rate of opioid overdose more than doubled.

No medication comes without problems, and opioids are certainly no exception. It is our hope that this writing does not scare you away from these very effective drugs—only that you be more cautious and aware. Even with all the side effects and addiction problems described above, opioids will work when nothing else can. Also, they can work in combination with other drugs. They are our strongest and most direct medication for pain.

...Glucocorticoids

Glucocorticoids (steroids for inflammation) are powerful medicines for inflammation. As such, they treat the pain and tissue damage caused by excessive inflammation, along with the pressure of swelling and edema. In some cases, they can act directly to decrease overactivity of certain cells in autoimmune problems and in certain cancers. They can be applied as creams for skin rashes or injected into an inflamed area (such as an epidural injection for spinal disc extrusion), or they can be used in pill form or even intravenously to treat things like intracranial pressure caused by a brain tumor and the severe headache that comes with it.

Steroids work by mimicking the natural stress hormone *cortisol*. If you are running away from a tiger or just running for your morning exercise, this hormone helps turn down your inflammation response and does many other things to get you ready for action. Normally, exercise (physical stress) helps metabolize this hormone, returning you to normal levels. It's normally part of our healthy stress-rest cycle.

If you think of the body under stress, you get an idea of some of the side effects and risks with glucocorticoids. In the short term, they can give a mild to severe manic feeling, the "prednisone high." If taken before bed, they can disrupt sleep or cause nightmares. In more severe cases, they can contribute to or even cause memory loss, psychosis, or delirium. They affect appetite, blood lipid, and blood sugar regulation. Long-term use tends to make people gain weight and lose muscle mass. There are other side effects. For more on this, see the information sheet from your loved one's pharmacist or the fact sheet on Drugs.com: https://www.drugs.com/drug-class/glucocorticoids.html .

For most patients in a caregiving situation, the benefits far outweigh the risks. **Dexamethasone and prednisone** are the most commonly used glucocorticoids, and most meds in this class end in the letters "sone" or "rone." When taking this medication orally, don't double-dose by also using a cortisone skin cream.

...Antidepressants

Antidepressants have proven to be effective in helping manage chronic pain. Depression and anxiety lower the pain threshold, and patients may benefit from the natural analgesia of having an improved mood and outlook on life.

These medicines may work independent of mood, however. Emotional and physical pain share many of the same neurons in the brain. Pain, especially uncontrolled chronic pain, tends to make the areas of the brain associated with emotional pain, depression, and anxiety more active. Antidepressant medications support neurotransmitters associated with control of those centers. The effect on norepinephrine has the greatest impact, but also altering serotonin and dopamine helps reduce pain symptoms. One group of medicines in this class is called *serotonin norepinephrine reuptake inhibitors* (SNRIs) like Effexor.

Another class of medicines called *tricyclic antidepressants* (TCAs) may actually stimulate our endogenous opioid (b-endorphin). We think this may be the reason antidepressant medications are often effective and are protective of the brain, even in doses much less than we would use for depression. Combining these with a Selective Serotonin Reuptake Inhibitor (SSRI like Prozac) may potentiate the TCAs' effect. TCAs often can help with sleep but may take 1–3 hours to cause sedation and also can cause "hangover" symptoms. Side effects include dry mouth, orthostatic hypotension (light headedness when first getting up), constipation, urinary retention, sedation, and irregular heart rate. *Avoid* these drugs with patients with heart disease, symptoms of enlarged prostate, and narrow-angle glaucoma.

...Anticonvulsants

Certain anticonvulsants are used to treat neuropathic pain. These drugs can decrease a nerve cell's ability to fire, which in turn reduces the sensation of pain. The two most commonly used are gabapentin and pregabalin.

They are processed by the kidneys and should be used with caution if renal function is impaired. Common side effects include confusion, dizziness, sleepiness, possible weight gain, and swelling. Pregabalin has the potential of causing euphoria, and as a result, it is a controlled substance. Pregabalin is also more expensive but is very effective and easier to dose, so it should be considered a first-line option for pain.

...Osteoclast Inhibitors

Osteoclast inhibitors are medications used to treat *osteoporosis* (low bone mass). They also can be used to treat symptoms associated with metastatic bone cancer by decreasing the cancer's breakdown of the bone. The medications block the activity of *osteoclasts*, the cells that normally break down bone, and at the same time support the activity of *osteoblasts*, the cells that help form new bone. These medications reduce skeletal-related events (SREs) such as fractures, structural instability, spinal cord compression, and *hypercalcemia* (too much calcium in the blood) that result from excessive bone breakdown. They also can be used to treat bone pain.

Denosumab (Prolia): This is a *monoclonal antibody* that inhibits osteoclasts by binding to a cell surface receptor, preventing the maturation of pre-osteoclasts into mature, active osteoclasts. It is used to treat bone pain and reduce SREs. This medication does not cause renal toxicity and results in a lower rate of hypocalcemia, but is much more expensive. It can be easier to administer; dose is a 60 mg injection every six months.

Bisphosphonates, the most commonly used group of osteoclast inhibitors, are usually well tolerated; most side effects are short term, such as flu-like symptoms and eye irritation. Expect to start with a low dose and frequent monitoring if there is impaired kidney function. This medication can also lower serum calcium level, so calcium and vitamin D levels should also be monitored. Rare events of *necrosis* (tissue death) of the jawbone have been documented, so people with a history of dental decay or recent oral surgery may not be candidates. This is also true to Denosumab.

Nonpharmacological Ways to Help Control Pain

Remember from this chapter's intro the concept that neurons are weighted switches? Anything that helps decrease the activation of neurons involved in the circuits of pain will decrease pain. You might say that this is mind over matter, and, in fact, it is. Then again, it's the simple biology of this complex system. If you read the preceding section, you learned a bit about how different medications work to decrease the activation. The concepts and practices in this section use the body's own mechanisms to turn down the gain on pain-associated neurons and tissues. As you read through some of these, you might remember your own experiences and the effects you felt on your pain perception.

A Sense of Control

Many years ago, the medical community began to figure out—again—that when patients had some control of their pain medication, it seemed to work better and they seemed to take less. In the 1970s the PCA pump (patient-controlled analgesia) was developed to put a button in the hospital patient's hand. That button would deliver a small dose of intravenous pain medication. People controlled their pain better, often with less medication.

You can help maximize this effect by fostering ways that your loved one can be active in controlling their own pain. Positioning for comfort (see Chapter 15, Basic Mobility and Transfers), pain-reducing exercises or activities (see below and Chapter 13, Exercise), and safe access to their pain medication are all ways they can gain active control.

The riskiest of these is self-medication. For as long as possible, Karen could keep her own pain medication and was trusted to self-administer. We recorded what she took and made sure she did not over- or underdose. When her memory became less trustworthy, she kept only a single dose, and we would replenish it as needed. When this became difficult, she got medicine by asking, with a double-check with the med log to make sure not to over- or underdose.

Exercise for Pain Relief

Exercise is a form of stress. The body needs a certain amount of stress, and certain types of stress, as part of the natural stress-rest cycle that keeps us healthy. All movement of the body is exercise, and there are different types of movements or exercises.

For pain we usually prescribe **gentle motion exercises.** This consists of gently, rhythmically moving a joint or whole body part through part of its natural motion. It stimulates the nerves in the area, hopefully in a nonpainful way, and helps with circulation, fluid movement, and muscle tension.

One example of this that we commonly use for the hip, knee, and back is called **heel slides.** Have the person lie comfortably on their back and gently slide one heel up toward their buttock, then back down, then do the same thing with the other leg. They can continue to alternate like this for 20–30 repetitions, then rest for 2 minutes. They can repeat this two to three times. If it is painful, it is not right and should be gentler or just not done.

Cardiovascular exercise need not be terribly strenuous to (1) stimulate the metabolism, bowel and digestive tract, and endorphin release; (2) help metabolize stress hormones such as cortisol; and (3) give a general sense of well-being. The most common form of cardiovascular exercise is walking (see About Walking in Chapter 13, Exercise). Whatever form of cardio you choose, it should not be unduly painful during or after.

Resistance training helps with metabolizing stress hormones, releasing endorphin, and giving a sense of well-being and control. To learn more jump to Chapter 13, Strength and Building a Basic Exercise Program. Here is another very gentle general exercise series done seated in a chair called sit and be fit http://www.sitandbefit.org/.

Stretching relieves excessive muscle tension, improves circulation, and releases endorphins. It too can help give a general sense of well-being. Your loved one can stretch by themselves, or a partner or caregiver can gently assist. Again, it should not be painful. For more specifics and good how-to, read Flexibility in Chapter 13, Exercise, and our basic exercise program. Here is another easy, basic guide from the Mayo Clinic with pictures http://www.mayoclinic.org/healthy-living/fitness/multimedia/stretching/sls-20076840?s=4.

The main rule to follow regarding any exercise is to **do what you can and not what you can't.** Remember that exercise is a stress on the body. Exercise should challenge the body a little, but not excessively. It will work best if exercise is taken when your loved one is feeling good rather than after the pain has set in. It does take energy, which must be considered if the person is having any difficulty with fatigue (see Chapter 18, Managing Discomforts.

Any **special problems** such as hip bursitis or difficulty breathing need be to adjusted and accommodated for. Karen's spine was very fragile, so she needed a supportive brace, and all exercise had to avoid excessive loading on her spine. A physical therapist, physiatrist, and maybe your loved one's pain physician can prescribe specific exercises to help relieve pain and others to help maintain or improve strength, function, and energy. Make sure that whoever is prescribing exercise knows the medical history of your loved one and is taking that into account when creating the prescription.

There comes a time in the dying process when any exercise is no longer appropriate. The simple effort of being is enough for the person. All I can say here is, that time will probably be obvious to you. Let them be as active as they can be. **Don't try to push them into activity and exercise,** but do not restrict them either. Let them do what they can.

Transdermal Electrical Neural Stimulation (TENS)

A transdermal electrical neural stimulation (TENS) device gives small to intense electrical stimulation to a region of the body. Generally we think they work by gate-control theory. The input from the neurons stimulated by the electrodes inhibits the nociceptive (pain) neurons at the spinal cord level, blocking the pain. These devices look something like a pager with wires for electrodes, and they are compact enough to wear on the hip or in a pocket. The electrodes look something like oversized round or square Band-Aids and can be worn for several days at a time.

TENS can be quite effective on low- to moderate-level pain associated with the muscles, a limb, or the spine. The devices are now not expensive; inexpensive ones range from $50 to $100 but can be much more. They are often available for rent or purchase through your loved one's physician or physical therapist. They are usually prescribed and administered by a pain specialist, physiatrist, or physical therapist, as settings and electrode placement are important and might be used in ways you wouldn't think about. In some cases, we use meridians or acupuncture points. Most of us in western medicine don't really understand this, but it does seem to work sometimes. This next piece by a Chinese medicine physician may help with understanding.

Acupuncture and Acupressure

By Gary Piscopo, ND, LAc

People are often intimidated by subjects like acupuncture, which involve having to wade into a whole different medical system—in this case, the traditional Chinese medicine (TCM) model. However, as a basic introduction to some of the mysterious concepts like *qi* and meridians, we can use an example that most people are familiar with: plumbing.

Everyone needs access to water each day of their life for drinking, cooking, bathing, and a host of other, less-vital reasons. Water is essential to life and has a number of important functions within our bodies. This is analogous to *qi*, or life energy, in the TCM model of acupuncture. In the Western world, a solution to having ready access to water is through the use of indoor plumbing. The water in a house does not go everywhere at once. Rather, it flows along certain channels called pipes. Likewise, the *qi* in your body follows along certain channels called *meridians*.

Along the pipes that exist with the walls of a house, special fixtures called faucets allow people to access and manipulate the water inside the pipes. Sometimes you might access the water to do work, such as filling a pot to boil water. Other times, you might want to access the water to prevent it from doing something harmful, as when you shut off the water to a toilet that is overflowing. In the same way, acupuncture points are used to manipulate the *qi* in the body. Sometimes we want to increase the flow of *qi* to a certain organ system, and sometimes we want to decrease it. Other times, there is an obstruction of *qi* and, just like a clogged pipe, we may have to manipulate a series of points to correct that problem.

With plumbing, you have to know something about how water flows and how plumbing fixtures work before attempting to do something like fix your toilet. Likewise, you need to understand something about *qi*, meridians, and acupuncture points before you try doing acupressure on yourself. Also understand that there are times when manipulating acupuncture points should never be done unless you have checked with a trained clinician. This includes when a person is pregnant, when a person has been diagnosed with cancer, when there is an acute medical emergency (like a heart attack) occurring, and in areas where the person has significant skin problems (like burns, infections, or new scars).

There are numerous ways to stimulate acupuncture points. The most common is through the use of **special sterile needles**, which is what acupuncturists use. To do this properly and safely requires years of study and a license. However, there are other ways to stimulate the acupuncture points that can be done by laypeople. One example is by using **special tuning forks**, as in systems like Acutonics or Acutone. This method requires only an introductory class and, of course, the tuning forks.

If you are working with an acupuncturist, they may be willing to show you how to use another method, called *moxibustion*. This method uses a rolled-up stick of an herb called mugwort to warm up acupuncture points in a specific way. While the professional use of moxibustion requires extensive training, simple interventions can be mastered in a single teaching session with an acupuncturist. It is not recommend to use moxibustion without the OK of a trained clinician, since there are times when it is not appropriate to use it.

The most common way for laypeople to stimulate acupuncture points, however, is with their **fingers**. This method is known in Japanese as *shiatsu*, and it has been used successfully for thousands of years. After a short introduction to this method, people can use it quite easily and usefully on their own.

To find acupuncture points, a **system of measurement** known as the "body inch," or *cun,* is used. One *cun* is proportional to the distance from one side of your thumb to the other side at the joint closest to the thumbnail. This allows you to measure distances proportionally, which is not possible with the standard inch since tall people and short people would have a different number of standard inches—say, from their pelvis to their feet. However, they have proportionally the same number of *cun* over the same distance.

For example, there is a well-known acupuncture point on the wrist that pregnant women often use when they feel nauseated called **Neiguan, or pericardium 6 (P6)**. This point is found about two *cun* above your wrist crease on the palm side, right between the tendons. Typically this point is stimulated from 30 seconds to 5 minutes on one side, then move to the other side if necessary. Some people respond best to simply pressing this spot, others respond best to rubbing either clockwise or counterclockwise. See what works best for you.

One of the most famous acupuncture-acupressure points for pain is **He Gu, or large intestine 4 (LI4)**. It is found in the depression between the thumb and the index finger, on the top of the hand. It is mainly used for headaches, jaw pain, migraines, and other head-related pain. It should not be used if the person is pregnant unless you are specifically instructed to do so by a trained clinician.

A very good point for strengthening the body and providing more energy is **Zu San Li, or stomach 36 (ST36)**. It has been called the "chicken soup point" because of its nourishing effects. It is found three *cun* below the kneecap and one finger breadth to the outside of the big bone in the lower leg called the tibia. It should be used cautiously in pregnancy, especially in the first trimester, unless specifically instructed to do so by a trained clinician.

Counterirritants: Ben Gay, Icy Hot, and Others

Creams that cool or burn or give some other type of sensation (such as Ben-Gay or Icy-Hot) also work by gate-control theory: They give the nervous system something else to think about, blocking pain at the spinal cord level. They can be effective with mild amounts of achy pain such as joint pain. Be careful that they do not irritate the skin. Try a little first and watch for redness or welting. Be sure to wash your hands after rubbing it on, and keep it away from the eyes or other areas of sensitive skin.

Music

Music offers much more than a simple distraction to help ease pain and anxiety. In study after study, it has been proven effective in at least temporarily lowering people's perception of pain and the physiological responses that go with it. Music therapists are now on staff in many hospitals and are on the care teams with palliative care and hospice. We seemed to gain wonderful benefit from the harp player who blessed us in some of our harder times. Somehow he connected with Karen and she melted into bliss. In fact, the whole room of caregivers and friends enjoyed the peaceful feelings and tranquility that filled the room. To find music therapists near you, see http://www.musictherapy.org/about/find/ or ask your loved one's nurse, doctor, or any part of their health-care team about music therapists. If they are anything like the good people I've experienced, they have a wonderful gift for you.

Whether you play an instrument or just the stereo, you can help pain with music. Choose pleasing melodies. Pleasing notes and melodies seem to stimulate dopamine release in parts of the brain associated with pleasure. This is good, as dopamine-based neurons and our pleasure centers are suppressed by persistent pain and depression. Music that doesn't work so well are songs associated with anger or angst, like some early rap or punk rock, songs with "red notes" (notes that do not seem to naturally follow in the melody, like some experimental jazz), or anything in particular that they do not like for any reason.

Familiar songs can stimulate memories associated with past pleasures and positive emotions. Let your loved one choose their favorite music. Almost any pleasing harmonious music works, of almost any style. It just needs to be something they like.

Invite your loved one to help make the music. Participating in the music, be it tapping a finger, humming along, or playing an instrument, increases their engagement in the music. Engagement amplifies all the effects described above. Engagement also activates their motor and/or speech centers and the *cerebellum* at the base of the brain, which is associated with timing and rhythm. Also, voice and movement associated with music are sometimes processed differently enough from speech and purposeful actions that people can sing and dance when they cannot speak or walk. How much your loved one can participate may surprise you both. For more information on music and pain, here is a PDF from the American Music Therapy Association http://www.musictherapy.org/assets/1/7/MT_Pain_2010.pdf.

Joy

Joy can be found anywhere. It is the smile on a child's face, a yummy bite, a hummingbird outside the window. It is in the moment. It is the opposite of pain. Inside the nervous system, joy actually is the opposite of emotional pain. It suppresses many of the circuits associated with pain while exciting opposing centers.

One example of this is the area just behind the prefrontal cortex called the *middle frontal gyrus* (MFG). For most people, the right MFG is associated with sadness, worry, and irritation. People who activate this more are more likely to be passive to life's difficulties and more prone to anxiety. The left MFG is associated with joy, contentment, and enthusiasm. Activating this region is associated with actively facing life's challenges and being more resilient to anxiety.

Like the rest of the brain and body, whatever you use gets stronger. Exercising your "happiness muscles" helps the body push back pain, anxiety, and depression. It also seems to help the immune system, the cardiovascular system, and the musculoskeletal system. Basically, it helps everything. Karen used gratefulness journaling and I used positive journaling (see Chapter 4, Dancing in the Rain: Healthy Habits for Caregivers) as a formal exercise, and the benefits were truly profound.

Joyfulness Meditation Exercise

Here is another short, easy exercise. It is a mindfulness meditation that focuses on joy in this moment:

1. Take a moment to notice any positive experience as it occurs.
2. **Remember all the sensations of it**—the sights, the sounds, the smells, how it feels in your body.
3. **Feel and enjoy the feelings it gives you.** Let those feelings linger for this moment.
4. **Let those feelings sink into your memory** for maybe up to 30 seconds.
5. **Inhale a deep easy breath.**
6. **As you exhale,** allow the feelings to spread throughout your body.

Meditation

Meditation is like lifting weights with your mind. There are many different exercises you can do, and each will make your mind stronger in some way. The type of meditations that have been used the most for pain control involve mindfulness. Mindfulness helps the most with mastery of emotion and sensation and has been used successfully to control even extreme levels of chronic pain. Again, I refer to the work of John Kabat Zin: http://www.soundstrue.com/shop/authors/Jon_Kabat-Zinn?gclid=CKKrs4_7qLYCFYdxQgodryMAjg. You will find a good discussion and how-to for mindfulness meditation in Chapter 4, Dancing in the Rain: Healthy Habits for Caregivers.

Body-focused meditation is a form of mindfulness in which focus is turned to each part of the body and flows up or down to encompass the whole body, relaxing each part in turn. It is almost always easiest to do with guidance. It is very effective for relaxation, but it may be difficult for someone to learn while they have pain greater than 3 out of 10 on the pain scale described in Measuring Pain earlier in this chapter.

Still, it can be tremendously powerful at controlling pain and, once learned and practiced, can work with higher pain levels. Here are guided body-focused meditation recordings available on the Web:

http://www.youtube.com/watch?v=obYJRmgrqOU&list=PL5602F9BEFDB2CFE7&index=26

http://www.youtube.com/watch?v=dbLzoOIuhhs

https://www.youtube.com/watch?v=IBwr1MOEmB8&index=2&list=PL5602F9BEFDB2CFE7

A Sense of Purpose

A sense of purpose adds more weight to all those things that are not pain. It activates so much in the brain that is not pain that it suppresses those pain signals, making pain less important. It helps the amygdala stay focused on positive motivations, decreasing anxiety while keeping the mind on other tasks. It activates the *prefrontal cortex* (reason) and the emotional centers on purposeful, positive tasks, as well giving a sense of control and well-being. It suppresses area CG25 and is protective against depression. If it is important, you are more likely to remember it, activating the cells in the *hippocampus* associated with memory creation. Activity and purpose also help block nonessential signals coming from the body. Purpose helps block pain at the spinal cord. All these centers that you use when you have important things to focus on get stronger while pain and anxiety fade into the background.

You can help your loved one by not protecting them from purpose or task. Help them engage in what they need to do while smoothing the physical and energy demands, keeping their physical demands to amounts they can handle; see Fatigue in Chapter 18, Managing Discomforts. You might be surprised that if they have purpose, they have more physical strength and more energy.

Perhaps you may help them find that purpose. Are there kids to connect with, a memoir to create, someone they can help or care for? Even if they can't physically help, perhaps they can hold a hand, listen, or just be nearby. Most people work best when they are not the center of their own universe. You know your loved one best. Think of the things they have done in their life so far. How may you help them live life on purpose now?

Gentle Massage

One of the best five dollars I ever spent was for a little wire head scratcher. A few strokes on the top of her head, and Karen would purr and coo. All pain in those moments would vanish and our world would fill with joy.

Neurologically the concept is simple. The scalp is very sensitive but most of the time does not get much stimulation. The gentle scratch of the head massager gives a huge sensory input to the brain stem, switching attention away from and essentially blocking the pain from ribs, spine, hip, or wherever else. It works for a little while until the body gets used to it and pays less attention. But while it works, you will be heroes.

A gentle foot massage or very gently and rhythmically moving the joints works in a similar way by a slightly different pathway. It blocks the pain at the spinal cord level. There is also something powerful about touch, connection, and feelings of appreciation and love that go far beyond simple gate-control theory of neuronal suppression. Above all else, gentle touch was our most important form of pain control.

Social Contact

Social contact can be a very powerful pain suppressor. Someone just being nearby is a strong distraction from the painful inputs, and it is even stronger if they are interacting with your loved one in any way. Connection and trust between living beings has its own properties, which in many ways can be more powerful than some medications. The interactions within our brains and bodies are complex, and research is just beginning to forge understanding of the amazing interplays involved in social contact.

Here is one example: Oxytocin, the cuddle hormone, is one of the stress hormones involved in pain suppression. Among other things, it suppresses the fear-danger activity in the amygdala. It is released in times of stress and pain, but it can be amplified when met with the social condition of love and trust by a series of complex chemical reactions in another part of the brain, the *nucleus accumbens* http://en.wikipedia.org/wiki/Nucleus_accumbens. It also makes us more open to loving and more likely to trust. Therefore, by just this mechanism love and trust beget comfort, which creates more love and trust.

Perhaps the best thing you can do is simply be there for your loved one. You don't necessarily need to be close by, though handholding was found to be more effective than just sitting close in some studies. Interact if they want to interact, but it takes energy and they might not have it to give right then.

Being around more people is not necessarily better. Karen and I are extroverts. We both gain energy being with others, and large groups were wonderful most of the time. Still, there were times when Karen wanted only one or two people around her. Introverts expend some energy being with more than just a few people, but being social is just as important for them and almost as helpful. They may want to keep their social support intimate; one or two close companions at a time might be best.

Be helpful when needed, but doting or being overly attentive could actually make them hurt more by focusing their attention on their pain or problems. Avoid excessive empathy, and don't try to get them to talk about their pains. Remember that nonverbal cues are pretty clear for most people, so try to leave all those "I'm so sorry" feelings at the door. You should leave your own problems at the door too. Unless they are really interested in you and you know they can handle it, they probably don't have room for your pain as well as theirs.

Simply be present. Be yourself and share in the love and beauty of the moments you have together.

Compassion

The major benefit of compassion is for the giver more than the receiver, which may be the other way around from how most people think it works. Giving compassion, connecting with someone (empathy), then giving them loving kindness floods our brains with positive emotions and activates many of the centers that are shut down by pain, fear, and anxiety. In many ways it is akin to gratefulness and joy.

Karen exercised her compassion and gratefulness muscles with gratefulness journaling (see Chapter 4, Dancing in the Rain: Healthy Habits for Caregivers). Not only did this help her quell her anxiety, it made a difference that was felt in our lives and in the lives of our friends. As the rest of her life fell away, her compassion grew. Just being with her was a joy. She became connection, love, our teacher, our Buddha in Pajamas. Whenever you choose to grow into a new challenge, you can never fully know all the gifts you might earn.

Compassion Meditation Exercise

You may also try this simple Karuna, or compassion meditation exercise:

1. **Take a smooth, easy breath**, inhaling to a count of four, then exhaling to a count of four.
2. **Focus your attention** on the person you are with or hold someone in your mind's eye.
3. **Imagine their feelings**, feel their feelings, breath as they're breathing.
4. **Now take a silent moment to wish them well in your thoughts.** You may wish them happiness and peace.
5. **Hold them in your heart**, as if your heart was giving them a warm, comforting, gentle hug.
6. **Breathe again**, in to a count of four and out to a count of four.

Interlude

Buddha in Pajamas

Her face relaxes. My shoulders relax. My soul relaxes. She smiles and the whole room lights up. She laughs and the whole room bubbles over with laughter. It's amazing how a good a simple sigh feels, especially when it's not your own.

We know, We <u>feel</u> how precious a simple smile is. Every little bit of good times is a great gift. Nothing is "for granted". Every bit of relief or joy is one more drop of wonderful life.

If you know life is short, each moment becomes more precious. If you know suffering and pain are close at hand, then happiness is such a wonderful gift. We are in the moment. We are giving.

We are all connected. We are social creatures. It's hard wired into us. If I watch you throw a ball, cells in my brain fire next to those that would fire if I threw the ball. If I see you smile, cells in my brain adjacent to those that signal smiling also fire.

We are all connected. She teaches us this. With each smile she gives a gift. We share her joy. We feel our connection. We again know the importance of the moment.

Chapter 18.
Managing Discomforts

As someone walks the path of an illness, they will undoubtedly face some bumps. In this important chapter, we hope to give you a quick reference guide for managing these problems using time-proven methods, best treatment practices, and just some darn good advice from professionals who have also been in your shoes as caregivers. Each symptom or problem is dealt with separately, so you may quickly access the solutions you need without paging through the entire chapter. You might just, in all that spare time you have, read this chapter before problems occur so you and your caregiving team can be ready to avoid or quickly smooth these bumps in your loved one's path.

Anxiety

Anxiety can be a nonspecific sense of angst. It is a fearful, uncomfortable hypervigilance. The funny thing is that once the brain is anxious, those feelings can become associated with *anything* the sufferer is focused on. If they spend time in a room with blue walls, that color of blue might become a trigger for the anxiety. If the sufferer is focused on a particular person, like their caregiver, that person might become the trigger for anxiety too.

When someone is very sick, there are a lot of possible things to be anxious about. Pain, difficulty breathing, unsteadiness (falling down), losing bowel or bladder control, losing control of one's life in general, and just being very sick and possibly dying are but a few possibilities. The disease itself, or the medications your loved one is using, might also interact to cause anxiety, even panic.

A Feeling of anxiety can run in the background of the conscious mind. It doesn't need to be related to what the sufferer is thinking or doing at the time. Gradually, though, it can increase as the brain builds more associations of angst with the common things around us—and angst colors our thinking.

Look for signs of anxiety early. It's easiest to treat before it becomes entrenched. With Karen, I noticed that she was white-knuckling the car-door handle if someone changed lanes 100 yards in front of us. This was not normal. This was the same girl who giggled with glee going 120 on the back of my motorcycle.

...Signs and Symptoms of Anxiety

Alert your loved one's medical team, especially anyone involved in prescribing medications. **Be specific about the signs and symptoms you are observing**. Write down things like these:

- elevated heart rate
- respiratory (breathing) rate
- muscle clenching
- jerking muscles
- emotional outbreaks such as crying fits
- confusion or other cognitive dysfunctions
- sedation

- vivid dreams
- hallucinations
- pain with touch or sensations that are normally not painful

Consider *all* the signs and symptoms you are seeing. It will give you a baseline and it might help the doctors hear you. These and others can add up to medicine interactions or other conditions that need to be medically managed. **Keep a medication log** (see Chapter 11, Medications). There might be a correlation between when a medicine is given and when symptoms peak. Report all the symptoms and signs to your loved one's prescribing doctors and nurses. Be ready to give them specific examples.

...Treating Anxiety

Look for and alleviate irritants such as uncomfortable clothing or positioning. Noise, harsh lights, strong smells, even negative irritating television can all contribute to their underlying feeling of angst. Sometimes needing to use the bathroom or being thirsty, hungry, cold, or hot can make someone uncomfortable enough to cause anxiety. Any source of pain or discomfort can make the symphony of stimulation in the brain turn to the negative and angst. The most common irritant in the very sick is an undiagnosed urinary tract infection (UTI).

Gentle touch, hand-holding, a quiet room, a puppy (or something or someone who gives a strong positive emotional response), gentle hugs, cuddling, a warm blanket, or a warm rice-bag hot-pack can all **help your loved one feel loved and calm.** Use anything and everything that works. Karen and I were able to treat her anxiety through a combination of approaches that included decreasing or stopping many medications, love and compassion, touch, mental exercises, exercise, and some new medications. Be careful though, because if the intimate approaches fail to work, they may become associated with the angst and become triggers themselves.

Calming Exercise

For mild to moderate anxiety, you may lead the sufferer through **mental calming exercises.** Try this four-count breathing exercise (also described in Chapter 4, Dancing in the Rain: Healthy Habits for Caregivers):

1. First calm yourself a little.
2. Then gently inhale smoothly while counting off four seconds in your mind.
3. Without pausing, exhale smoothly, also counting four seconds silently in your mind.
4. Continue this for three more breaths, in and out.

This exercise is often calming and centering. It allows your loved one a moment to step out of the scene and helps activate their *parasympathetic* (calming) nervous system. Now, ask your loved one to take another moment to see this scene simply as an observer. They may notice their body's reactions or environment. Ask them to feel their heart beat. Notice their temperature. Are their hands cold? Are they clenched? Have them notice the scene around them. They may find it amusing or ridiculous. They may sense the scene more fully. Ask them to take notes of their own signs of stress. Simply taking a moment to notice activates their *prefrontal cortex* (rational mind). Now it can help them return to the situation and help them make more rational decisions and take calmer actions.

Meditation (see Chapter 17, Pain Management) is an incredibly powerful tool for anxiety if they have been practicing and are pretty good at it already. It can be remarkably difficult to do once they're anxious, though, so learning it while anxious may be out of reach.

Anxiety Medications

Benzodiazepines can be very effective and may help the sufferer be calmer and regain control. These medications bind to gamma-aminobutyric (GABA) type-A receptors in the brain, which increases the potency of these inhibitory neurotransmitters. Activating these receptors reduces anxiety and causes muscle relaxation and sedation. We also discuss benzos in the Chapter 14, Sleep) as they can be used to put someone to sleep and make them sleep longer.

Benzos come in several strengths and duration of effect. Most of us have heard of **Valium (diazepam)**. This is a long acting benzo. **Lorazepam (Ativan)** and **alprazolam (Xanax)** are shorter acting forms. As a general rule, it's best to use short to intermediate-acting medications to avoid or limit excessive daytime sedation. Your loved one's doctor may recommend these or other benzodiazepine medicines.

Do be aware that the benzodiazepines may have anxiety and delusions as a side effect, especially when mixed with morphine-based drugs, see Delirium: The Hard Road at the end of this chapter. Other common side effects include amnesia, confusion, loss of coordination and balance (increased risk of falling) and respiratory and cardiovascular depression. All benzodiazepines can accumulate in fat tissue, so regular use of higher doses can build up a reservoir of medicine, triggering side effects, especially in obese patients. Caution should be taken when using these medications in the elderly, and long-acting benzos should be avoided. **Temazepam (Restoril)** is usually well tolerated by elderly patients)

With all that said about side effects, especially more anxiety and delusions, benzos are still a first-choice medication for anxiety. Don't be afraid to use them, as anxiety can be more difficult to treat than pain and can make pain worse.

...Managing Your Response to Their Anxiety
Be careful about telling someone that you think they're anxious. Once they're anxious, it is difficult to hear it without feeling like you're judging them. You may cue a treatment such as medicine or the calming exercise (described above) toward their elevated heart rate instead of speaking of their anxiety.

If you do become a trigger, consider removing yourself from the situation for a while. Let their feelings disassociate from you before you return. If you are a trigger, removing yourself is the compassionate thing to do.

Most of all, **don't take their anxiety personally.** Consider again that the angst they are directing at you may be from an underlying process. Unless you've been standing over them with a pitchfork, it might not be anything you are doing. Love and compassion may be the best medicine and may help you both through this difficult time.

For more on related issues, see Delirium: The Hard Road later in this chapter.

Fatigue

Fatigue is the most common symptom in many diseases, including cancer. Just to make matters a little more complicated, fatigue can also be an additional secondary symptom of associated problems as the body goes through the disease process. Sure, we experienced the pressure of fatigue as Karen's body was usurped by growing tumors, but the disease also attacked her bone marrow, where blood cells are made, giving her anemia. The persistent tiredness was only compounded by energy-sapping pain, the sedation of the pain medications, and then chemotherapy and radiation. This is just what we experienced—your loved one's case might include a host of other factors, including problems with any organ associated with energy: the heart, the lungs and airways, the brain (the most common problem being depression), a thyroid imbalance, an electrolyte imbalance, and just plain deconditioning (losing cardiovascular conditioning). Some describe fatigue as more of an issue than pain when dealing with disease.

...Treating Fatigue

As a physical therapist, I've been helping people deal with the problem of fatigue for a long time. Even in the depth of all that Karen and I faced, we dealt with it. So will you. This section provides some tips and hints that may help. First, look to treat the things you can.

Dehydration is one of the more common problems facing the sick or elderly. If you suspect mild dehydration, adding a few glasses of fluids per day may turn that around. For more severe cases, medical help may be needed.

Electrolyte imbalances are easily treated by supplementing whatever is low. A routine blood test will show it. Calcium, magnesium, and potassium are the most common culprits. A little (a pint or two) of your typical sport drink usually contains enough electrolyte replacement to bring most people back into balance. Pedialyte will have a little more as well. If you suspect an electrolyte imbalance, it is of little harm to give a sport drink even if they don't need it, but be careful in cases with edema or congestive heart failure, as salts may make these conditions worse.

Low vitamin and mineral levels also can give fatigue. B12 is a common suspect here. Anemia may be related to iron deficiency. Natural sources include most meats and dark green leafy vegetables. For more on nutrition, see Eat Right in Chapter 4, Dancing in the Rain: Healthy Habits for Caregivers, and Chapter 12, Food and Nutrition. Good nutritional balance helped Karen's anemia immensely, but it sometimes wasn't enough. She was given medications to help stimulate her bone marrow and eventually was given a transfusion. All this helped her fatigue.

Remember, when supplementing fluids, electrolytes, or vitamins, you are "trying" these things to see if they help. If they don't help, don't continue to push them.

Medical management of fatigue can be simple or a tricky business. If **low thyroid** is the problem, a simple test will show it. Synthroid, which functions as a synthetic thyroid, can help restore normal metabolism and energy. There are other drug-based strategies to boost energy, but each drug comes with its own issues and difficulties. **Psychostimulants, corticosteroids,** and **megestrol acetate** are some of the more commonly used drugs, and they seem to give variable success. There are others as well, depending on the particulars of the case. Seek consultation with your loved one's physician team and pharmacist about the risks and benefits of each.

...Managing Their Fatigue

Adapt their lifestyle a bit to accommodate a lower energy level. They probably won't be able to, or want to, do as much with a day. **Plan a bit less activity** in a day, but do plan activity. Most people have a time of day when they have the most energy. For Karen it was the afternoon. For others, it's the morning. Try to plan activities in this time and allow your loved one to cancel if they just don't feel up to it.

This includes emotional and mental activities as well as physical ones. Remember, the brain is a hungry machine and it takes a lot of energy. It also needs exercise. You might notice diminished concentration and decision making as the brain tires. Honor this and let them rest when they need to.

Use microresting. In other words, help them to rest whenever they can wherever they can. If there is a quiet moment and a comfortable place, help them use it.

Try to **keep overall activity level of big days and smaller days fairly close to each other** in volume. In my PT clinic, to help give values to this concept, we put a measurement on activities using the *metabolic equivalent of a task* (MET). One MET equals the effort required to sit or lie down quietly. Hiking would be 6 METs, while grocery shopping would be 2.3 METs. Multiply METs by the time spent on the activity, and you have MET hours. For a list of MET values, see http://appliedresearch.cancer.gov/atus-met/met.php.

Karen and I generally tried to keep the activity level of our big days no more than 50 percent more than that of our rest days, and vice versa. We never actually calculated the METs for Karen, but some people do find the structure of this system helpful; either way, you get the idea. Allow one or two days of relative rest following a bigger day, but not more than three rest days.

Exercise is still helpful in maintaining or even building your fatigued loved one's strength and endurance. The big lesson here is to have them do what they can and not what they can't. Effort level is relative. For most people, 20–30 minutes per day of moderate cardiovascular exercise is recommended, even when very sick. For most people, this would be exercising to a heart rate that is 60–70 percent of their age-adjusted (220 minus their age) projected maximum (equivalent to zone 2). For most healthy people, this means walking at a brisk pace, and for fit people, easy running. For Karen, when things were good it meant walking up stairs or hills and doing strengthening exercises. When things were difficult, it could mean just walking in the house with support. Either way, Karen did what she could. For more information, see Exercise Concepts in Chapter 13, Exercise.

Shortness of Breath: Dyspnea

Ever have that feeling like you just couldn't catch your breath? Perhaps you just sprinted downfield to the goal or swam that extra half pool length underwater and came up gasping. As climbers, we would sometimes get the sensation of unquenchable breathlessness as we headed higher into the thinning air. For a healthy person, usually the feeling passes in a few minutes, but if you can remember the feeling, you might imagine what it feels like for someone who is sick and suffering from dyspnea. It's distressing just to think about, isn't it?

There are many reasons why dyspnea can occur. Basically, anything that impairs the ability to breathe air into the lungs, exchange carbon dioxide and oxygen, exhale the lung air, circulate oxygenated blood, and perceive that oxygenated blood is adequate can contribute to the feeling of shortness of breath.

...Treating Acute Dyspnea

As with any of the conditions discussed in this chapter, **any sudden or dramatic change should cue you to contact your loved one's health-care team immediately.** Several conditions that could cause dyspnea need to be treated right away by medical professionals. Get help! Call your loved one's doctor, your hospice nurse, or 9-1-1. Even if shortness of breath does not come on suddenly, if they are breathing very poorly, are looking blue, or are unconscious, get help.

It is common toward the end of life for a person to become short of breath as the body shuts down. When the primary goal of care is comfort, we can use medications that will reduce suffering and the feeling of shortness of breath. If the goal of care is extending life, more-aggressive interventions such as a ventilator will be used. Any discussion about breathing distress wouldn't be complete without mentioning again the importance of your loved one having provided caregivers with **clear advance directives.** If the person you're caring for goes into respiratory distress, any interventions need to be performed *now*. But at the same time, caregivers and rescuers need to be able to honor your loved one's wishes regarding CPR, ventilation, artificial life support, and other heroic measures. The POLST, living will, or advance directives need to be known and posted. For more on this, see Advance Directives in Chapter 6, The Notebook of Important Papers.

...Treating Mild to Moderate Dyspnea

So let's say you walk into the room and notice that they just don't seem to be breathing really well or they are bent over in their chair, hands on knees breathing, but still in distress. You ask if they feel out of breath, and they nod yes, but they *are* breathing. They are conscious and their eyes are clear. They are not blue but still they are in distress. What do you do?

First, don't panic. They are getting enough oxygen to not be in danger. **If they are on oxygen, check these things:**

- Is the machine on?
- Is oxygen flowing? If not, is the hose kinked?
- Is the cannula positioned where they will breathe in the oxygen? If it's in their nose but their nose is stuffy, perhaps put it on their chin at their lower lip.
- Is the oxygen level OK, or can you increase it?

Generally we use as little supplemental oxygen as it takes to make them comfortable and get good profusion (above 95 percent oxygen saturation). When I was in school, I learned that anything above 3 liters per minute could burn and damage the airway or lungs. Now we've learned that this doesn't really seem to be the case and not to be afraid of this. However, nurse Mary says there is little reason to go above 4–6 liters per minute by cannula.

Now, think about what you know about them. Your knowledge of **their health history** is key to helping you know what's going on. Consider questions like these:

- Do they have a history of **chronic lung problems** and shortness of breath? What might be making it worse now? Look for the obvious.

- Do they have a history of right-sided heart insufficiency or **congestive heart failure** (CHF)?
- Do they have a history of **poor kidney or liver function** or considerable edema?
- Might they have a **respiratory (lung and airway) infection**?

Any of these conditions could give more fluid in the lungs. If they are lying down, move them to **sit up supported,** which is usually an easier position to breathe in. Make sure if you do this that their back is supported and they are not slumped over. This is so their chest can be open and fully expanded to inhale.

Pursed-lip breathing often helps. Ask them to purse their lips as if blowing out a candle. Exhaling with a bit of back pressure against pursed lips helps to gently open and relax the lungs and bronchioles.

If their dyspnea is still severe, call the professionals. Among other things, they can listen to their lungs and tell you what positions are best to help the lungs drain and open.

Do they have a history of anxiety or distress? **Anxiety or panic** can cause the perception of breathlessness. It can also cause the bronchioles to constrict and breathing to become shallow. Might something be making them uncomfortable and making their anxiety worse? Can you address what that might be? Pain, constipation, or urinary retention can cause anxiety and contribute to the feeling of not getting enough air.

You can use any technique discussed above to help them. Sometimes **opening a window** or turning on a fan gives a feeling of more air, calming the person, letting the bronchioles relax and dilate, and causing their breathing to deepen and normalize. It all can help. While you're doing this, **keep yourself calm**; they will feel your emotion in your actions and the tone of your voice. Your calm will help their calm.

There are several **medications** that help with coughing, drying secretions, fluid volume in the body, and anxiety. There is also a cocktail of opioids, and perhaps opioids and Ativan, that seems to relax and regulate the breathing. This is usually employed when people are near the end-stage of their disease when the primary goal is comfort. The hospice nurse did this for Karen, and it worked wonderfully. This is definitely a "don't try this at home, kids" item. There are guidelines in the medical literature and quite an art to it. We did a lot of high-end home care for Karen, but still I would seek a very experienced professional for help with medications for dyspnea.

Do they have a history of **aspiration** (breathing fluid or food into the airway)? It is common for people to lose control of the swallow reflex. Did they eat or drink lately? Are they gasping a little, wheezing, or trying to cough? Perhaps they have a history of aspiration but haven't eaten or drunk anything recently. It is quite possible to aspirate on the body's own mouth, nose, and/or throat fluids, which sometimes slowly drain into the lungs, even while they're asleep.

Positioning them forward, leaning over a large pillow or couch cushion, will often help them cough it out. If they are breathing, the Heimlich maneuver is not something you want to do, especially if they are frail. We used the over-the-cushion method for Karen and made a little video to teach our caregiving team https://www.youtube.com/watch?v=E1MEARcZt8s&t=133s. For more on aspiration and clearing the airway, see Swallowing Issues in Chapter 12, Food and Nutrition. For more on postural drainage, see this page by the National Institute of Health http://www.nlm.nih.gov/medlineplus/ency/patientinstructions/000051.htm.

Swelling and Edema

Swelling is a general term for any enlargement of a body part. Generally here we are talking about a whole limb, or limbs, the abdomen, or even in the face and around the eyes. There are several types, which look and feel different, relate to different causes, and have different treatments to consider.

Inflammatory swelling is caused by an inflammatory process. It is usually angry-looking—often reddish, warm to the touch, and usually tender. The most common problem if a whole limb or body part looks like this is infection or *cellulitis*. Seek medical attention. Proper diagnosis and treatment, probably with antibiotics, is what is most likely needed. Don't wait. Call your loved one's doctor today.

Edema is caused by excessive fluid in the tissue. It is usually not red or warm and may not be markedly painful. It often has a boggy, fluid-filled feel if you squeeze the limb a little. Edema is caused by a mismatch of the amount of fluid coming out of the arteries to the body and the amount of fluid going back up the venous and lymphatic vessels and returning to the heart. Anything that affects this balance—more fluid coming out than going back—results in edema. Edema can affect any part of the body but is most often apparent in the lower legs, feet, and ankles. These parts are the farthest from the heart and usually are also the lowest. Water flows downhill, and this dynamic is true for body fluid too.

Edema is **a sign of an underlying problem**. If possible, the best way to address it is to figure out and address that underlying problem. Consult your loved one's health-care team. Treatment may be as simple as changing their diet, helping them get a little physical activity, or perhaps changing a medication.

For more on causes of edema, try this website as a starting point for your own research http://www.medicinenet.com/edema/article.htm. Generally we see **two types of edema:** pitting and nonpitting.

...Nonpitting Edema

Nonpitting edema is swelling that is not inflammatory, but if you squeeze the limb, your finger does not leave a dent or pit. If it is tender, especially in the calf, and especially if it is one-sided, call your loved one's doctor and get a proper workup and treatment, because the most common cause here is a **deep vein thrombosis (DVT)**.

Whenever the blood stops moving, it begins to clot, which is a lovely property for sealing wounds and beginning the healing process, but it is big trouble within the veins or arteries. Do not massage or pump the limb with muscular action like ankle pumps, because you do not want to "throw the clot," sending it somewhere it could cause more serious problems. A good medical workup includes a thorough physical exam and health history and perhaps a Doppler examination where the doctor can listen to their veins with ultrasound.

There are noted **risk factors for DVT** and a diagnostic risk criteria called Wells' Criteria for DVT. Oh, yes: DVT may also have pitting edema, so tenderness and risk factors are the biggest clue. If your loved one has two or more of the following, they have high risk; take two points off their risk if an alternative diagnosis is more likely:

- active cancer
- bedridden more than three days or major surgery within last four weeks
- collateral veins apparent (nonvaricose veins, which are not the usual)

- swelling in the entire limb
- localized tenderness along the deep vein system (for example: calf, back of the knee, back of the thigh)
- pitting edema more on the symptomatic side
- paralysis or immobilization of the limb
- previous DVT

Another possible cause for one-sided or bilateral nonpitting edema is **early-stage lymphatic insufficiency**. The lymph system is the tissues' drain system, a series of perforated channels that drain fluid back to the heart. These channels or vessels have small one-way valves and nodules of white-blood-cell reservoirs called lymph nodes. The lymph system is important to the immune system as well as for body fluid balance and drainage.

Nonpitting edema can occur in the early stages of this condition, but the affected area is usually not tender and there is not necessarily the risk factors listed above. If there are known lymphatic damage problems, such as with cancer surgery involving the lymph nodes or radiation to a drainage area, this condition becomes more probable. Exercise, periodic elevation of the area, compressive and lymph edema dressings, lymphatic drainage massage, and salt management are the **key treatments** here. There's more about treatments under Pitting Edema, below.

Hypothyroidism (low thyroid) also may cause swelling under the skin, giving nonpitting edema. This is usually symmetrical, nontender, and not severe.

...Pitting Edema

With pitting edema, if you squeeze the limb for a second or two, your finger does leave a dent. This indicates that there is excessive fluid in the tissue, between the cells. It can be quite severe and even cause the skin to weep fluid, leading to skin breakdown and wounds that can be very difficult to heal. The choice of treatment strategy should be somewhat linked to the cause and mindful of the loads that returning the fluid might place on the body. The basic treatment strategies are as follows.

Treatment Strategy 1: Returning the Fluid to the Heart

Be careful with returning the fluid to the heart, especially if there is any weakness in the heart. Watch for any heart signs such as chest pain or heaviness and for coughing or difficulty breathing. The first destination for all that fluid after the heart is the lungs. If the abdomen is distended, watch for this worsening. If they have to pee, that's a good sign. That's where the fluid is supposed to go: through the heart and lungs to the kidneys and on out of the body.

Elevation: Elevating the limb or body part above the heart, or at least not below it, allows gravity to take effect and the fluid to naturally head downhill. Simple, eh? Consider elevating the limb for 30–60 minutes several times per day. Try to be mindful not to compress the vessels that run down the back of the leg over any sharp edge, such as a hard chair seat.

Pumping exercises: Both the veins and the lymph vessels have one-way valves, much like tiny heart valves. As the muscles pump and the body moves, these vessels are squeezed and pumped much like the heart. In PT we like to say that the calf is the "heart" of the lower leg. One simple exercise is to pump the foot up and down, flexing at the ankle to get the calf to work. Try sets of 20 to 30. This works well in conjunction with other treatments like elevation and compression. Don't forget to work the toes too. The deep vessels run right next to the long toe-flexor muscles in the lower leg.

Exercise: Movement is life for the body. Exercise works in the same way as specific pumping exercises and usually works very well in moderate cases without severe medical complications. Easy walking for 20–30 minutes, partial squats or sit-to-stands, or gentle weight-lifting pumps existing fluid and stimulates the cardiovascular system for several days. Typically we prescribe 20–30 minutes twice a day at a moderate level of whatever the person can do safely. Hopefully it is something that they also enjoy and that gives them social stimulation as well. One of the best exercises for this is **swimming or water aerobics.** Moderate levels work best. Exercising aggressively can give a mild inflammation response in the muscles and/or give more cardiac output than the return flow can handle, making the swelling worse over time.

Compression: Compressive garments such as **TED (thrombo-embolic deterrent) hose** give more positive pressure to the limb, literally helping to squeeze the fluid back into the vessels. TED hose are a strong, usually white elastic stocking. They come in many forms and differ on pressure, depending on what's needed. They are pretty much standard issue in the hospital when edema and DVT are a risk. Custom-fitted stockings are often stronger but must be prescribed and fitted. Your loved one's nurse or PT can help with this.

There are also **pneumatic leg sleeves** that have a pumping action. Progressive or sequential pneumatic pumping action takes this idea one step further by squeezing different compartments of the air bladders sequentially up the leg. **Ace-bandage wraps**, if applied correctly, work well; specific edema wraps are less elastic and somewhat more effective when edema is severe. Your loved one's PT can help with these and may be able to teach you to apply them. **Lymph edema garments** often have specific patterns of compression channels to encourage lymph flow. This is also the realm of PT, nursing, or an orthotist specializing in lymph garments.

Sequential compression massage: This is what it sounds like. Elevate the limb above the heart and wrap your hands fully around the limb, more distal (at the end of the foot or hand) first, and give a gentle squeeze for about 10–20 seconds. Move your hands up so they still cover some of the area you just squeezed. Repeat this all the way up the limb. Repeat the whole process three times or more. You should be able to see the limb volume decrease gradually. **Warning:** Do not try to press in hard enough to make a big dent, which stretches out the adjacent tissue with the fluid you are displacing.

Lymph massage: Lymph massage is a very specific set of massage techniques that very gently pump and stimulate the lymphatic system. It is effective for lymph edema as well as general pitting edema. Rather than trying to explain the technique here, it might be easier to link to one of the many videos produced that show how to do it. Try this video for self-massage of the upper leg http://www.youtube.com/watch?v=4vLN1WRg_Eo.

Treatment Strategy 2: Decreasing the Amount of Fluid

Salt: Managing salt intake is powerful medicine here. It is salt, or sodium, that draws fluids into the bloodstream, giving more fluid volume to the blood and causing more edema. Managing salt intake means a bit more than keeping the salt shaker off the table. Salt is a very strong flavor. Most processed foods and restaurant meals are loaded with it. Take time to read the labels. For specific low-salt menu ideas, try this Web page from the Mayo Clinic http://www.mayoclinic.org/healthy-living/nutrition-and-healthy-eating/in-depth/dash-diet/art-20047110.

A healthy diet and plenty of water: Eating a healthy diet and drinking enough water is the first line of defense for many things, including edema. Drinking an extra glass or three of water a day helps your loved one pee off more salt. A healthy diet with more fresh, home-prepared foods—including fresh fruits and vegetables, adequate protein, good fats, and less salt than is in pre-prepared or processed foods—helps in many ways. Good whole foods help to clear toxins from the blood and give less toxic load on the liver. Cooking at home usually means using less salt (at least you get to control the amount), and you can substitute savory spices for salt. Fresh whole foods also have more vitamins and nutrients in the form we were made to absorb, improving the health and function of everything. For more on this, see Eat Right in Chapter 4, Dancing in the Rain: Healthy Habits for Caregivers.

Diuretics: These are drugs that make you pee. That's why they're called water pills. Generally they open the channels a bit wider in the microtubules of the kidney. Furosemide (Lasix), torsemide (Damadex), and butethamine (Bumex) act on the upper portion of the tubules, while hydrochlorothiazide (HydroDIURIL) and metolozone (Zaroxolyn) act on the lower portion. The two different classes can be used together.

Itching

Itching is not necessarily an issue of dry skin; it could be a side effect of medications (such as opioids or aspirin), an allergic reaction (especially anything new over the last week, including foods, medicines, adhesives or other medical products, and skin products), a metabolic or hematologic (blood-related) issue, an infection, or a skin condition. The skin is the body's largest organ, and there is a lot that can affect its sensation and create the perception of itching. Successfully addressing the symptom depends on the underlying cause.

Dry skin: If the skin is red, dry, or fragile, it may very well be just a case of dry skin. Moisturizers work well here, but not the usual lotions a healthy person might use, because they are often mostly water and usually have perfumes and alcohol, which all can irritate fragile skin more. Serious dryness requires an emollient and moisturizer. Nurse Mary says good 'ol petroleum jelly (Vaseline) is the best bang for the buck. She also likes Aquaphor as well as baby oil. These are greasy, but a little bit used after a bath on damp skin works well.

Skin conditions: Dermatitis is usually recognizable by its appearance. There are many different causes and appearances, but most are characterized by spots, marks, or rashes. A consultation with a dermatologist is a good idea, since trying to treat with over-the-counter products can mask the symptoms and prolong the condition rather than treating the underlying cause.

Allergic reaction: If dermatitis is related to an adhesive or other product on the skin, it will most likely show where that product was used. Discontinue that product immediately. There are a few strategies to help soothe the skin and decrease the histamine (allergic) reaction. Cooling agents such as calamine lotion or menthol cream may help with a mild itch. Antihistamines may be helpful, but be careful here, because anti-itching drugs such as Benadryl can cause agitation and/or confusion, especially when interacting with other drugs. Topical steroids such as cortisone cream are very effective, but again be careful here. If your loved one is taking an oral or injected steroid, the effects are additive, and the addition of a topical steroid may be too much. Another old-fashioned remedy is the oatmeal bath; Aveeno makes a product for this http://www.aveeno.com/product/aveeno-+soothing+bath+treatment+.do or you can make your own. I found pretty good instructions on Wikihow http://www.wikihow.com/Make-an-Oatmeal-Bath.

Metabolic or medication related: Itching in the absence of skin conditions may very well be metabolic (related to the blood, liver, kidney, or thyroid) or a side effect of medication, especially morphine and all the other opioids. A thorough review of the body's systems and the medications your loved one is using might be warranted. Sometimes switching to another type of opioid or backing down on the opioid use while compensating with a different type of pain management can help. In the case of morphine, it is associated with histamine release, so antihistamines might be effective. Also, tricyclics such as Doxepin might also help by blocking histamines. For more on pain medications and their side effects, see Chapter 17, Pain Management.

Psychogenic: Itching can also be in the person's head (*psychogenic*). All sensation is a perception and interpretation of neurons firing. The brain has the power to create most any sensation without a direct cause from the tissues of the outer body. Treatments that are soothing to the skin may help here. The nonpharmacological treatments for pain might also offer some relief here. See Nonpharmacological Ways to Help Control Pain in Chapter 17, Pain Management.

Don't scratch: In any case, the last thing you want them to do is scratch. If they do have dry, fragile skin or their health is compromised enough to need caregiving, scratching will most likely result in skin breakdown and wounds. Light tickling or touching might help with some immediate temporary relief, but seek to find the cause and treat it with the other interventions listed above as soon as possible.

Muscle Spasms and Myoclonus

First, if your loved one is suffering a muscle spasm *right now*, they need right-now relief, so this section starts out with treating spasms, then discusses underlying causes as well as myoclonus.

...Treating Muscle Spasms

For right-now relief, a **long, slow stretch** is the best medicine. If you don't know the stretch for that particular muscle, your loved one might do well to move the body part in the opposite direction that the spasm is pulling it toward. It may take holding the stretch up to 2 minutes.

Stretches

The most common muscles to spasm, and the stretches for them, are shown in the pictures in this section.

Calf: There are two muscles in the calf—the gastrocnemius, which starts above the knee and so is stretched with the knee straight (fig. 25), and the deeper soleus, which comes off the lower leg bones and so is stretched best with the knee bent (fig. 26). If your loved one can stand, the standing calf stretches work better than doing them lying down.

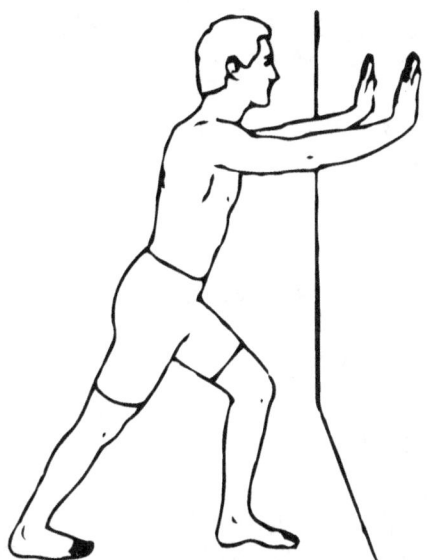

Figure 25. Standing calf stretch for gastrocnemius: press the heel down and rock the hips forward

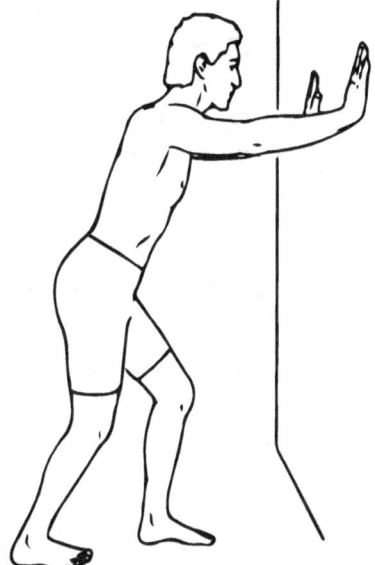

Figure 26. Standing calf stretch for soleus: press the heel down and rock the hips forward.

These two calf stretches (figs. 27 and 28) can also be performed with the assistance of a caregiver with the person lying down. Remember to use gentle, firm, steady pressure.

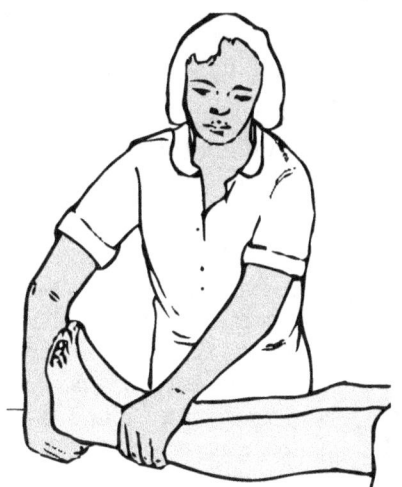

Figure 27. Supine calf stretch for gastrocnemius: cup the heel and pull the ball of the foot up.

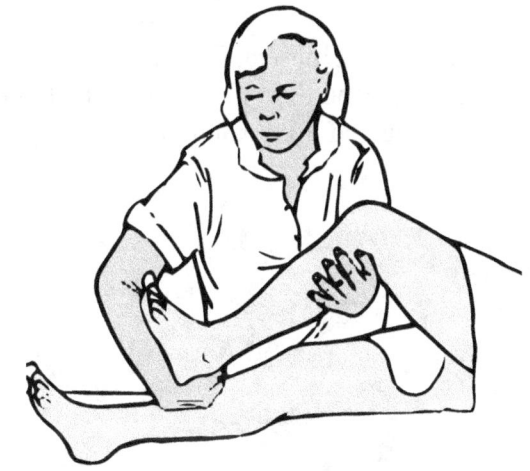

Figure 28. Supine calf stretch for soleus: cup the heel and pull the ball of the foot up.

Hamstring: There are two sides to the hamstring group (figs. 29 and 30). If the spasm is more to the outside of their leg, have them turn the toe in; if the spasm is more to the inside of their leg, they should turn the toe out.

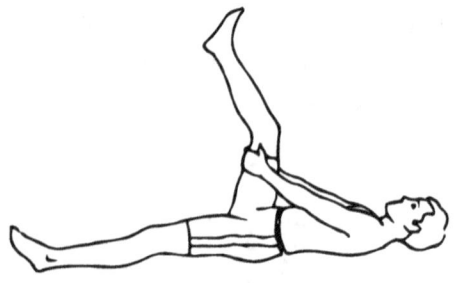

Figure 29. Supine hamstring stretch: bring the knee toward the chest, hold behind the thigh, then gently straighten the knee, raising the heel toward the sky.

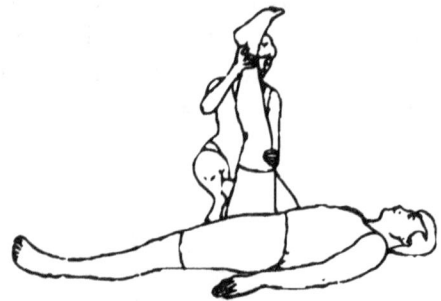

Figure 30. Assisted supine hamstring stretch

If they also have sciatica, do not use these stretches, as they also stretch the sciatic nerve. Use direct pressure instead.

Quadriceps and rectus femoris (long quadriceps): Three of the four quadriceps muscles come off the upper leg bone, while one comes off the pelvis. To stretch the first three muscles, bring the heel toward your bottom (fig. 31).

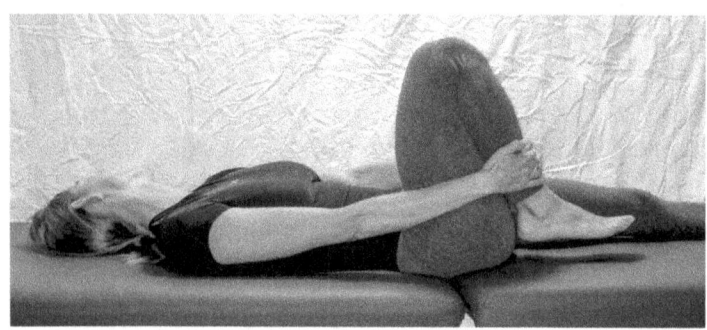

Figure 31. Supine quadriceps stretch; for more thigh emphasis, slide your hands further down the shin toward the foot

For the last muscle, the rectus femoris, have your loved one lie on their side or stomach and bend their lower leg at the knee, then bring the upper leg down and back, straightening and even extending the hip (fig. 32). Be careful to not let their back arch or hips twist.

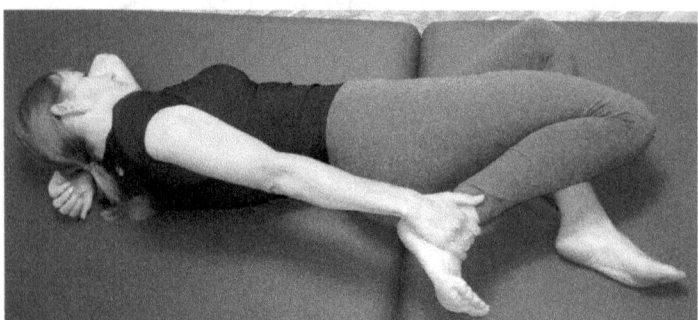

Figure 32. Side-lying quadriceps–rectus femoris stretch: Bring the heel toward the buttock as far as is comfortable for the knee. For more emphasis on the rectus femoris, then bring the knee back, extending the hip. Be careful not to extend or twist the low back.

Low back: This looks much like the quadriceps stretch but for more low-back emphasis, allow the pelvis to roll to flatten the back. You can also have them do both legs at once for the low back.

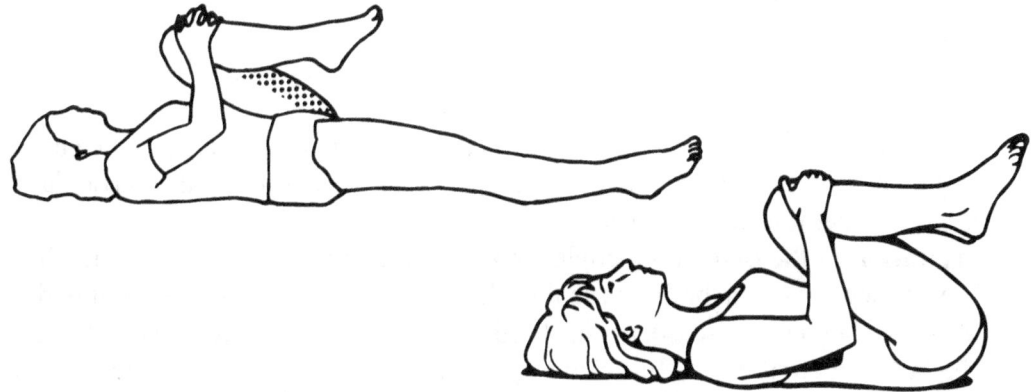

Adductors: These muscles run on the inside of the thigh, sometimes referred to as groin muscles. Having your loved one lying on their back with knees bent, they should lean their knees out, away from each other (fig. 33). Some adductors cross the knee; to stretch these, straighten the knee.

...Preventing Muscle Spasms

Wow, now that *that's* over, let's talk about what's behind the problem. As a physical therapist, I often hear the question, "What causes muscle spasms?" My usual answer is a thoughtful "Ummmm." There are so many different things that can result in muscle spasms that there is not any one useful answer. Basically the answer is, anything that disturbs the metabolic balance of the muscle or its motor nerve, all the way up to the brain. That's a lot of possibilities.

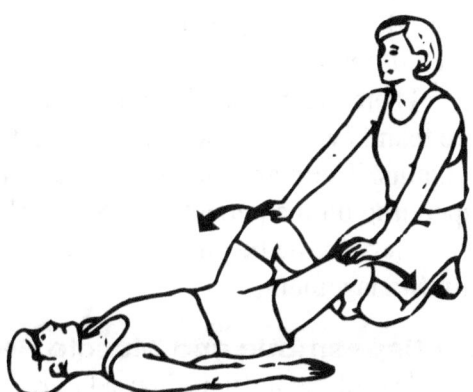

Figure 33. Supine adductor stretch: Gently press the knees apart. This can be done one leg at a time and/or with the knees nearly straight.

For the athlete, the usual suspects are fatigue, dehydration, electrolyte imbalance (often potassium or sodium), and mineral imbalance (often magnesium). For the frail or ill, we need to include problems with the kidneys, liver, thyroid, peripheral nerves, spinal cord, brain, and a very long list of medications. That's even more possibilities. If the person you're caring for is experiencing muscle spasms, you might not be able to pin down the exact cause. Consider treating the easy and obvious possible causes first:

- **Dehydration** is number one. If it's possible to do without causing swelling and/or breathing problems, have them take in more fluids. A couple pints usually are enough to help. See Swelling and Edema and Shortness of Breath: Dyspnea earlier in this chapter for more information on swelling and breathing problems.

- **Magnesium deficiency** is easy and safe to address with a magnesium supplement.
- **Potassium deficiency** can be addressed with diet. Bananas contain potassium, but be careful as they are quite binding and may make constipation worse. Other good potassium sources include avocados, most fruit (including raisins and prunes), dark-green leafy vegetables like spinach, potatoes with the skin, and mushrooms.
- **Sodium and chlorine deficiency**—two more necessary electrolytes—can be relieved by having a little salt. A small bag of salty potato chips can work wonders. Often a sports drink such as Gatorade will do the trick, but be careful if they have edema, high blood pressure, or weakness of the heart, particularly CHF or other reasons to restrict salt.
- **Irritation in the body.** For people who have a neurological disorder affecting the connection of the brain to the muscle, such as a spinal cord lesion or end-stage Alzheimer's Disease, a muscle spasm might be triggered by something in the body that irritates. A full bladder, a lump in their seat, or anything painful could give spasms. Anything that sooths the nervous system helps in general. We got great relief with just being social, having a good head scratch, and giving a very gentle massage to Karen's feet and hands.

Talk with your loved one's health-care team about other possibilities, especially problems with major organ systems and medications. If muscle spasms happen more than just a little bit, definitely alert the health-care team. Even if the spasms are mild, they might be a sign of medicine interactions or other problems that need to be addressed.

There are medications that can help. Again, talk with your loved one's health-care team. We've included here a brief discussion of antispasmotic and muscle relaxants. There are also other classes of drugs which their doctor may prescribe depending on the patient and the problem. You may find more on benzodiazepines in Anxiety in the beginning of this chapter, and Pain Medications in Chapter 17, Pain Management.

...Antispasmotic and Muscle Relaxant Medication

This class of medications is used to reduce muscle spasm. Most are centrally acting, directly affecting the brain and spinal cord. We still do not completely understand the mechanism of action of these medications other than a general understanding of certain receptors stimulated and the effect of muscle relaxation and often sedation.

Baclofen: This centrally acting muscle relaxant inhibits spinal-cord reflexes by inhibiting monosynaptic and polysynaptic spinal reflexes. It is often used to treat symptoms caused by multiple sclerosis and spinal-cord injuries and diseases.

Cyclobenzaprine (Flexeril): This centrally acting (brain/spinal cord) muscle relaxant potentiates norepinephrine and binds to serotonin receptors, reducing spasticity.

Metaxalone (Skelaxin): This medication's mechanism of action is unknown but it depresses central nervous system activity. It is often well tolerated and less sedating.

Methocarbamol (Robaxin): This suppresses central nervous system activity.

Tizanidine (Zanaflex): This inhibits motor neurons by stimulating alpha-2 receptors, which can reduce spasticity.

...Myoclonus

Myoclonus is when the muscle spasm, or involuntary muscle contraction, is briefer and more shock-like. There are lots of examples of this that occur in normal healthy people, such as hiccups or sleep jerking. Caregivers need to be especially aware of myoclonus because it is one sign of a type of opioid toxicity related to a hyperexcitability of the nerves. If the person you're caring for is on opioids, don't brush these symptoms off. Myoclonus can be very serious and can worsen into constant severe jerking, as well as delusions, hallucinations, and what we call "the hard road" (for more on this, see Opioid Toxicity under Delirium later in this chapter.

Hiccups

Karen would take out a dollar, hold it in front of me, and say, "I'll give you this if you can hiccup again." That was the hiccup cure she learned, and sure enough, I could rarely earn that dollar without faking the next *erp*.

Pretty much everyone has had a case of the hiccups. Usually it's no big deal; they either go away on their own or the dollar, gargling upside down, scaring the bejeezus out of someone, or some other creative cure works its miracle. Most "cures" usually involve some interruption in the breathing, a distraction or change of attention, or anything that stimulates the *phrenic or vagus nerve*. There is no great evidence that one method is any better than another.

Sometimes, however, especially late in life, the hiccups can be severe or go on and on and on. If they last longer than 48 hours, they are labeled "**persistent hiccup**." Usually by that time, most of the "cures" you know have been tried at least once. Nurse Mary says, "We usually go to the meds" in cases of persistent hiccups.

There are several **medication approaches** out there. Antipsychotics like chlorpromazine (the only FDA-approved drug for hiccups), anticonvulsants (see Pain Medications in Chapter 17, Pain Management), or antispasmotics like Baclofen (see above) are sometimes used, but so are a pretty big variety of other things. Each case is different.

The **possible causes** and the person's current medication list need to be considered. In other words, see your loved one's doctor about this one. Also, consider again that any severe, sudden change in symptoms, including the hiccups, warrants notifying their health-care team. Even the silly little hiccup can be one sign for some other more serious medical issues.

Dizziness and Wooziness

For most people, the terms *dizziness* and *wooziness* are somewhat interchangeable. For me, and for this writing, we can make a very important distinction. Let's call wooziness that swimming-in-the-head feeling you might get when you get up too fast or before fainting. And let's say that dizziness is that head-spinning sensation of getting off a spinning carnival ride. But there's more to both of these sensations than this.

...Wooziness

When people are sick, what we're calling wooziness is most often some combination of orthostatic hypotension, hypoxia, and/or medication side effects or interactions. **Orthostatic hypotension** is that drop in blood pressure to the head we all feel when we get up too quickly. When you're sick, it might take much longer for the heart and blood vessels to adjust to the change.

To compensate for this, we ask people to **get up more slowly or in stages.** You might ask the one you love to try sitting up in bed first, just raising the head of the bed or propping up on pillows. They may try making circles with their feet or bending and straightening their knees a few times to help get the blood moving. Usually within 30 seconds to 2 minutes, they are ready to sit at the edge of the bed. A couple easy breaths and shoulder rolls help get things moving some more. In another 30 seconds to 2 minutes, they might be ready to stand and feel OK. If you can take their blood pressure, you might find it's dropped 10–20 mmHg on each rating as they sat or stood up. If this remains low when they are lying down, consult their health-care team.

Hypoxia is a drop in the amount of oxygen in the blood. You might see this as paleness in their face, especially in the edge of the eyelid or fingernail. A pulse oximeter is that device they put on your finger in the hospital to measure the redness—and, thus, the amount of oxygen—in the blood. These devices are now small and inexpensive. You don't necessarily need one, but your loved one's nurse or PT probably has one. We like to see their oxygen saturation rates above 90 percent before they get up.

Getting up in stages helps here too. There also are several techniques to encourage more efficient breathing. **Pursed-lip breathing** is one of my favorites. This is simply to purse the lips on exhale as if blowing out a candle, to create some back pressure. Breathe in through the nose if possible, then exhale slowly against this back pressure. It should take a few seconds. Another technique is a **four-count breath** (three if breathing in deeply makes them cough). Simply inhale for a count of four and exhale for a count of four. Repeat this four times. This is the same Calming Exercise described earlier in this chapter. You can use the two techniques together. I usually see this raise the oxygen saturation 2–6 percentage points. **Supplemental oxygen** has become common in palliative and hospice care. Our hospice team installed a machine in our home before we knew we needed it. Here is the video of the instructions we were given on how to use it https://www.youtube.com/watch?v=YvbSuA_AGZs&t=34s. For more on hypoxia, see Shortness of Breath: Dyspnea earlier in this chapter.

Medications: Your loved one might expect some wooziness if their pain or anxiety medicine dose was recently increased. Getting up in stages helps for this too. It is only a compensation, though. Even if the symptoms are mild, it is best if you and your loved one's health-care team can figure out the source of the problem and address the cause. Many medications can result in wooziness alone or as an interaction. If your loved one is experiencing new or severe wooziness, consult the health-care team right away.

...Dizziness

That head-spinning sensation of getting off a spinning carnival ride—dizziness—we can attribute to a **problem with the sensations of balance**. A healthy person's brain deciphers and compiles signals from three distinct sources: (1) the vestibular organs of the inner ear; (2) vision, especially peripheral vision; and (3) all the billions of receptors throughout our joints, muscles, tendons, skin—the whole-body (*somatosensory*) system. We can rely on just one system if the other two systems are not conflicting. If they are conflicting ... well, ever been seasick?

Signs and symptoms of dizziness include:

- a room-spinning sensation
- *nystagmus*—the eyes flick back and forth as if you're just getting off a carnival ride; this might occur with turning or tipping the head
- nausea, especially with movement of the head
- profound loss of balance, especially in the dark or in visually busy situations
- bumping into walls
- falling down

There are many different problems that can disrupt any of these systems. It is important to get dizziness checked out and properly diagnosed. Also, protect against falls. There is much to do for fall prevention. Please see Home Safety and Physically Helping Your Loved One Move in Chapter 15, Basic Mobility and Transfers. In the meantime, here are some tips to help compensate for each system.

To Help Them with Their Vestibular Balance

An otolaryngologist or ear-nose-throat (ENT) doctor works with the vestibular system and balance disorders in general. This is most likely the type of doctor your loved one will see to gain an accurate diagnosis and begin treatment. A vestibular-trained PT or physiatrist can help compensate for and treat certain types of vestibular disorders and other balance disorders.

To Help Them Better Use Their Visual Balance

- Keep the lights on if they are getting up.
- Be careful in visually busy places; a lot of movement in the peripheral vision is confusing to the visual balance.
- Be ready to catch the fall if there are visual cross cues, like a bus or train that moves in the peripheral vision, making it look to the brain like the world (not the vehicle) is moving.
- Avoid glasses that block the peripheral vision.

To Help Maximize the Balance Sensations from the Body

- Have them watch their feet while they perform 10–20 slow, purposeful ankle circles.
- Gently stretch the calves; this is best if done with them standing.
- If they can do this with minimal symptoms, they can try looking to the side with their eyes, then slowly turn their head toward what they are looking at, keeping their gaze focused. Try this 6–10 times on each side several times each day. They can slowly increase their speed as this becomes easier without symptoms. This also might help the body learn to compensate for vestibular loss.
- If they are having an episode of marked dizziness, sometimes maximizing the sensation of being grounded in the rest of the body helps. If they are standing, leaning their back against the wall and resting their hands on the wall will give their brain more sensation of being stationary. Focusing the gaze on an object and slow, calm breathing also helps.

Constipation

Constipation is a common problem in the healthy population and much more common in people who are frail or ill. The National Institute of Health (NIH) defines constipation as fewer than three bowel movements a week or movements with hard, dry, small stools, which makes them painful and difficult to pass. **Three major factors contribute to constipation:**

1. hard or dry stool
2. weak, slow, or ineffective peristalsis—the smooth-muscle contractions in the intestine
3. clenching of the pelvic-floor muscles

The most common problems for the types of patients who need caregiving are mostly due to the first two factors.

...Preventing Constipation

For most people, a combination of **adjusting the diet, exercising, and having a bowel medication program** can keep things in balance. How to Use Nutrition to Keep the Gut Balanced and Moving in Chapter 12, Food and Nutrition, explains quite a bit about fiber and other dietary considerations, with plenty of links to more information about adjusting the diet.

Nurse Mary recommends **fruit as a great source of fiber** that is gentle on the system—but avoid bananas, especially green ones, as they can be very constipating. Increasing fiber gradually may improve constipation in a patient who continues to take in enough fluid and remains active. However, a sudden increase in fiber can make constipation worse and also cause gas and bloating, especially with low activity and decreased fluid intake. Increasing your loved one's daily regular prune intake by three to five dried prunes or one cup of prune juice can be very effective for acute constipation.

Preventing constipation should start as soon as a narcotic or other constipating medication is prescribed. The prescribing physician or health-care team will often prescribe a regimen that might include **bowel stimulants** such as Senna, **softeners** such as Doss, and recommendations for different types of **fiber, fluid intake, and exercise.** Senna (Senokot) and bisacodyl (Dulcolax), bowel stimulants that trigger contractions of the intestinal muscles, are recommended daily when the patient is using narcotics regularly; they counteract the effects of narcotics on the bowel. Dulcolax is often used in the form of a suppository. Do not let your loved one go off the regimen once the glorious movement is achieved. If they are continuing on the constipating medication, all the factors that stopped them up are still there, even if they had a good movement this morning.

Over time, people develop a tolerance for the pain control of narcotics but, unfortunately, not to its constipating effect. If the narcotic dose is increased to keep pain under control, the Senna dose may need to be increased as well. To make things just a little more complicated, **bowel medications can become less effective over time** and may need adjusting, even if the other medication stays the same. This is where keeping a medication log (see Chapter 11, Medications) and creating a carebook (see Chapter 1, Building a Caregiving Team) can help you.

...Treating Constipation

It is important to differentiate prevention from treating acute constipation. Once things are stopped up, the strategy needs to change. If your loved one is having discomfort such as gas pains, bloating, and nausea along with no bowel movement for three or more days, they have a case of **acute constipation.** If your home treatments are not comfortably effective within 24 hours, you need to contact your loved one's doctor or nurse, as this condition can be more than uncomfortable—it can lead to impaction, which can be life threatening and not a nice way to go.

Once constipation occurs, increasing soluble fiber may only make the problem worse; all that bulk has nowhere to go. Increasing any bowel-stimulant medications such as Senna can cause increased cramping and pain. What is needed is something to **relieve the blockage.** There are quite a few treatments. Nurse Mary finds that polyethylene glycol (Miralax) works well in most cases. She also recommends an enema (see below) as one of the quickest, most effective, and safest treatments in severe cases.

Over-the-Counter Treatments

Prunes and plums are loaded with both soluble and insoluble fiber. They also contain the natural peristalsis stimulant and natural stool softener *sorbitol*, which works by drawing water into the intestines. Increasing their daily regular prune intake by three to five dried prunes or one cup of prune juice in one day can be very effective. (Prunes or prune juice can also be used daily as part of the prevention program.)

Polyethylene glycol (Miralax) works by drawing water into the colon. This is a great medication, very effective and generally the one recommended first. Both Miralax and milk of magneisa (MOM) work in the same way, though MOM is a bit more likely to cause bloating, cramping, gas, and thirst. Miralax is gentler but also more expensive than milk of magnesia.

Stool softeners such as Colace, Doss (docusate), or Surfak also add moisture to the stool. They are often used in conjunction with senna for narcotic-related constipation and can be used to prevent constipation unrelated to narcotics. Prolonged use can cause electrolyte imbalances, but they do not cause the cramping and bloating that many other laxatives do.

Saline laxatives such as magnesium citrate are a type of salt that work to somewhat violently pull water from the body into the colon. They are commonly used prior to surgery or procedures like colonoscopy for which the bowel needs to be completely cleared of stool. It is usually used for constipation in severe cases, as it works so strongly and quickly and can continue to work for 12–24 hours. It will keep the person near the bathroom, and it can cause serious side effects, including dehydration. It is recommended that they drink a large glass of water immediately after taking this. The one time we used this concoction, Karen drank it literally sitting on the toilet. It should not be used on a regular basis, or they can become dependent on it and be unable to have a bowel movement without it.

Enemas work by flushing out the colon, bringing water into the colon from outside the body. They usually work immediately, are short acting (once it's done, it's done), and do not risk dehydration, electrolyte imbalance, or cramping. They are a safe, effective choice. We have provided a superfantastic, absolutely brilliant how-to at the end of this section for your reading pleasure (see below).

Prescription Medications

Prescription medications are generally used when the over-the-counter treatments do not give relief. There are many, often with several names for the same one or similar ones. Here are some of the most commonly used and well-trusted prescription medications:

Lactulose is a form of sugar that pulls fluid into the colon, helping with chronic constipation. It is also used for other conditions such as liver disease. It can cause diarrhea, nausea, and cramping, and patients often do not like the taste or syrupy texture. This medication is very effective, although it does not work quickly and can take up to 48 hours to work initially.

Opioid antagonists: Methylnaltrexone bromide, alvimopan, and naloxone are some of the newer (and very expensive) drugs that counteract the effect of opioids on the bowel without affecting analgesia (pain control) or precipitating withdrawal. These drugs cannot cross the blood-brain barrier, so they can often have opioid antagonist effects throughout the body, counteracting effects such as itching and constipation, but without affecting opioid effects in the brain. Unfortunately, their effect is not perfect and they may increase pain under some circumstances. At this writing, these medications are currently used as a last resort for treating constipation.

Treatment of Pelvic-Floor Muscles

For problems with clenching of the pelvic-floor muscles or a discoordination between the smooth muscles of the colon and the anal sphincter, the strategy is completely different, because these muscles usually function quite automatically. This condition usually needs to be diagnosed by digital exam (doctor's finger). The Mayo Clinic literature also discusses several imaging studies that may help confirm and further define the root causes. They also recommend a treatment protocol that relies heavily on biofeedback to retrain the muscles. For more on this, I refer you to their web page http://www.mayoclinic.org/medical-professionals/clinical-updates/general-medical/retraining-pelvic-floor-muscles-correct-chronic-constipation.

...Performing an Enema

An enema, though awkward and potentially quite messy, is the gentlest, safest, and most effective way to relieve acute constipation. Nurses recommend it when conservative measures fail and before more-severe methods such as ammonium salts. Personally, it was a scary prospect for me, and finding myself headed to the store for enema supplies was more awkward than going for wine coolers or tampons. But I got over it, and therefore so can you.

Gathering Supplies

Enema bag or enema kit: Nurse Mary recommends the old-fashioned heavy rubber hot-water bottle type still available in most drugstores. It holds about a quart and is durable and easy to use. There are enema kits too; Fleet is one popular brand (if you can say "popular" and enema in the same sentence). It is a 4.5-ounce premixed bottle with a prelubricated applicator. If you're getting this, buy several. They are cheap; you might use them later, and you might need more than one now. Also, if you get the Fleet, you can skip the next two items.

Mineral oil: Nurse Mary recommends about 2 tablespoons per quart of warm water. This helps to lubricate the bowel and make things flow more easily.

Lubricant: KY Jelly or another water-based lubricant works best. A dab on the applicator will do.

Latex gloves: Nurse Mary recommends triple-gloving each hand. That way, if you need to, you can dispose of the outer gloves and easily be clean and still double-gloved.

Toilet paper: Duh.

Chuck pads: Lots of them, especially if you are using the standard method of having your loved one lay on their side.

Portable commode: It will likely be easier to get your loved one from the bed to a nearby commode than to the toilet in the bathroom.

A toothpick: I'll tell you about that later.

The Sequence

The usual method is to have the patient **lie on their side on the bed,** with the commode nearby. We recommend that with this method you use chuck pads or other waterproof barriers on the bed, around the commode, and on the path from the bed to the commode. Then follow these steps:

1. Fill the bag with 1 to 1.5 quarts of warm water. Test the temperature on your wrist as you would for baby formula to be sure the water is warm but not hot.
2. Add 2 tablespoons of mineral oil, seal the bag, clamp the hose, and mix.
3. Lubricate the applicator with a dab of water-based gel and insert the applicator you-know-where.
4. Ask the patient to "hold it" as you unclamp the hose and slowly elevate the bag or bottle 1–2 feet above their abdomen. The higher you elevate the bag, the more water pressure it will give. Keep it comfortable, ok?
5. Empty the bag or bottle, having them continue to "hold it." Reclamp the hose to prevent backflow.
6. Remove the applicator and help your loved one get onto the commode. This is where it may get messy, as holding a quart or more of water may be more than just a little difficult.

Nurse Mary suggests having them **sit on the commode or toilet** to apply the enema to minimize the messiness. This method works well with a bag, but not the bottle-type kits. Here's the sequence for this method:

1. Fill the bag with 1 to 1.5 quarts of warm water. Test the temperature on your wrist as you would for baby formula to be sure the water is warm but not hot.
2. Add 2 tablespoons of mineral oil, seal the bag, clamp the hose, and mix.
3. To insert the lubricated applicator, you will have to ask them to stand up a little (or help them with a sit-to-stand transfer).
4. You still need to ask them to hold it, to allow time for the water to soften the stool. Raise the bag to their chest height. Setting it on a countertop or the toilet tank works well.
5. Empty the bag or bottle, having them continue to "hold it." Reclamp the hose to prevent backflow.

6. Once the bag or bottle is empty or things start moving, you can remove the applicator from behind, again standing them up a little so that you can gently pull out, not up, on the applicator tube. Have them stay on the toilet for 10 minutes or so. This allows the stool to soften, or if they already went, it allows time for the second wave.

Cleanup

Lightly moistening the toilet paper makes cleanup more comfortable and thorough. Baby wipes work well, but are not flushable.

This is also a good time to check for redness or skin breakdown around the nether regions and sacrum. Apply any barrier creams (see Wounds or Ulcers later in this chapter), but avoid lotion on the anus other than Preparation H or those prescribed for the anus. The skin is different there and quite a bit more sensitive.

Troubleshooting

If the bag or bottle is not emptying: The little holes in the applicator may be clogged. Reclamp the hose, remove the applicator, poke the holes in the applicator clear using the handy toothpick, and test to make sure you got the applicator cleared. Do this with the applicator above the sink or toilet and keep the bag at the same level as the applicator when you start to unclamp the hose, so it doesn't squirt all over when you unclamp the hose.

The bag is empty and nothing happened: Check to make sure the applicator is in the anus; this is especially an issue if you use the sitting method (you might just be emptying the bag into the toilet). You might need more liquid; this is often the case when using the small premade bottles. Otherwise, you can refill the bag and do the sequence again. Sometimes it takes more than one quart. Just be aware of making them uncomfortable with volume. If they are having increased pain or severe cramping, stop. Allow time for them to empty the bowel of fluid and try again a little later.

Diarrhea

Diarrhea can be one of the most difficult conditions to cope with and treat. It is not only inconvenient and embarrassing, it can cause **dehydration, electrolyte depletion, and skin breakdown.**

There are many causes of diarrhea, and it is important to rule out certain causes, such as an **infection**, which can be caused by taking antibiotics. If your loved one has an infection such as *Clostridium difficile* (*C. diff*) and they take an over-the-counter antidiarrhea medication, this can cause serious complications. Diarrhea can also be caused by **chemotherapy and radiation**, especially to the pelvic area.

...Treating Diarrhea

As a general rule, if diarrhea lasts more than three days, your loved one should see their health-care provider. Up until that point, there are some strategies you can try at home:

- **Keep them hydrated** with drinks such as Gatorade, Pedialyte, and clear juices. Avoid caffeinated beverages, milk, creamed soups, carbonated beverages, juices with fruit pulp, and alcohol.

- **Feed them the BRAT diet:** bananas, rice, applesauce, toast. Less-ripe bananas can be especially helpful for treating diarrhea, as they tend to bind the food-and-waste mass in the gut.
- **Protect their skin** by cleaning with baby wipes with aloe or baby oil after each toileting.
- **Help them take warm baths or sitz baths** (a kit for this can be purchased) several times a day, and use Desitin or vitamin A&D ointment on skin around the anus after each bowel movement.

If the diarrhea is persistent, there are several **over-the-counter and prescription medications** that can be helpful, but these should be used only with your loved one's health-care provider's approval. If the cause of the diarrhea is not what the medication treats, such as an infection, it could make things much worse.

When you take your loved one to their provider, bring **a log of how often they're having diarrhea** and other details, such as whether they are having cramping and what they are eating and drinking, if it happens right after they eat. It may be difficult to recall this information when they see their provider, so this is another situation when keeping a medications log and using basic charting techniques are helpful (see Chapter 11, Medications).

Also, their provider may ask for a **stool sample** so it can be tested for infections and other problems. They should give you instructions for this if they ask for it.

Wounds or Ulcers

By Seth Fader, D.O.

A **wound** is a disruption of tissue due to external violence such as sudden trauma or surgery. In contrast, an **ulcer** is a breakdown in the skin with loss of surface tissue; it is a disintegration of the components of the skin, causing a chronic condition. Most skin injuries treated in wound care are actually ulcers. The most common types are *venous pressure ulcers, diabetic pressure ulcers,* and *arterial ulcers.*

...Pressure Ulcers (bed sores)

Pressure ulcers are **focused areas of skin and underlying tissue damage** resulting from pressure between a firm external surface and an underlying bony prominence. The compressive forces cut off the blood supply, starving the tissue of oxygen and nutrients. At the same time, metabolic waste builds up, causing further damage.

People who are immobile or have lost sensation (such as diabetics or after a stroke) are at **high risk** for developing pressure ulcers. In addition to immobility, shear and friction forces (such as sliding on bed sheets, etc.), moisture (such as from incontinence), and malnutrition can combine to escalate skin damage. Pressure ulcers can be very painful and can become life threatening. The keys to treating a pressure ulcer are prevention and early detection.

Prevention

Proper positioning is essential for anyone who stays in bed a lot. Almost all pressure ulcers (95 percent) occur over a few bony spots or prominences (fig. 34): the base of the spine (*sacrum*), the prominence near the top of the femur (*greater trochanter*), butt bones of the pelvis you sit on (*ischial tuberosity*), back of the heel (*posterior calcaneus*), and outside anklebone (*lateral malleolus*), elbow, and back of scalp (occipital region).

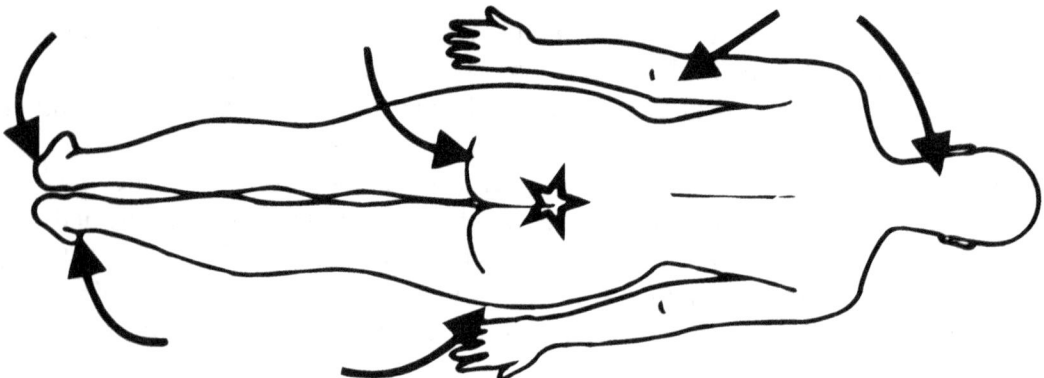

Figure 34. Locations of most pressure ulcers.

Look again at Positioning for Comfort in Chapter 15, Basic Mobility and Transfers; now consider those bony prominences. Most people like to sit up in bed. This puts more pressure in their tailbone, especially if they tend to slide down. Can you pad under their legs and buttocks to form a bucket seat, keeping the pressure off their ischial tuberosities, tailbone, and sacrum? Can you place a pillow under their calves to float their heels in the air? Still, they need to move. If they are now lying on their side, can they be lying three-quarters toward their side or three-quarters toward their stomach, supported by pillows or a rolled blanket to keep the weight off the ischial tuberosity? Can a pillow between their knees and calves help keep their feet off each other? Now that you know the basic principles, you can be creative in how you position, pad, and support.

Minimize wrinkles in the bed sheets as this creates a small pressure area. It also may trap debris which can lead to infections. Be aware of pressure from casts, splints, shoes, or other medical devices such as their wheelchair, as they may cause an ulcer. The same positioning principles apply here as with positioning in a bed.

If they have incontinence, you should have a skin protecting treatment plan such as moisture-barrier lotions and gentle skin cleansers. Incontinence and Peri-care in Chapter 16, Hygiene, will provide you with good management techniques.

Good Nutrition helps prevent ulcers by supporting a healthy immune system (see Eat Right in Chapter 4, Dancing in the Rain: Healthy Habits for Caregivers). A consultation with a registered dietician will help ensure your loved one's daily nutritional needs are met. Look to Chapter 15, Basic Mobility and Transfers, to help with transferring and positioning techniques, as well as support surfaces and mattresses. Nurses and/or therapists can help you here, as well with instructions for specific techniques and recommendations for equipment.

Early Detection and Stages of Ulcers

Take every opportunity you can to check their skin. People at risk should have daily skin checks. Moving them in bed, bathing, toileting, changing clothes, and changing the bed are all good times. Pay extra attention to those areas of bony prominence in Figure 34 above. You may need to 'sneak a peek' into the upper part of the gluteal cleft (yes, that is actually the proper name of the butt crack) to visualize the lower sacrum and tailbone. The first sign of a pressure ulcer is **red skin. If that turns white with pressure** (*blanchable erythema*), it is irritated but not yet an ulcer. At this point you may avoid the ulcer by giving extra attention to keeping the pressure off this area and by using a barrier cream. For specific products, consult with your loved one's nurse or pharmacist. Nurse Julia prefers types with zinc oxide.

If red but intact skin does not blanch with pressure, it has become a **stage-one pressure ulcer.** In individuals with darker skin, the ulcer may appear purple or blue rather than red. The skin will likely be warm to touch and more sensitive, unless there is impaired sensation.

A **stage-two pressure ulcer** is a loss of the outer layer of skin, or a blister. A **stage-three pressure ulcer** is complete loss of the skin layers down to the fat layer. The deepest stage is **stage four, exposing muscle, tendon, and bone**.

Some pressure ulcers may at first be unstageable based on how they look. Intact skin may hide deeper injury, especially if it is heavily bruised or there is a large blood blister. **If you suspect an ulcer, alert your health care team right away. The ulcer should be evaluated by a health care professional trained in wound care.** There are different types of ulcers and wounds and different treatment protocols depending on all the issues a person might have.

Treatment: General Ideas

There are sound basic guidelines that can be applied to most wounds and ulcers. Keeping the wound or ulcer clean and moist enough without being too wet are key. Good old soap and water will work well for cleaning most wound/ulcers and surrounding skin. Even better are gentle wound cleansers available in spray bottles. There are several brands on the market (just type wound cleaners into your search engine). Avoid using hydrogen peroxide or betadine on open wounds. They kill bacteria but they also injure tissue, slowing the healing process. Once clean, some wounds will require debridement which is removal of dead tissue. This can be a delicate art so often it should be done by your wound care specialist.

Keeping the injury moist enough without being too wet depends a lot on dressings. Your health care team should guide you as to what dressing they're using and why. If a wound is draining, the dressing will need to be very absorbent such as foam dressings that can act like a sponge but not stick to the wound bed. If the wound is dry, the dressing should add moisture such as hydrogels which are composed of water and glycerin. Many wounds need topical gels applied to the wound bed, this can be a simple sterile clear gel. A very versatile product that I like is Leptospermum Honey (such as brand name MEDIHONEY GEL). This product derived from honey can be used on most wounds such as burns, ulcers, surgical and other traumatic wounds. It should be avoided for people who are allergic to honey.

As important as proper dressing selection is deciding how frequently the dressing will need to be changed. Very moist draining wounds will likely need dressing changes once or twice daily. Some wounds will do well leaving the dressing on for two to four days. Again, the wound care specialist will guide you on how often this needs to be done. Any wound dressing that is leaking fluid must be replaced since there is a breach in the barrier protecting the wound from infection.

There is a misconception that wounds should be dry and leaving scabs on helps. Healing tissue likes a nice clean surface free of dead tissue and also a moist, warm (body temperature) environment for cells to replicate. Fluids produced at the wound site help naturally clean the wound. The exception to this rule are heel wounds. Dry closed scabs on the heel often should be left alone due to a poor blood supply. Removing the scab may extend the size of the wound.

The other exceptions to this are infections and very deep wounds or ulcers. In these situations, they may need to be left open to drain. This means different types of dressings and may mean a drain line or even a drain pump. This is not something that you as a caregiver will be managing without express instructions from your care team.

As a general rule, wounds caught early should heal over two to four weeks. Ulcers can take some time to heal but should be at least 30 percent smaller in a month. If a wound is not closing, the wound specialist needs to reevaluate the protocol. Based on the health of the individual there are some wounds that will never heal and the goal may be to maintain the wound and reduce pain.

Now that you know some of the general guidelines let's discuss more about those different types of ulcers and some of the specific strategies for treatments.

Venous Pressure Ulcers

The most common pressure ulcer is the **venous stasis ulcer**, accounting for at least 70 percent of ulcers medically treated. Although arteries and veins have the same layers of tissue, veins have much less smooth muscle and connective tissue and are therefore vulnerable to being stretched and dilated. Over time this causes leakage of fluids into surrounding tissue, which triggers inflammation and damage. White blood cells release destructive enzymes. This, combined with impaired blood flow to the skin, triggers skin breakdown. Red blood cells rupture and stain the skin. This chronic inflammation changes the appearance and texture of the skin, causing a condition called *lipodermatosclerosis*.

Venous ulcers usually **form below the knee**, often in the region of the inner anklebone (medial malleolus). These ulcers are shallow, with irregular roundish borders and often heavy drainage which wets the borders and wears them away. These ulcers are both painful and very vulnerable to infection.

Special treatment for a venous ulcer includes all things which assist the veins and lymph vessels in moving fluid back to the heart. This relieves the excess pressure in the skin, allowing it to repair. All the things which help with pitting edema (discussed earlier in this chapter) may also help here. The **mainstay treatment** for venous ulcers is compression therapy.

Prior to beginning compression therapy, it is important to assess the state of the arterial blood supply to rule out peripheral arterial disease. Compression applied to a limb with poor arterial blood flow can lead to loss of blood flow to the limb.

Dressings used over the venous ulcer need to be able to absorb drainage and must be changed when saturated with fluid. **Multilayer compression therapy** may be very effective initially, but it should be evaluated and changed twice weekly. There are several options for administering compression; the health-care team makes decisions based on the patient's needs. If the venous ulcer is not responding to treatment, then infection should be suspected and treated. As a caregiver you can watch for signs of infection: bad smell, pussy or yellow drainage, red angry looking skin around the wound, and/or a mild fever.

Once the ulcer is healed, compression socks should be used daily. There is a high rate of recurrence after healing. If the patient is healthy enough, surgery such as **laser ablation** of the leaky veins can dramatically reduce symptoms and may cure the ulcers completely.

Diabetic Pressure Ulcers

Of the 20 million people in the United States who have diabetes, 15–25 percent will develop ulcers on their feet or legs. Diabetes attacks the nervous system and the vascular system, altering sensation, blood flow, and the musculoskeletal system. The damage to multiple systems makes diabetic patients uniquely **vulnerable to forming ulcers at pressure points** such as the heels and balls of the feet (metatarsal head). Diabetes can gradually change the shape of the foot and ankle, called **charcot foot**, http://care.diabetesjournals.org/content/34/9/2123 creating more pressure points and areas of skin breakdown. These ulcers often recur in the same area. Since the immune system and circulation are compromised, diabetic ulcers are often infected.

Prevention is critical. This includes daily skin checks, fitted shoes, and soft orthotics. White socks help a person see signs of bleeding and fluid leakage too. Patients with well-controlled blood sugar are far less likely to develop such ulcers. High-risk patients may require orthopedic or vascular surgery to prevent future skin damage. Diabetic ulcers are difficult and treatment is complex. Even with good care, 15–25 percent lead to amputation. This makes diabetes the number-one cause of nontraumatic amputation in the United States. If your loved one has diabetes and you see signs of an ulcer, get help. Get treatment now.

...Arterial Ulcers

Arterial ulcers are a result of **diminished arterial blood flow**, which starves the tissue of vital oxygen and nutrients. Ulcers from arterial insufficiency occur most often in the lower leg, and the initial trigger of the ulcer is often minor trauma such as bumping a lower leg on furniture. We usually see them over the outer anklebone (lateral malleolus), shin, or toes. The diminished blood flow results when arteries are damaged by *atherosclerosis*: hardening of the blood vessels, which starts from elevated cholesterol and is escalated by stress, smoking, hypertension, diabetes, obesity, and advanced age.

The ulcer is usually quite painful and may be worse when elevating the leg. Usually the wound is first small and shallow and gradually becomes worse, forming a round lesion, usually with little bleeding or drainage. Because the blood flow is poor, **infection is a big risk,** so arterial ulcers can lead to gangrene and may lead to an amputation.

Treatment

Unlike venous ulcers, arterial ulcers should not be treated with compression therapy since this will cut off an already compromised blood supply. This is also true for elevating the affected limb. **Regular exercise** has been shown to improve arterial insufficiency by creating collateral circulation around the blockage, helping to restore blood flow. This takes a little time, though (weeks), so patience and persistence are important, as well as good wound care. Some patients are candidates for vascular bypass surgery or stenting to restore blood flow.

...Skin Tears

Immobile or elderly patients often have thin, fragile skin. This puts them at risk for skin tears such as scratches or cuts. This type of wound commonly occurs on the forearms or lower legs, areas vulnerable to "bumping injuries." Long-sleeved shirts and long pants may provide enough protection to reduce the incidence of such wounds. Bringing wound edges together when possible is often desirable to reduce healing time. Keeping it clean, covered, and not too dry or wet usually helps it heal.

...Reopened Surgical Wounds

A surgical wound can sometimes split open again. Many factors can contribute to this, such as tension at the closure site, infection, malnutrition, smoking, impaired immune system (diabetes, steroid use), or loss of blood supply. Reopened surgical wounds need to be **evaluated by the surgeon** to decide if they should be reclosed or left to heal on their own.

Infections and Compromised Immune Systems

By Rosalind Billharz, PhD (Microbiology)

We live in a world teeming with microorganisms too small to see with the naked eye. While bacteria, fungi, viruses, protozoa, prions, and helminths all have the potential to cause disease, the vast majority of these microbes are harmless to humans most of the time. In fact, we derive great benefits from them. Bacteria in the human gastrointestinal (GI) tract play an important role in digestion, vitamin production, and the immune response. We even ingest these "good" bacteria in the form of probiotics (see Balancing Intestinal Flora in Chapter 12, Food and Nutrition). Similarly, bacteria adapted to live on human skin outcompete harmful microbial pathogens, thereby preventing infections. Normal microbial flora inhabiting human skin and the GI tract outnumber human cells about ten to one.

Without the beneficial activity of these microbes, we as humans would not be alive today. We will never live in a sterile world, nor would we want to. So how clean is clean enough? For most people with a normal healthy immune system, we need only to prevent exposure to known pathogens. Simply said, wash your hands after using the toilet, and stay away from people if you are showing signs of an illness. If you have a fever, runny nose, or cough or know that you were recently exposed, it might be best to stay home.

Things change if you are in contact with someone with a compromised immune system. The first line of defense in our immune system is our skin and the fluid systems around our eyes nose, mouth, and airway. If you or your loved one has a break in the skin, this is a portal for infections. If it is on your hands, use gloves and wash your hands frequently. Use a moisturizing lotion to prevent cracks in your skin. If your loved one has a wound or ulcer, wash your hands and use gloves before touching anything around the lesion. Applying a small amount of antimicrobial cream (enough to cover the wound but not enough to wet the surrounding healthy skin) and keeping the wound covered with a clean, dry dressing helps. Keep sheets and clothing in the area clean and dry.

The secondary immune system involves our white blood cell and antibody system. As we begin to talk about care for *immunocompromised patients* (people with a compromised secondary immune system), a basic understanding of the microbial world is essential for establishing the hygiene "best practices" necessary to protect them from infection.

Not all patients are immunocompromised in the same way or for the same reasons. An individual's genetics, age, disease progression, drug regimen, and presence of other infections—for example, human immunodeficiency virus (HIV) or hepatitis C virus—can all dramatically impact that person's immune response. Nevertheless, several **common-sense measures** are appropriate when caring for *any* immunocompromised patient. These habits are simple, inexpensive, easily taught, very practical, and reasonably effective.

...Hygiene Best Practices

The goal of implementing hygiene best practices is to **reduce and/or prevent infections**. Often, the microorganisms living in or on the patient are the source of infection. Other times, microorganisms in the environment are to blame: they can be ingested with food, inhaled from the surrounding air, or introduced via invasive medical devices like catheters.

The Importance of Hand Hygiene

Human hands connote care and healing, so it is somewhat ironic that poor hand hygiene on the part of unwitting caregivers is often the cause of disease transmission. This is especially true as caregivers go from room to room and patient to patient. **Good hand hygiene** is one of the best things a caregiver can strive for to protect the patient. The Centers for Disease Control and Prevention (CDC) have published a free *Guideline for Hand Hygiene in Health-Care Settings*: http://www.cdc.gov/mmwr/preview/mmwrhtml/rr5116a1.htm This document is a lot to read but it does give a good "best practices" for hand washing and cleaning. Here's the basics.

Hand washing with antibacterial soap and warm water, followed by ethanol- or chlorhexidine-based hand-sanitizer use, is preferred to the simple use of hand sanitizer alone (although caregivers should always carry hand sanitizer). Caregivers should always wash their hands before and after preparing meals and after using the bathroom. Contact with animals or other sick patients also calls for hand washing, as does any significant time spent in public spaces where doorknobs, handrails, touch pads, and elevator buttons are rarely sanitized.

Develop a hand-washing routine, such as singing "Happy Birthday" (perhaps not audibly), which is helpful in ensuring each hand-washing session lasts long enough to be effective. Avoid excessively long fingernails and/or false nails, and clean under nail beds carefully (scrub brushes are sold for this purpose). Use warm, not cold water. Wash forearms as well as hands. Use a clean towel to turn off the faucet and to handle doorknobs when exiting a bathroom. Because frequent hand washing and use of hand sanitizer can dry the hands, opt for a nongreasy hand lotion to prevent hands from chapping or cracking.

Encourage the immunocompromised patient to follow diligent hand-washing guidelines both before and after use of the toilet to minimize urinary tract infections. Encourage the patient to close the toilet lid before flushing.

Insist that visitors wash their hands with soap and water before spending time with the patient. Make sure the hand-washing area is visible to caregivers, visitors, and the patient. Keep it stocked with liquid soap (bar soap is not as hygienic), clean towels, and hand sanitizer. Place hand sanitizer in multiple locations around the living area. Use signage liberally to gently remind visitors that hand washing is not optional, and include instructions for effective hand washing directly above the sink. In cases where the patient is extremely immunocompromised, it may even be worth offering visitors disposable latex or nitrile gloves (although these gloves usually do not ship sterile from the factory).

Personal Hygiene Precautions

In addition to following good hand hygiene, immunocompromised patients should consider certain other aspects of their personal care. They should generally **avoid nonessential invasive devices or procedures** (for example, tampons, suppositories, enemas, douches). They should limit **nail care** to gentle filing and cuticle care; artificial nails are not advised. Because of its propensity to flake off and spread bacteria, nail polish is also discouraged. Have them keep a personal box of nail-care utensils that they do not share with others. Similarly, they should avoid public manicure-pedicure salons. Also have them avoid sharing makeup, eye drops, lip balm, etc. For shaving, electric razors are recommended because they are less likely to break the skin.

Dental care is more complex for the immunocompromised patient. Have them use a toothbrush with soft bristles and store it in a cupboard or with a toothbrush cover so that toilet aerosols cannot reach it. They should not share a toothbrush with others, and they should clean or swap the toothbrush for a new one frequently, even weekly. Most dishwashers can effectively sanitize a toothbrush. Take care, too, when scheduling dentist visits. Even a simple cleaning or minor procedure can lead to infection in the immunocompromised patient. Consult with your loved one's doctor before scheduling a dental procedure.

Visitor Guidelines

Visitors can unintentionally cause harm by exposing the immunocompromised patient to pathogens. Ask visitors to call before arriving, and employ good signage to educate visitors about the importance of removing their shoes at the door and washing their hands. Gently but firmly refuse any visitor with obvious symptoms of illness, even a minor head cold. Children and adults who were recently vaccinated should not visit immunocompromised patients, as live vaccines (including those for influenza, measles, rubella, chicken pox, mumps, and polio) can be contagious and cause harm to a sick immunocompromised patient.

Food and Water Guidelines

Food is not sterile, nor was it ever intended to be. In fact, we would not have beer, wine, chocolate, yogurt, soy sauce, sauerkraut, cheese, sausage, and countless other foods without bacteria and fungi. Humans ingest microbes in their food with every meal. Thus, the goal of preparing food for the immunocompromised patient is not to serve sterile (that is, microbe-free) food but, rather, to **minimize the risk that microbes in the food will cause illness and/or infection**. Common sense goes a long way.

Keep a clean kitchen, and regularly sanitize surfaces with a 10 percent bleach solution or a comparable disinfectant. Dedicate a separate cutting board for raw meat and another for fresh produce, and do not cross-contaminate them. Opt for dishwasher-safe cutting boards. Cook food well-done, especially meat, eggs, and seafood. Wash fresh produce thoroughly, peeling fruits and vegetables when possible. Avoid bringing the patient to salad bars and buffets.

Purchase pasteurized food whenever possible, including beer and honey! Refrain from cutting off moldy food sections and eating the remainder—think cheese. It is far safer to discard the entire food if any part of it is moldy. Pay close attention to "sell by" and "use by" dates on foods. While immune-competent individuals can often get away with consuming foods past these dates, this is not a safe gamble for the immunocompromised patient.

Store prepared food wisely. Use shallow covered containers to refrigerate food, and do not leave food at room temperature for more than two hours if it normally requires refrigeration. Do not leave open or prepared foods in the refrigerator longer than three days.

As a general rule, **avoid herbal supplements**. They are not typically regulated by the FDA, and their use can be counterproductive to other drugs a patient is taking. Herbal supplements can even be toxic. Always seek the opinion of the patient's physician before using an herbal supplement. The **probiotics** industry is also poorly regulated by the FDA, and many products on the market make false or exaggerated claims as to their effectiveness. Physicians often will recommend probiotic use following treatment with a broad-spectrum antibiotic, but patients with blood cancers should not use probiotics. As in the case with herbal supplements, seek the advice of your loved one's physician before including probiotics in a patient's care.

Drinking water from the kitchen tap is generally very safe in the United States, Canada, and Europe. The same cannot be said for well water, which should be tested for safety annually if the water will be used by an immunocompromised patient. Public drinking fountains often harbor microbes, as do the produce misters at grocery stores. These microbes may not be pathogens, but the immunocompromised patient should avoid them.

Swimming poses certain risks for the immunocompromised patient. Lakes, ponds, rivers, and oceans all contain microorganisms with the potential to cause disease. Public pools and hot tubs are usually treated with chlorine-based disinfectants, which tend to be very effective. Nevertheless, patients with a weakened immune system are often advised to **avoid public pools and hot tubs**, as cleaning and maintenance guidelines vary and may not be followed or enforced. Swimming is also problematic for patients with exposed tubes or catheters, which should never be submerged in water.

Keeping Sex Safe

The term "safe sex" takes on a whole new meaning for the immunocompromised patient. Patients with low platelet or white blood cell counts may be advised against intercourse, but this will vary on a case-by-case basis. Those who do engage in intimacy should avoid sexual practices that promote oral exposure to feces. Male partners of male patients should use condoms, which can also minimize exposure of the nonpatient to chemotherapy drugs. Use of lubricants is helpful in both sexes, to minimize irritation and/or tears in the lining of the vagina and/or rectum. Urinate after sex if possible to reduce the risk of a urinary tract infection, and clean the genital area very well both before and after intercourse.

Caring for Pets and Livestock

Certain animals should be avoided by the immunocompromised patient in every circumstance. These include farm animals, reptiles, birds, fish, and rodents. Cats with claws should also be avoided. In general, patients should minimize time spent with cats and dogs and follow strict hand-washing guidelines after handling these pets. Sick pets, particularly pets with diarrhea, should be removed from the home until they are healthy. Vacuum cleaners with HEPA filters will trap fungal spores, dust mites, and bacteria brought in by pets. Last, cleaning of litter boxes, cages, kennels, and aquariums should be relegated to a healthy person, not the patient. In fact, patients should never handle urine or fecal matter of any sort.

Precautions When Traveling Away from Home

Immunocompromised patients should **avoid crowded public areas**: as a rule of thumb, if they are within an arm's length of others, consider the area crowded. They should avoid small closed spaces where germs can accumulate, such as a crowded elevator or reception area. Airplanes use HEPA filters to recirculate cabin air, but it is important to recognize that respiratory viruses are too small to be trapped by the pores of a HEPA filter. Therefore, these viruses will continue to circulate with the rest of the plane air. When in the car with the patient, recirculate the cabin air and keep windows closed. Have them use an N95 respirator mask when visiting care clinics or other public places.

They should also wear this respirator when gardening and **avoid digging in soil** or mulch, as it is rich in microorganisms that could potentially cause harm to the immunocompromised patient. Generally speaking, patients should wear masks if they come within two football fields of a construction or digging site.

Minimize the risk of falls both at home (see Fall Prevention in Chapter 15, Basic Mobility and Transfers) and while traveling. Falls frequently lead to cuts or open sores, and these in turn allow opportunistic pathogens the chance to establish an infection. Stairs, slick surfaces, and uneven ground can all promote falling. Consider installing extra handrails in the home; have the patient take the elevator instead of the stairs when away from the home; and encourage a patient to choose common-sense footwear to avoid falling.

...Signs and Symptoms of Infection

As a rule, infections that are treated early are most likely to heal, with a minimum of "collateral damage" to the patient. *Do not hesitate* to call a nurse or doctor if any of the following signs or symptoms occurs:

- fever above 100.5°F (38.05C), with or without chills
- signs of inflammation at a wound: excessive heat, tenderness, redness, swelling
- sore throat
- new cough
- abnormal urination: frequent, burning, urgent
- any other sign or symptom that may indicate infection, such as sinus pain

The chart in Figure 35 lists some of the more common biological agents that cause infections in immunocompromised patients. While it is not an exhaustive list, it may be helpful for both patients and caregivers who wish to better understand the specific risks associated with different parts of the body.

Figure 35. Causes of Common Infections

Location of Infection	Common Infectious Agents
Surgical wounds	*Staphylococcus aureus* ("Staph".; including MRSA) *Escherichia coli (E. coli)* *Enterococcus* species (including VRE)
Lungs (pneumonia)	*Klebsiella pneumoniae* *Pseudomonas aeruginosa* *Staphylococcus aureus* (including MRSA) *Enterobacter* species *Escherichia coli*
Intravenous catheter	*Staphylococcus epidermidis* *Staphylococcus aureus* (including MRSA) *Enterococcus* species (including VRE) *Candida* species
Urinary catheter	*Escherichia coli* *Enterococcus* species (including VRE) *Pseudomonas aeruginosa* *Klebsiella* species

MRSA = Methicillin-resistant *Staphylococcus aureus*
VRE = Vancomycin-resistant *Enterococcus*

Source: Mechanisms of Microbial Disease, *4th ed., by Engleberg, DiRita, and Dermody (Lippincott Williams and Wilkins, 2006).*

You don't need years of medical-school training to provide excellent care! Often, caregivers for the immunocompromised patient are partners, friends, and/or family members with little to no formal training in health care. Hopefully this section will encourage those who worry that they will not be capable of handling the logistics of caring for their loved one on a day-to-day basis. When it comes to reducing the risk of infection in the immunocompromised patient, practical common sense will serve you well. An awareness of the abundance of microbes in our environment and in our bodies is the first step. Practicing excellent hygiene and educating others will follow naturally from this heightened awareness.

Also referenced for this section: The Johns Hopkins Hospital Patient Information Pamphlet "Care at Home for the Immunocompromised Patient" (revised/reviewed June 2012).

Delirium: The Hard Road

When we first began to talk about delirium, nurse Mary said simply, "We call that the Hard Road." It's still assumed by many seasoned caregiving professionals that the Hard Road is inevitable—it just happens sometimes. All we can do is manage it as best we can and keep the patient as safe and comfortable as possible.

While this may be true for many people, there is a growing body of evidence and medical literature challenging this belief. In some cases, delirium may be preventable. The key is to recognize the signs early, get at the root of the problems, and treat the problems more than the symptoms. At this point in this book, you are probably sick of reading that the list of contributing factors is long. Well, it is. Sorry. Still, it is not an impossible list, and many things can be done in a shotgun approach that are pretty safe and not too difficult to do.

Karen walked more than a few feet down the Hard Road. My mom was full in. With Karen we were lucky, probably because I was quite aware of the signs after the experience with my mom, and early on we alerted our medical team. By reading this chapter, you too can be aware of the early signs.

...Signs and Symptoms of Delirium

1. The most basic signs of delirium are changes in cognitive function in one or more of five different areas:
2. Difficulty either staying attentive and focused or switching focus
3. Short-term memory loss
4. Anxiety or mood changes
5. Changes in sleep patterns, especially sleeping during the day and waking during the night
6. Difficulty with basic motor tasks such as writing a sentence or tracing a shape

Delirium may manifest in different ways, and your loved one's illness and some of the normal responses to the medication they are on can also give some of these signs, so the signs are often misinterpreted. Here are some pointers:

- **Delirium differs from dementia** in that it fluctuates much more. It can come on quickly, sometimes in hours, whereas dementia may take years. It often comes and goes over the day, whereas dementia progresses fairly steadily over months and years.

- **Delirium differs from psychosis** in that psychosis rarely affects peoples' sense of time and place. They usually know what day it is and where they are, even if they are telling stories of spacemen.
- **Delirium differs from drowsiness** associated with most medication, which usually stabilizes after 7–10 days of a steady dose. Delirium worsens.
- **Delirium differs from depression** in that delirium is associated more with cognitive impairment.
- **Delirium's presentation may change through the day,** at times agitated and psychotic with hallucinations and other times quiet and just out of it, seemingly depressed.
- **Different causes of delirium** may be associated with specific signs and symptoms. More on that below.

...Looking for Causes

So let's say you begin to notice increased signs of anxiety (beginning of this chapter). Perhaps you also notice some disassociation or confusion: Your loved one is confused about what day it is or whether it's morning or evening. Perhaps they tell you of feelings of disassociation or hallucinations. Perhaps they've recently lost their ability to write or repeat a few words you just said.

Call their doctors, particularly the ones prescribing medications. They should rule out some of the easy causes, such as:

- dehydration
- vitamin deficiency
- metabolic imbalances such as electrolyte imbalance or low blood sugar
- low or very high blood pressure
- low oxygen in the blood
- infection
- the results of organ failure, especially the liver or kidneys
- medication history: look in depth for unwanted side effects, toxic reactions, interactions; more on this below

Their doctors might do brain imaging such as an MRI (magnetic resonance imaging) or a CT (computerized tomography) scan, and they might do an EEG (electroencephalogram). Typically delirium presents with low EEG, though it is usually diagnosed bedside by physical exam.

...Medication Problems

As for medication issues, there are many drugs that can cause or contribute to delirium. The three most common culprits for causing delirium in the very sick or dying are **opioids, benzodiazepines, and steroids.**

The important thing is to notice the signs early and alert your loved one's healthcare team. If they do not review the medication list thoroughly and simply try to manage the symptoms with more drugs, consider getting a second opinion. Early and thorough treatment of delirium is the key.

Opioid Toxicity

Our medical community is making better efforts to control pain these days. In this effort, we are using more opioids. We now recognize opioid toxicity as one of the major contributors to the Hard Road. Like all these contributors, catching it early is critical.

Besides the signs and symptoms at the start of this section, opioid toxicity may make nerves in the brain and body hyperexcitable. This means they fire when they are not supposed to. One sign of this is muscle spasms and, more directly, muscle jerking: **myoclonus** (earlier in this chapter). Another is **itching** (earlier in this chapter); you might also notice **bronchospasms**—kind of like asthma in someone who doesn't have asthma.

Other signs of opioid toxicity include **hyperalgesia** (sensation that should normally be comfortable, like light to medium touch, is painful) and **allodynia** (all-over body pain). This is a particularly tough paradox for some clinicians, as the patient complains of more pain, requesting more pain medicine. Farther down this same road lie hallucinations, delirium, and seizures. If you see these signs, especially coupled with the other signs of delirium, contact your loved one's doctor right away. Let them know of all the signs you are seeing.

Normally morphine and most of the drugs derived from it are metabolized in the liver and excreted by the kidneys. The breakdown process has multiple stages. The molecules from these intermediate stages are called metabolites. Problems with the liver or kidneys, or with decreased blood fluid volume to these organs—as with dehydration, congestive heart failure, or other severe cardiovascular disease—may lead to more of these metabolites in the system. Certain metabolites—morphine 3 glucuronate and morphine 6 glucuronate—are thought to be the primary contributors to opioid neurotoxicity. If their **liver or kidneys slow down**, you can expect more chance of toxicity even if their opioid dose hasn't changed.

Increasing fluid intake may help clear the metabolites if the kidneys and heart are working well enough.

Decreasing opioid dosage needs to be done carefully so as not to send them into withdrawal. **Changing the type of opioid** can often change the metabolite picture and solve the problem. Figure 36 is a basic chart of the three main classes of opioids.

Figure 36. Three Main Classes of Opioids

Opioid Class	Drugs
Phenanthrenes	Morphine Hydromorphone Oxymorphone Codeine Hydrocodone Oxycodone Levoraphanol
Phenylpiperadines	Fentanyl Remifentayl Meperidine Sufentanil
Diphenylheptanes	Methadone Propoxyphene

Treatment may include a combination of changing the class of opioid and decreasing the overall equivalent dose. If a decrease is made, your loved one will need other ways to manage pain. For more ways to manage pain, both with and without medications, see Chapter 17, Pain Management.

Benzodiazapines—The Paradox

Benzodiazepines are one of the drugs of choice for anxiety and agitation. The most common drugs in this class are lorazapam (Ativan) and diazapam (Valium). There are others; please see Benzodiazapines in Chapter 14, Sleep, for the other drugs in this group, their uses, and their side effects.

If you have ever used benzos or seen them in use, you know how sedating they can be. The **sedation effect** alone can contribute to the disorientation that is such a feature of delirium. On the other hand, benzos can allow someone to relax enough to reorient. This is part of the paradox of benzos: we often use them for the anxiety associated with disease, declining mental function, and opioid use, as well as the agitation in active delirium, but they can cause more of these symptoms or, simply, cause delirium.

Like opioids, benzos are broken down in the liver and excreted by the kidneys. Any problems with these organs may lead to a **drug buildup.** A person may also experience a buildup of the many different intermediate forms the drug molecule goes through as it's broken down. There's a fairly wide range of problems and other drugs that may interfere with steps in the breakdown process, and some of the intermediate forms affect the body and brain. This is a second source of benzo-caused delirium.

Also like opioids, benzos are physically addictive. As a person continues to use the drug, some **dose escalation** occurs (they need more of it to gain the same effect). This can give more intermediate forms in their system. Also, if the person suddenly stops the drug, they may experience withdrawal. Delirium tremens (DTs) is the classic withdrawal sign. It is similar to alcohol withdrawal and has such street names as pink elephants, the shakes, and the horrors because it often has hallucinations and sometimes violent shaking. You could call this the third source of delirium from a drug we often use to treat the problem it is supposed to help. Backing off the use of benzos must be done carefully under physician supervision both to prevent withdrawal and to address the reasons the benzos were given in the first place.

Steroid-Induced Psychosis

Glucocorticoid drugs, or steroids for short, refers to a class of drugs that mimic one of our body's stress hormones, cortisol. **Prednisone, cortisone, hydrocortisone, and dexamethasone**—as well as several others—are all in this class. These drugs are one of our strongest, safest ways to shut down our inflammation response. They are often used to treat the pain, swelling, and tissue damage associated with excessive inflammation.

They are stress hormones, however. One of the first side effects people often notice when they initially start on them is the **prednisone high**. They feel great. They suddenly have lots of energy, they talk a mile a minute, they are ready to get things done. This is the manic phase or, if not too excessive, hypomania. Onset of **mild hypomanic symptoms** in the first few days of increased dosage is not uncommon. This often decreases over a few days and people return to normal.

The more serious symptoms might follow the hypomanic symptoms or may come on almost any time later.

The flip side to the prednisone high is distractibility, restlessness, insomnia, anxiety, and fear. In the longer term, this can develop into more pronounced mania and/or periods of indifference, lethargy, and depression. Other long-term side effects include an increased or even insatiable appetite, weight gain, and eventually diabetes. The **cognitive deficits** that began as mild difficulty in remembering words can grow into confusion, psychosis, delirium, or dementia.

Treatment: The good news is that these effects are pretty much reversible by decreasing the dose. Doses below 40 mg per day or equivalent of prednisone had minimal risk. Risk went up in the elderly, in women, and in those also using a tricyclic antidepressant.

Be careful in helping your loved one to go off these drugs too, as **rapid withdrawal may also give symptoms.** If going off the steroid is more dangerous than the symptoms they are causing, there are other ways to manage the symptoms. I liked this article best http://www.the-rheumatologist.org/details/article/867939/When_Steroids_Cause_Psychosis.html. Partner well with your loved one's medical team. Again, keeping a medication log helps (see Chapter 11, Medications).

...Hospital Shock

A word about what we call "hospital shock": It can be incredibly disorienting to injure yourself or become sick enough to wake up in a hospital bed or nursing home. Sometimes that itself gives a delirium we call **hospital shock**. Suddenly your loved one feels awful and they are in a strange room with all sorts of new people who seem to change each shift. They may have their sleep disturbed by a roommate or by the necessities of medical monitoring. Their safe, familiar environment is gone.

It's not uncommon for people to become disoriented, and it's sometimes difficult for them to come back to the reality they know and love. One of the best things you can do is to be there when they wake up. Visit often. Hold their hand. Talk to them even if they are unconscious. Bring pictures and familiar things from home. Read the list in the next section below.

...Managing the Hard Road

Sometimes, despite everyone's best efforts, there are problems with the brain that are beyond treatment. Delirium can still happen. The hardest part for most caregivers is that their loved one is anxious and agitated. Sometimes the best you can do is help minimize their anxiety (earlier in this chapter) and keep them comfortable and safe. This section provides some tips to help.

Help Them Keep Hold of or Regain Hold of Reality

- **Help them use eyeglasses or hearing aids**, if they have them. Getting them clear sensory input helps.
- **Help them reorient to time.** A clock they can see, a calendar, a date book, a written schedule for the day all help.
- **Introduce visitors** even if they know them. You might need to introduce yourself too as you walk into their awareness.

- **Bring pictures and familiar things from home** if they are in an unfamiliar place, like a hospital. Waking up in a hospital or nursing home is disorienting enough. A few pictures from home can help give comfort and grounding.
- **Tune the radio or TV to something they like.** Understand that understimulation can be as hard on them as overstimulation. Sometimes a radio with their favorite music helps. Usually I'm not a fan of mindless daytime TV, but tuning to one of their favorite movies might bring joy and grounding.

Keep Them as Comfortable as Can Be

- **Minimize excessive noise and glaring lights.** Warm yellow light (like an incandescent bulb) works much better than glaring white light (like the old fluorescent bulbs).
- **Keep the temperature where they like it,** where their home is usually. Oftentimes older people like it a bit warmer than you or I might. Blankets or a warm rice-bag hot-pack work well for warmth. A cool washcloth on the forehead works well to cool.
- **Look for things that might make them uncomfortable or cause pain.** Common problems are poor positioning or postures (see Positioning for Comfort in Chapter 15, Basic Mobility and Transfers), knotted or twisted bedding, urinary retention, constipation (earlier in this chapter), and developing pressure ulcers (earlier in this chapter). That said, try to minimize poking and prodding, especially at odd hours or off their schedule.

Keep Communication Clear, Concise, and Kind

- **Simple one-step messages** in short, clear sentences work best.
- **Face to face** works best. Try not to talk across the room or behind them.
- **Write it down** if it's something you want them to remember. Write it large enough for them to read it (when they are doing better) and put it where they can see it.
- **Bring it into *their* field of vision** if it's something you want to show them.

Keep Them Safe

- **Keep them from falling out of bed.** If they are at risk of falling out of bed, it might be easiest to put the bed on or very close to the floor. This will make it harder for them to get up, though. Sometimes we put a mattress in front of the bed so if they fall out, they get a soft landing. Be very careful with the bed rails if they're using a hospital-type bed. People in this state can get themselves twisted in the railings.
- **Have someone with them all the time** if that's needed. A small number of familiar people work best. For more on resources here, see Chapter 1, Building a Caregiving Team, and Chapter 2, Calling in the Pros.
- **Keep them from falling.** Please read Fall Prevention and Physically Helping Your Loved One Move in Chapter 15, Basic Mobility and Transfers.

A Few More Thoughts on Delirium

There are medications to treat different symptoms and aspects of delirium. Specific lists or recommendations are beyond the scope of this writing and are best left to the good judgment of your loved one's health-care team. These medications can be very helpful. **Do seek help.**

Toward the very end of life, some delirium is common. This is often not preventable but **part of the normal process** as the body and brain begin to shut down. The same tips in this section will be helpful at that time, but there are other things to consider too. For more on this, please read Chapter 20, Near the End.

Delirium is one of the hardest things you and your loved one may face together. Remember the person you love as they were when they were healthy. Now they may be confused, agitated, scared, or angry. It is just a result of parts of their brain not working well. They are still in there. You still love them. Try to make this as easy on both of you as possible. Good luck to you and to the person you love.

Chapter 19. Dementia

Now that we are all living longer, dementia has become one of the most prevalent and most difficult reasons someone will require caregiving. Western medicine has made tremendous strides in treating heart disease, cancer, arthritis, and many other ailments, but we are still in our infancy in understanding the brain. Currently there are more than 60 different known diseases that all give rise to the experience we collectively call dementia. Alzheimer's is the most common and most widely known, but it is but one disease, and there are many. The signs and symptoms may differ, as may the underlying pathology, and the treatment for one disease may be disastrous for a different one.

If you notice a change in your loved one's mental status, please seek medical help. The most common things people notice early on involve problems making new memories. This means remembering things that happened recently, like breakfast or a visit from Aunt Hilda. Another problem might involve finding words or recognizing familiar words. They might also have difficulty with focus, either switching away from something or maintaining attention. These things combined make it difficult for them to follow a story. You might notice they repeat things, like the same question, or are waiting for Aunt Hilda when she visited yesterday. They might also have difficulty reasoning or solving simple problems. We often consider dementia as affecting at least two of these areas of mental function enough to affect their daily life. Usually with dementia the onset of these problems is gradual.

There are things besides brain disease that may change someone's mental status. **Medication interactions or reactions**, **infection**, and **metabolic problems** such as dehydration are some of the most common problems affecting mental function. These tend to come on more suddenly. Any **lesion in the brain**, such as from a tumor, damage from a stroke, or multiple sclerosis, or even a history of multiple concussions or brain trauma all affect brain function. Grief, depression, social isolation, poor sleep, and just plain lack of stimulation may also affect memory and cognition. None of these things are dementia, and each is treated differently, so it is important you do not try to diagnosis this yourself, and certainly don't label someone without a clear diagnosis.

Diagnosing Dementia

Most of the time, people never discover the exact pathology of the brain disease giving them dementia symptoms. The fallback diagnosis of Alzheimer's Disease or just "dementia," or even the older diagnosis of "senile dementia," is all they ever learn about it. To gain a more exact diagnosis, you and your loved one may need to seek out a practitioner with special interest in **geriatric neurology**. This may be difficult to find in some parts of the United States. The Alzheimer's Association http://www.alz.org/ or your local Area Agency on Aging http://www.n4a.org/ may be able to help you locate an excellent physician in your area. Having a more exact diagnosis may help with knowing what to expect, selecting better medicines, and better tailoring non-medicine-related treatment and coping strategies.

Even if you don't visit a specialist or gain an exact diagnosis, most practitioners have tests and tools to measure mental functions. Some of the more common tests include these:

- Mini Mental State Exam (MMSE)
- Montreal Cognitive Assessment (MoCA)
- St. Louis University Mental Status (SLUMS) exam

The SLUMS exam is quite simple (one page) and is not proprietary, so anyone—even you—might use it to gain some idea of whether or not there is a problem http://www.elderguru.com/download-the-slums-dementia-alzheimers-test-exam/. Keep in mind that, if you do use this, it does not diagnose—it only gives you an idea that there is a problem. Also, practicing the test will make anyone better at it, improving their score without changing their mental function, so don't give it very often.

...Types of Diseases Causing Dementia

Before we discuss specific diseases, it might be helpful to discuss the basic types. These are protein-based dementia, vascular dementia, mixed (protein and vascular), and alcohol-related dementia.

Protein-based Dementia

When something goes wrong with one or more of the **complex protein molecules in the nervous system**, dementia can result. Alzheimer's Disease, Lewy Body Dementia, Pick's Disease, and Huntington's Disease, are all protein based dementias. Parkinson's Disease may also have at least some protein-related causes. The signs and symptoms of these diseases and their progression vary widely, but these diseases all tend to be progressive and many have, at least in part, a genetic component.

Vascular Dementia and Vascular Cognitive Impairment (VCI)

These conditions are caused by **injuries to the blood vessels supplying blood to the brain**. This could involve multiple strokes, injury to the small vessels, or vascular disease in the small or large vessels. Some of these diseases are lifestyle related and can be somewhat reversible, while others may be genetically or environmentally related and may be progressive.

Mixed Dementia

This condition is **some combination** of the above types.

Alcohol-Related Brain Disorder (ARBD)

This condition is caused by **regular excessive drinking**. We have all heard that alcohol kills brain cells. This disease is the end stage of that process. Excessive drinking is also associated with increased rates of Alzheimer's Disease and vascular dementias. People who tend to drink too much also collect other risk factors, including lack of exercise, poor nutrition, obesity, poor sleep, and smoking. Something else about alcoholism is that it often causes a lack of vitamin B1 (thiamine), giving another form of dementia called Korsakoff's Syndrome. Paradoxically, it seems that one or two drinks in a night seems sparing to the brain, as it is associated with lower rates of dementia. (Other brain-damaging substances such as methamphetamine may also give rise to dementia, but those folks have yet to get old.)

...The Most Common Diseases Causing Dementia

There is way too much to write on each one of these diseases. Rather than write ad nauseam on each, here we simply list them, give a little information to help you tell them apart, and give links to their descriptions, including pathology, symptom pictures, prognosis, and treatment, as well as some resources.

Alzheimer's Disease

Alzheimer's is the **most commonly diagnosed dementia**, and it's often the fallback diagnosis for anyone who exhibits memory and cognition problems. Usually the onset and progression are slow, over years, and the ability to record new memories is affected first. The **first-line medications** here are cholinesterase inhibitors (which increase acetylcholine in the brain), and the most common one of these is Aricept.

The **Alzheimer's Association**, which offers the most comprehensive resources for any of the dementias, gives a basic description of Alzheimer's http://www.alz.org/alzheimers_disease_what_is_alzheimers.asp. This resource is also helpful for all of the dementias, offering support, advocacy, and local resources as well as good information.

Vascular Dementia

Without diagnostic imaging, it might be difficult to tell the difference between Alzheimer's Disease and vascular cognitive impairment (VCI). The person with VCI may show more difficulties with problem solving and maintaining or switching attention than a person with Alzheimer's, who may show more early problems with memory creation, but people with VCI may show memory problems too. **Neuroimaging** like MRIs often show a difference. The main drugs that are helpful for Alzheimer's are not yet specifically approved for VCI, but there is some evidence they may help a little.

The Alzheimer's Association website also gives good information and support for vascular dementia http://www.alz.org/dementia/vascular-dementia-symptoms.asp. You may also find information with the **National Stroke Association** http://www.stroke.org/we-can-help/survivors/stroke-recovery/post-stroke-conditions/cognition/vascular-dementia and the **American Heart Association,** which offers links to many scholarly articles http://www.heart.org/HEARTORG/search/searchResults.jsp?_dyncharset=ISO-8859-1&_dynSessConf=-2823687402485562717&q=vascular+dementia.

Parkinson's Disease and Parkinson's Associated Dementia

Parkinson's Disease tends to be a movement disorder before anything else. The early symptom is usually tremor. As the disease progresses, it makes controlling muscle tension and initiating or stopping a movement more difficult. This may progress into the movements of speaking, swallowing, and breathing. Cognition and memory can be affected but aren't always. When this occurs later in the process, we call it Parkinson's Disease Dementia or Parkinson's Associated Dementia. Parkinson's Disease affects the dopamine-producing cells first, and **Levodopa** is the mainstay in treatment. The main challenge in medication management is keeping the right level of dopamine assistance onboard. **Exercise** is key in treatment here; please see Exercise and Parkinson's Disease in Chapter 13, Exercise.

The **Wikipedia description** on Parkinson's Disease is pretty comprehensive but a little thick in the reading https://en.wikipedia.org/wiki/Parkinson's_disease. Of the several major groups offering support and research funding, the most influential three are the **Parkinson's Disease Foundation** (founded in 1957) http://www.pdf.org, the **American Parkinson's Disease Association** (founded in 1961) http://www.apdaparkinson.org, and the **Michael J. Fox Foundation** https://www.michaeljfox.org/, which focuses more on research but does offer information, a blog, and support.

Lewy Body Dementia

Lewy Body Dementia (LBD) is much like Alzheimer's but is **differentially diagnosed** by how the symptoms are presented. Patients tend to exhibit Parkinson's-like movement problems first, then dementia symptoms within one year. If it takes over a year for dementia symptoms to appear, the diagnosis is Parkinson's Disease Dementia. They also may have trouble interpreting visual information and have visual hallucinations and delusions, confusion, and varying alertness and may act out dreams (REM sleep disorder).

Aricept is still a key **drug treatment**, and Levodopa may help the movement problems, but other dopamine agonists may increase confusion, hallucinations, and delusions. Selective serotonin reuptake inhibitors (SSRIs) may help with the associated depression, but older antidepressants may cause problems. Many antipsychotics, benzodiazepines, and anticholinergics should be avoided.

Lewy Body Dementia Association https://www.lbda.org offers information and links to local resources and support in your area. **Alzheimer's Association** http://www.alz.org/dementia/dementia-with-lewy-bodies-symptoms.asp also offers a good description, as well as some ways it's differentiated from other dementias.

Frontotemporal Dementia

Pick's Disease is one type of frontotemporal dementia. This is another type of dementia for which the proper diagnosis is important. Because the brain's frontal and temporal lobes are affected, the early signs are difficulty with language, difficulty with initiating movement, and impulsive behavior and/or apathy, more than memory problems. Poor judgment, gullibility, and difficulty reasoning or planning also can be early signs. (You probably think you have it now, don't you?) **Neuropsychological testing** and a PET scan (positron-emission tomography) might confirm the diagnosis.

The usual **treatment** for Alzheimer's Disease, cholinesterase inhibitors (Aricept), can throw these people into more agitation, even delirium, and they may not recover once the drug is withdrawn. Benzodiazepines are also a problem and may increase behaviors as well as harm memory and motor function. There are problems with other drugs too. I found this site to be readable and immediately helpful http://memory.ucsf.edu.

Treating and Managing Dementia in the Early Stages

Because neurons in the brain are so interconnected, and because they require stimulation and use to stay healthy, anything you can do to improve brain function is sparing to neurons and helps brain health in the longer run.

...Medications

Many medications don't just relieve symptoms, they help preserve neurons and maintain brain health. **Aricept** is one of the most commonly prescribed medications in this group, but there are many others. Your geriatric neurologist can help you sort out the risks and benefits of each. Please be careful with medications, though, because sometimes it is important to have the diagnosis right. If you look through the descriptions of the five most common diseases causing dementia, listed above, you will notice that sometimes a drug that is helpful for one disease may be tragic for another. The details of each medication is beyond the scope of this writing, but the links provided on each disease listed above will help you learn more.

...Brain Preservation

There are many, many activities that have proven to help cognition, memory, and brain health in general. Much of this is discussed in Keep Your Brain Healthy in Chapter 4, Dancing in the Rain: Healthy Habits for Caregivers. Below is a brief list of **strategies and activities** you and your loved one can do to help their mental function and function in general:

- Participating in social interaction and engagement
- Being in an environment where they feel loved, connected, and happy
- Feeling love for others
- Taking on important and challenging tasks

Regarding this last point, as a member of the caregiver team, you can help by *not* doing everything for your loved one, yet still showing them love and encouragement. **Let them challenge themselves.** Let them figure it out. Let them lead. This might be a little more challenging for you than for them. Patience, my friend; you might be surprised by what they can do. That said, beware of letting them fall into frustration or become defeated. Try to exercise the art of helping them succeed on their own. If you have kids, you probably know this art.

Healthy Habits for Brain Health

The nervous system is the most changeable tissue in the body. It responds more and faster to exercise than do muscles, joints, or any other tissue. Exercise and a **health program for the brain** includes physical exercises, but it also includes all things healthy you might do with the nervous system. Here's a start:

- **Eat well,** especially omega-3 fatty acids. For specifics on this, see Eat Right in Chapter 4, Healthy Habits for Caregivers.
- **Get daily cardiovascular exercise.** This actually helps with generating BDNF protein (brain-derived neurotrophic factor), which helps the brain make new connections as well as helps excite and oxygenate the brain. Plus endurance exercise helps vascular, blood, and general health.
- **Do moderate weight lifting** two days per week to help generate a different BDNF protein that is complementary to the one from cardiovascular exercise. Strengthening exercise also helps preserve mobility and general functional ability. For more details and a good how-to, see Chapter 13, Exercise.

- **Get good sleep.** For more on this, see Chapter 14, Sleep.
- **Get daily exposure to sunlight.** This helps excite the brain and helps with sleep regulation.
- **Do specific cognitive exercises,** such as sudoku and other cognitive games; check out this workbook from Dr. Winningham full of healthy brain games http://www.activityconnection.com/ccbook/.
- **Try dual tasking:** Mix physical exercise with cognitive exercise. Most sports have a mental and physical component. Be creative in choosing or creating things your loved one can do, such as a scavenger hunt.

For lots more ideas, practical advice, and resources, visit http://www.robwinningham.com/. This author also has another book, *Train Your Brain: How to Maximize Memory Ability in Older Adulthood*, available on Amazon https://www.amazon.com/Train-Your-Brain-Maximize-Adulthood/dp/0895037831?ie=UTF8&*Version*=1&*entries*=0.

Prehab

"Prehab" is what I call preparing for what's ahead and making life as good as can be as the disease progresses. Here are some ideas:

- **Play games with different mobility assistive devices.** How about a wheelchair race? Or obstacle courses on crutches or a walker? Maybe on one foot if using two feet seems too easy. Learning the basic skill and feel of using an assistive device now, when the body is stronger and memory and learning work better, will make using one easier if they actually need it later. Perhaps this sort of game could be combined with a scavenger hunt to maximize dual tasking. You can be creative here.
- **Exercise into basic functional movements** such as the squat, getting up from a lunge, or getting up off a low mat or the floor.
- **Practice mindfulness** and begin guided meditation training; see Mindfulness Meditation in Chapter 4, Dancing in the Rain: Healthy Habits for Caregivers.
- **Reduce or mitigate long-term stress and anxiety.** See Chapter 4, Dancing in the Rain: Healthy Habits for Caregivers, and Anxiety in Chapter 18, Managing Discomforts.
- **Develop good exercise habits.** Make it a conscious habit, such as "I exercise after (or before) breakfast."
- **Develop good social habits and strengthen the social fabric.** Does your loved one have a card-playing group? A stitch 'n' bitch (that's what a friend of ours called her sewing group), or any other posses or gangs? Can you help them create any new ones? Can they strengthen their relationships with their children, their grandchildren, or even great-grandchildren? The connections they have now will make life much better later.
- **Create a written record of the things that have been important to your loved one throughout their lifetime.** What was their favorite music at each decade of life? What sports did they enjoy doing or watching? Gather their old pictures, favorite movies, and best stories. Know who they loved deeply and who gives them some stress still. Know some of their more difficult experiences or memories. This intimate act will help you get to know them

better now and later may help all their caregivers know better who and where they are as they walk this path.
- **Create a memory book.** This is the scrapbook full of photographs, newspaper clippings, and text balloons that they might write for themselves. This is a good tool for preserving old memories and also a wonderful thing that they can create for their family, kind of a picture book of their lives.
- **Help them do their best to gain a healthy and forgiving attitude,** especially toward themselves and toward all whom they love. Here is an excellent TED talk on this by Alanna Shaikh https://www.ted.com/talks/alanna_shaikh_how_i_m_preparing_to_get_alzheimer_s

Managing Dementia in the Middle and Late Stages

In mid- to late-stage brain-disease dementia, it is still important to keep your loved one as engaged and functionally active as possible.

Physical exercise still helps, both cardiovascular and resistance training, but exercises may need to be made much simpler for them. See Exercise and Dementia in Chapter 13, Exercise.

Cognitive training may need to be adapted. The *Cranium Crunches Workbook* has exercises and games for multiple different levels http://www.activityconnection.com/ccbook/.

Do continue to exercise their **executive function** for as long as possible. Any exercise or activity that demands attention, impulse inhibition, problem solving, mental flexibility, planning, and/or social interaction helps. Can they do simple tasks such as help fold laundry or help with meal preparation (careful with those sharp knives)?

Their **familiar and favorite music** can have tremendous benefits. Please look into this lovely film on music therapy called Alive Inside https://www.youtube.com/watch?v=IBwr1MOEmB8&index=2&list=PL5602F9BEFDB2CFE7

Try to **understand their world**. To help with this, it might help you to have a little better understanding of how the brain works and how someone with brain disease might experience their world.

...Understanding How Memory Works

Most things we think of as a memory are encoded by the hippocampus deep in the brain. Certain cells create an echo, firing a chain of neurons in a certain pattern, strengthening their connection. This can go on continuously (while you sleep too) for up to a couple days. Each time the pattern fires, the neurons' connection gets a little stronger.

A memory is not a unique recording, like a tape recording (remember those?), but a set of linked subprograms that probably already exist in the brain. Objects, words, concepts, emotions are all subprograms. Every time you remember something, you replay these links.

The initial linking exists in a short-term way. We might call this **working memory.** Usually we can hold three to seven things in working memory for a couple minutes. As more items come into working memory, older items (unless rehearsed in the mind) will be pushed out. For a memory to be held and encoded into long-term storage, it must be strongly held in the mind for at least a little while. Distraction is the natural memory eraser.

Memories initially live in the hippocampus. After about five years, they begin to reside more in the cortex. This may be why people with brain diseases like

Alzheimer's, which damage the hippocampus early, seem to lose their more recent memories first while older memories remain intact.

Procedural memory—habits and motor learning—works somewhat differently, so it can remain intact much longer in most brain diseases.

Putting These Concepts to Practical Use

So how can you use these concepts with your loved one?

- **Give instructions in simple steps.** Working memory is small, remember? Unless you are trying to challenge and exercise their working memory, don't give too many things at once.
- **Let them know that you will ask about this later,** if it's something important you want them to try to remember. Don't you always study harder if you know there will be a quiz? Letting them know there will be a quiz may cue them to pay more attention and rehearse it in their short term memory enough to help it record into long term.
- **Have them write things down in a notebook.** The act of writing something demands that they hold it in their mind longer and activate it through several parts of the brain. It also gives them a written record in their handwriting so they may refer to it later.
- **Let them work things out a little for themselves.** If they have to figure something out a bit on their own, they are paying more attention and recruiting more cells. Avoid frustration; try to keep the challenges doable for them. Set up the challenge and cue them so they don't fail at it more than twice.
- **Have them rehearse and repeat.** If memory is difficult, using the exact same cues and sequence will help. You might make a video of your training so the other caregivers may do the training the exact same way. See Producing and Publishing Training Videos in Chapter 1, Building a Caregiving Team.
- **Avoid agitation and distraction.** These are natural memory erasers.

Training the Memory in Late-Stage Dementia

Spaced retrieval is a memory-training procedure we use for people who have some but very poor new-memory creation. The concept is simple: we repeatedly give them a quiz, doubling the time between quizzes each time they get it right. We begin by setting up a cue for which we teach them to give a specific response: "When I say 'Get up,' you say 'Get my walker.' " We repeat this several times with them, then let them begin the response on their own. We begin with a short interval, say 10 seconds, then double it to 20 seconds, then keep doubling the time every time they get it right, for up to a couple days. Of course there is an app for this: Spaced Retrieval Therapy by Tactus Therapy http://tactustherapy.com/app/srt/ gives an app that will cue the user for time and the cue used.

Procedural memory—memory for habits and motor sequences—remains intact for most people until very, very late in the disease process. This means that, even though they seem to have no new memory creation ability, they can still learn. This could be something like "After breakfast I go to exercise class" or "I set my brakes before getting out of a wheelchair." To use procedural memory, it helps to perform the task the exact same way with the same sequence and the same cues. It usually takes about 100 repetitions for the memory to begin to engrain. Creating a video of the sequence and cues will help here too.

...Helping Them Orient

In late-stage dementia, it may be more important for caregivers to try to understand what your loved one might be experiencing. Consider where they are, who they are, and who they once were. If their ability to make new memories is limited, they are in their experience, right now. Each moment may be, for them, like waking from a dream. They will need **familiar anchors** to help them orient:

- **Clocks and calendars** help.
- **A set routine** helps.
- **Familiar objects, smells, sounds** all help.
- **The memory book** you created together will help (see Prehab earlier in this chapter).
- **Having people around** who can understand them and seem friendly and helpful, even if your loved one doesn't recognize them, helps the most.
- **Giving them references to things that are familiar** to them in their present mind helps. This is where your understanding of the music they enjoyed, the events in their life, and the people they loved at each decade in their life helps.

Retrogenesis is a phenomenon that sometimes happens in the later stages of Alzheimer's and other dementias. The pattern of neural destruction takes out more recent memories first and works its way back. Imagine what it might feel like if your most recent memory is from 1963 and you wake up to find yourself in this modern world. To them, if that is their most recent intact memory, it *is* 1963. Now think how disturbing it might be to tune into Fox News or hear the latest hip-hop from someone's iPad. Anchors from the time they're remembering can be tremendously calming. If you can figure out *when* they are, you might find old movies, favorite songs, even commercials that will help them anchor and find comfort. That iPad might not seem so weird if it's playing their favorite *I Love Lucy* episode.

...Communicating Strategically

They may have trouble communicating what they need or what might be troubling them. **They may have trouble understanding you.** If they have trouble moving their head or eyes, you will need to be in their field of vision if you want them to attend to you. Get down to their eye level. Think about their sensory perceptions:

- **Seeing:** Do they need glasses to see clearly? Are the glasses clean?
- **Reading:** Do they need big, thick writing to see written words? Can they still decipher words?
- **Hearing:** Can they hear you OK? Do they use hearing aids? Do they hear better on one side than the other?

Consider their thought-processing speed. Speak in clear, simple sentences in your normal speaking voice and speed. Give them time to process your sounds into ideas. If you must repeat yourself, use the same words, the same way. Don't paraphrase yourself—that is just new sounds that they have to process all over again. You may need to keep questions simple with yes-or-no answers or simple choices.

Keep in mind that your nonverbal communication may be more powerful than your words. Look at your own posture. Feel your own voice. If you want them to be calm, you may need to calm yourself. Soften your shoulders. Let that tightness come out of your throat. Even if you're getting completely exasperated, it won't help anyone to be sharp with them. Take a breath. Step outside yourself. Practice your own mindfulness.

Distraction is one of the most helpful tools. What works so well with little kids and Congress can work well here too. If they are perseverating on something, try pulling out one of their old pictures: "Is that Uncle Harry next to that big Cadillac?" Funny videos work well too. A cat knocking something over is funny no matter your age or mental state.

Don't be afraid of telling a little white lie if it is meant to help them. Perhaps they don't want to go to the doctor that morning. Maybe, if you ask, they may want to go somewhere else, such as a favorite restaurant: "Well, get your hat, let's go" will get them out the door, even if you know it's impossible to take them to that restaurant. Chances are, by time you get to the doctor's office, they will have forgotten all about not wanting to go there.

...Managing Unwanted Behaviors

People in general can say and do things that are just plain difficult to take. People with a brain disorder, who may have difficulty creating new memories, difficulty thinking outside themselves (empathy), or difficulty with executive functions—impulse control, attention, problem solving, mental flexibility, planning—can do preposterous things. Does your loved one hit, spit, or just scream out all night? If not, you might just consider yourself a little bit lucky.

How do we deal with these problem behaviors? First, look again at the list in Brain Preservation earlier in this chapter for preserving mental function. Cognitive games, exercise, social time, and mindfulness all help tremendously to strengthen executive function, which is probably your loved one's best tool to help them control outbursts. It also helps relieve boredom and break mental or emotional perseveration that can lead to anxiety and more unwanted behaviors. In fact, everything discussed in Brain Preservation can help. Music therapy has been shown to help with agitation, spitting, and hitting behaviors. Daylight and exercise both help with sleep and thus unwanted night behaviors. They also help with anxiety.

Avoid arguing or escalation. It certainly doesn't help them, and remember: you're arguing with someone with a brain disease. Don't you feel silly? Even if you're not arguing with words, is your nonverbal communication threatening? Are your shoulders tight? Is your voice sharp or overly controlled? Are you towering over them or in their space? Double-down on watching your own emotions and how you are presenting yourself to them. This is especially challenging when they just peed in the oven, but it will only agitate them further. Try to find the humor in it all. By the way, if they are absolutely wrong about reality, you don't need to correct them. That may further agitate them, and it usually doesn't work anyway. In fact, we usually deflect questions that may escalate.

Look for things that may be causing agitation or perseverations. Are they as physically comfortable as can be? Is their bedding in a knot? Could they have an undiagnosed infection? Listen to them. Listen to more than just their words; try to "decode" what might seem like nonsense or out of context. There may be something in their reality that is disturbing to them. Can you help them work out the problem? Wandering behaviors often are the result of a sense that something needs to be done somewhere. Can you help them be comfortable here? Sometimes they are just having trouble getting oriented. Look again at retrogenesis in Helping Them Orient above.

Sometimes people are just ornery and may act out to get attention. Don't just give them attention when they are misbehaving, it only serves to reinforce the behavior. Try to keep your attentiveness even, no matter how mad you are.

It might help you to know that memory and intelligence are not quite the same thing. Memory is part of intelligence, but not all of it. Just because someone has difficulty creating new memories doesn't mean they cannot grasp difficult concepts, understand people, or love. You may find that as your loved one's brain changes, **their abilities change, sometimes revealing sides of them no one knew existed.**

For more information about managing dementia, dealing with both the difficult and the sometimes surprising behaviors, as well as great advice for the caregiver to take care of themselves in the unique situations brain disease brings, I love the work of **Elaine Sanchez** http://www.caregiverhelp.com/. You will find videos, books, and other resources. For more tips and resources, I also like https://www.caregiver.org/caregivers-guide-understanding-dementia-behaviors.

...Using Monitors and Alarms

Karin, the most wonderful professional caregiver who was there for my mom, said, "It's best if you never need to use any kind of monitor or alarm to help keep someone safe. If you can hold hands, be there with them, that's best." What she says is true, but it's not always possible. If someone needs 24-hour monitoring or if they have a tendency to wander off, some simple devices may give both you and your loved one a longer leash from each other and help give comfort, safety, and more of a feeling of independence.

A simple baby monitor, the kind they sell in most department stores or baby-care stores, allows a caregiver to hear if a sleeping person awakens or begins to try to get up. We found it best to have a wearable receiver. It's important to check the range to be sure it would work in your house.

Pressure sensing pads placed in the bed, on the floor, or on the seat of a wheelchair activate if a person takes weight off (or puts it on, for the floor pad), which alerts caregivers to assist someone who is trying to get up on their own when they shouldn't. We commonly use them in nursing homes and memory-care centers to help prevent falls. The **Alzhiemer's Store** http://www.alzstore.com/browse-alzstore-s/1898.htm has a wide arrange of products that might fit your specific needs.

Any alarm-type monitor you use should signal the caregiver through a pager-type device, I believe. Alarms that make noise might annoy or agitate your loved one. Often, if someone is confused or agitated enough to wander, the usually shrill sound of an alarm only agitates further. As for devices that put timers on stoves, our fireman friend finds that most people disable them, so he doesn't recommend them.

For people who have a tendency to wander off, there are several types of products and services which may help. The Alzheimer's store as well as other vendors offers **door alarms, and personal alarms** that signal when a person has wandered out of their designated range. You will also find GPS locators and less-expensive ID-type products.

MedicAlert with Safe Return http://www.alz.org/care/dementia-medic-alert-safe-return.asp is a piece of metal jewelry that has your loved one's information and a call-center phone number. This device relies on someone in the community, including police and fire department people, to find the person and call in. The caregiver also may have an ID tag that identifies them as the caregiver. This tag cannot be handed off between caregivers, but there can be up to three emergency contacts listed for the person. There is a low annual fee for the service.

A simple generic medical alert bracelet can also be found on e-Bay or Amazon. There is no backup service or call center, but you can engrave your loved one's name and an emergency contact phone number onto it. Also https://www.medicalert.org/product/catalog/medical-ids

...Taking Care of Yourself

Caring for someone with dementia is probably one of the most difficult of all caregiver situations. Give yourself plenty of room. Look again at all the information in Chapter 4, Dancing in the Rain: Healthy Habits for Caregivers. Again, look into http://www.caregiverhelp.com/. Consider that these diseases are often gradually worsening and long in their progression. **It is best if you have a caregiving team**, if you have support, and if you are not too stubborn to reach for outside caregivers for help. If you haven't done so, read Chapter 1, Building a Caregiving Team.

So, someone in your family has dementia. Is there a genetic component? Perhaps. In many of the more than 60 different types of dementia, there is a genetic component. Should you freak out every time you forget your car keys? Probably not. Genetics may determine half of our path, but what we do with our bodies and our brains determines the other half. The very same concepts and activities that help your loved one in the early and middle stages of this disease (see Brain Preservation earlier in this chapter) can help you prevent dementia's onset or at least give you more healthy time.

Physical exercise, both cardiovascular and strength training, plus cognitive challenges, a sense of purpose, connection, and love all serve to strengthen your nervous system against disease and decline. Keep your friends and family close, stay on your sports team, and accept the challenges that lay before you, and you can help give your body the input it needs to stay strong. Rest and sleep well, meditate, and exercise the patience it takes to solve the difficult problems in life, and your brain will continue to function well.

If you are still worried about it, take the SLUMS test yourself (see Diagnosing Dementia earlier in this chapter). Record your score, then give good effort to practice all those things in this chapter and look into the brain games described here and in *Train your Brain*, under Brain Preservation earlier in this chapter. Take the SLUMS test again next year. Good luck. Even if you don't live longer, you will probably live better for the practice.

Chapter 20.
Near the End

"Oh God, I want this to end! ... Oh God, I really don't want this to end!!!"

At some point the body begins to shut down. It's hard to know exactly when this will happen, but I think you will know when it's happening. There are physical and emotional changes.

Physical Changes

Most people in this process will have a lot less energy. They may sleep more, all day and through the night. They may be difficult to rouse at times. They may go through periods of confusion. If they are sleeping through the night, let them sleep in the day if they need to. You can be with them. Hold them, comfort them, gently stroke their hair, say all those loving, soothing things that need to be said. Even if they are unresponsive, they might hear you. Listening is one of the last senses to be lost.

If they are confused, you can help them reorient by simply being there, being loving and calm, and letting them know that it's OK. Remind them who you are, speak of familiar things. Remind them of the time of day, where they are, and who is there with them. Think of it as if you were being awoken from a dream in a dark room: "Honey, it's me, Dave. Jayne is here, it's almost lunch time" says a lot to give people footholds to this reality.

This helps if they are restless too. You also might lightly play some music they like, read them a story, or just be with them, giving them soothing touch. As with anxiety, consider things that may be making them uncomfortable. If they are trying to push the covers away, perhaps they are too warm, or if they're tugging at them, too cold. A warm pack or cool washcloth on their forehead might help worlds here. Are they clean and dry? Are their pain medications on track? Do all those things to keep them as comfortable as can be.

Metaphysical Changes

Sometimes the discomfort might not be physical. They may feel that there is something left unsaid or undone. Can you help them here? Is there something that they feel needs to be that you can help them with? Now is your time.

It's not uncommon for people near the edge of life to see things you cannot see or seem to speak with people who have died already. You don't need to contradict them or try to explain this. It is real to them and common enough to be considered normal. I believe there is a certain magic in all these things we don't understand yet. For me it is OK to not understand. If it frightens them, comfort them. You are warm. You are here. If they are of Faith, this might be a good time for their minister to visit.

It's common for people to begin to pull away from all those around them. This didn't happen for us, though we expected it. Karen always loved all her friends around and loved the party. Some people, especially those more introverted in their orientation, may close their circle. They may need to, one by one, say good-bye. You can honor this. It is OK to say good-bye, to let go and give them permission to let go.

As the Body Shuts Down

Near the very end of life, the circulation and metabolism slow. They will probably no longer be hungry or thirsty. Let them lead here. Don't try to force food or fluids. Food may be impossible for them to digest, and fluid may only contribute to pooling in the lungs or backing up the heart. The dehydration that occurs naturally may help them produce more endorphins, helping them be more comfortable. This is one place where IV fluids or a feeding tube may actually make them less comfortable.

You can help by keeping their mouth and lips moist. They may like ice chips or a little water, juice, or sport drink on a sponge popsicle. A little lip cream or petroleum jelly might help moisten the lips. As they take the step down in function, it is very important to switch their medication away from pill form to patches, liquids, IV, or other forms. Sometimes they will lose their ability to swallow.

Their hands, arms, and then feet and legs may become cool. You may notice the color of their skin changes: their underside becoming darker and perhaps spotty, while their upside may become more ashen as their circulation moves more to their core. Help them stay warm with light, fluffy blankets. We generally don't recommend warm packs here. Without the circulation, they are more prone to burning. Warming your hands on a warm pack, then gently touching them might be terrifically soothing.

Their breathing pattern may change. They may begin tummy breathing, shallow breaths, or not breathing for short periods, sometimes up to a minute. They may also develop some gurgling as fluids pool in their throat or lungs. If they are on IV fluids, this will probably happen more. This isn't usually distressing for them. It may help to slightly elevate or turn their head. Sometimes their nursing team will administer atropine or other drugs to help.

You might notice that the color of their urine changes, becoming dark like tea. This is normal as the circulation to the kidneys slows. They may become incontinent as the muscles of the pelvic floor relax. Simply keep them as clean and dry as you can while protecting their dignity and comfort (see Incontinence and Peri-Care in Chapter 16, Hygiene, Bathing, and Toileting).

Leave Nothing Unsaid

Sometimes people near the very edge will have a sudden burst of energy and alertness. This can be horribly confusing for loved ones, as they feel the person may be making a miraculous recovery. You might best use this window to help resolve any issues they may have—to hug, to kiss, to do all that needs to be done. To leave nothing unsaid.

One of the greatest gifts you can give is to release your loved one from all their concerns of this life, to let them know it's OK to let go. Saying good-bye in a loving and honorable way, acknowledging all their gifts, may be your ultimate gift of love.

In the last few hours of life, people tend to gather in what we call a "vigil." Below are the words of our caregiving team, from our time with Karen. It was one of the most powerful events in all of our lives.

If everyone is loving and respectful, there is no wrong way.

You will find your way.

Our Vigil
Time with Karen, My Lifeline Post May 29, 2013

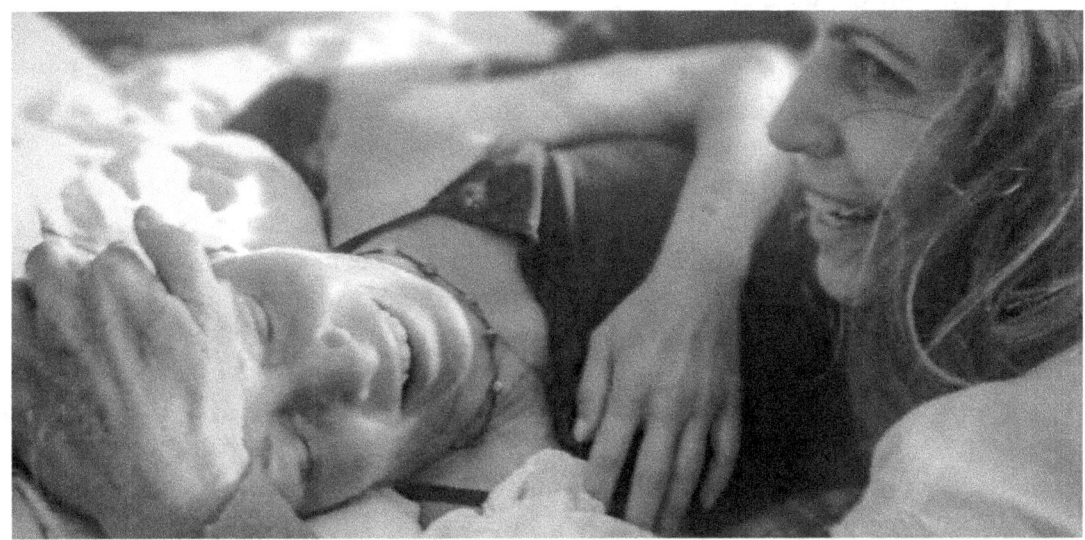

Figure 37—Karen with Paula (and Dave's hand)

Paula here, Dave's sister.

Dave and Karen asked me to write the next entry. Sorry I have taken so long. I've been here almost two weeks and leave tomorrow. In that time we've had two outings—one to retail therapy at the junction (Dave missed that one) and the other the incredible Chihuly museum, both last week. Karen made us cry showing us her favorite Chihuly exhibits, just telling us how much she wanted to share the experience with us. There are so many facets of Karen. She is up and down, of course. This week she still wanted to go on outings, but it's been a smaller window, too small to actually go.

Each increment of change makes us sad. It is a strange sensation: laughing and snuggling in the awake time, and yet seeing that what makes her laugh is less and less sophisticated, sometimes even just sounds or words.

Thanks to good advice, we are fast-tracking the transition from pills to patches and liquids, as much as possible, preparing for when she cannot swallow. Her pills are now fed to her on a spoonful of yogurt or pudding or very thick soup. Her liquids are thickened with this stuff called Thick-It, to the consistency of honey, to cut down on matter going down the wrong pipe. She must eat and drink with great concentration and lack of distraction, no longer able to party with a beverage in her hand.

Today (Tuesday) starts with Karen being unresponsive and incontinent for the first time since I've been here. Dave has hooked her to oxygen and tells me she's improved in the last half hour. I stay with her while Dave showers, starts laundry. I hold the oxygen nozzle near her mouth. Her first motion is to wave it away, but after a bit we are sharing tokes on it and laughing. So she is better for the moment. Not much better, but better enough for us to all be happy, exhausted, bewildered.

The hospice nurse comes later in the morning and tells us Karen's eyes are more yellow and her feet are more chronically swollen than they were Friday, both indications of a poorly functioning liver. We tell the nurse that Karen has bounced back before. The nurse tells us as gently as possible that the liver doesn't bounce. The news is brutal, frightening, but the same dire situation happened two and a half weeks ago when Julia was here, and Karen bounced back. Not as high a bounce, of course, which we know with a large part of our minds, but of course there is a part that can't comprehend any of this at all.

Still, I had thought Dave was wrong this time, that with the liver in so much decline that Karen wouldn't rally. The nurse was trying to get us ready for the next stage. But then the long, beautiful spring evening happens and people start arriving. And more and more people, until the house is filled with boisterous and quiet joy.

Karen, apparently sleeping, receives continuous loving attention and touches. At one point, several of us are piled on the bed with her—Dave and us girls, all of us petting her until Ronnie, the little boy from up the street, comes in from the back deck to say good-bye. Karen sits up, brightens, listens to the boy describe his play, gives him her full attention, and comments. Dave and I just stare at each other. This is the pillow, he says, the pillow of love in action, all her loving friends making her journey so much more enjoyable.

After talking with Ronnie, Karen requests the wheelchair, the bathroom, and after that she is energetic, hungry, thirsty, and bright. She must be a cat, for this is yet again a new life. I'm in bed scribbling this, and the party and laughter go on over my head. Karen appears to be in no hurry to leave this world, at least not right now.

Thank you to all you angels, not just for taking such loving, thoughtful care of Karen, but because you are all the pillow of love for Dave, too. I know both Dave and Karen are so grateful, so surprised, really, at such sustained capacity for feeling and action. I am so moved by you all.

...Dear Friends, My Lifeline Post written late May, posted June 4, 2013

Marc Fendel and Jayne Simmons here.

We had an amazing weekend at Dave and Karen's. The sun has been out in Seattle, and the house was filled with beautiful music and nonstop visiting with old friends and even a few new faces too. Marc and his uncle and cousin played music for Karen early in the afternoon, then old friends Paul and Susie headed up the sing-along, while their amazing kids ran around and the hummingbirds dive-bombed each other and probably mated in the bushes. Scott and Leona visited from Bellingham with their 18-month-old and other beautiful news in the circle of life. And the three-year-old "Fire Chief Ronny" arrived on his truck in full attire to pay a visit. Having all these kids around at this time reminds us that the circle of life continues and *love* is the thread running through this party we call Karen Morgan's life.

Friday she showed us her spunky, amazing sense of humor once again when she woke up from a nap, looked at the broken clock across the room, and said "It's still ten minutes to eight." Still cracking jokes through the pain! (We changed it to 4:20 and the thing gave us quite a chime performance!)

During what turned out to be a party this Sunday, I (Marc) got a chance to hop up on the bed and hold Karen's hand. I told her I loved her. She barely responded, but said "I love you too." I told her that I'd be coming back tomorrow to make some strong coffee and that we'd enjoy some "coffee sips." She smiled that glowing smile we all are so attracted to. Later, Dave gave her kiss-sized sips of margarita—she was surprised a bit, but when he asked if she wanted more, she smiled, opened her mouth like a little bird, and nodded her head yes!

Yesterday Karen enjoyed some of the beautiful weather outside on the porch and even ate a bit of soup, which hasn't been happening very much in the last few days. She seems to be comfortable now after a really rough afternoon and night.

Even though Karen is mostly sleeping today, her beauty shines through the pain—she continues to amaze and inspire me every day that I am here. (She heard me sneeze the other day and said reflexively "bless you" and even tried to clap her hands after the songs on Sunday!) She thanks us, but we are the ones to be thankful that she allows us to share this sacred space and time.

There are a few things that we should be aware of. If you are visiting or are a caregiver, we are asking folks to please wash your hands when entering the house. There will be some hand sanitizer close to the front door. Also, if there are lots of people here, please keep conversations quiet, positive, and to a minimum, or step outside and enjoy this glorious weather. Please check the carebook for updates when you are here.

Most of all ... Send or bring your love to Karen!

...My Lifeline Post May 30, 2013

I hold her in my arms. She is slowly slipping away. Her good times now are not so good. We did not make it out of the house today. We did not make it out of the house yesterday either. She is very sleepy now, probably 16 hours a day now. Still She loves. Still she smiles. Still She is Love.

We have so much to learn. We have so much to learn.

...Morning, My Lifeline Post June 3, 2013

I hold my ear close to her mouth to catch her whispered words. "I love you," she says as we hold each other.

...Vigil, My Lifeline Post June 5, 2013

Karen did not wake up yesterday. We worked to keep her airway clear. We hold her in our arms and say all those things. Nothing is unsaid now. Her breaths are short and shallow. The on-call nurse arrived quickly about 5:30 a.m. Her pulse was 155 but blood oxygen saturation only 85 percent. She is cold and hot at the same time. "Soon," says the nurse, "probably today."

After pulling myself together, I wash her. We change her clothes. She is so pretty. Her cat rests on the bed with her and nuzzles her thigh. Crows keep visiting the house, looking in the window but saying nothing. The phone keeps ringing. Wishes of Love. Wishes of Love.

My sadness pulls away as I hold her hand. Words from a teacher of hands-on physical therapy techniques come into my mind: "Put your heart into your work." The instructor was talking about posture—but, then again, she wasn't.

As I look at her, pure love, helping her walk this journey, the pain that has enveloped my head for the past two days subsides. My heart is here. We are here now. We are with you.

Walk Gently.

Today is a good day ...

—Dave

...From Mary Lou, My Lifeline Post June 5, 2013

We are waiting. The house is full of love. Karen is sleeping peacefully. The nurse has told us that Karen will likely pass into pure spirit before the next sunrise. We are all still drawn to her and want to share our love, but the house can't fit all the love that's out there.

For people who wish to gather, please find each other at the first/westernmost fire pit on Alki Beach (the one closest to the Statue of Liberty). Sunset is always a natural time. Bring candles, chocolate, wine, and love to share. You're welcome to come to the house if it's important to you. Dave just wants to be sure he can keep his heart and mind where it needs to be—with Karen—and the house can be a peaceful place.

...1:42 a.m., My Lifeline Post June 6, 2013

"Nothing is unsaid now" John "t-shirt":

> That is the grace of having time to say good-bye, despite the pain and hardship. Pain and hardship are temporary and can be borne by people such as these. Peace and communion, not everyone gets, but we got it in spades.
>
> The courage, love, and brilliance of both Karen and Dave created this uncommon community. You are with all of us, Karen. Your spirit has shaped us and will echo for generations.

Epilogue

Karen Morgan beat cancer.

In the most surprising way, despite a grave diagnosis, she went on to a full and wonderful life.

She went on to become a shining beacon of love and strength to all who knew her and helped care for her. She was the center of our Framily, our Buddha in Pajamas. By sharing her journey, she gave each of us gifts that we continue to revel in and pass forward. She, in her way, performed the most graceful and wonderful backflips. And each of us is richer in our lives for being with her and with each other during this precious time.

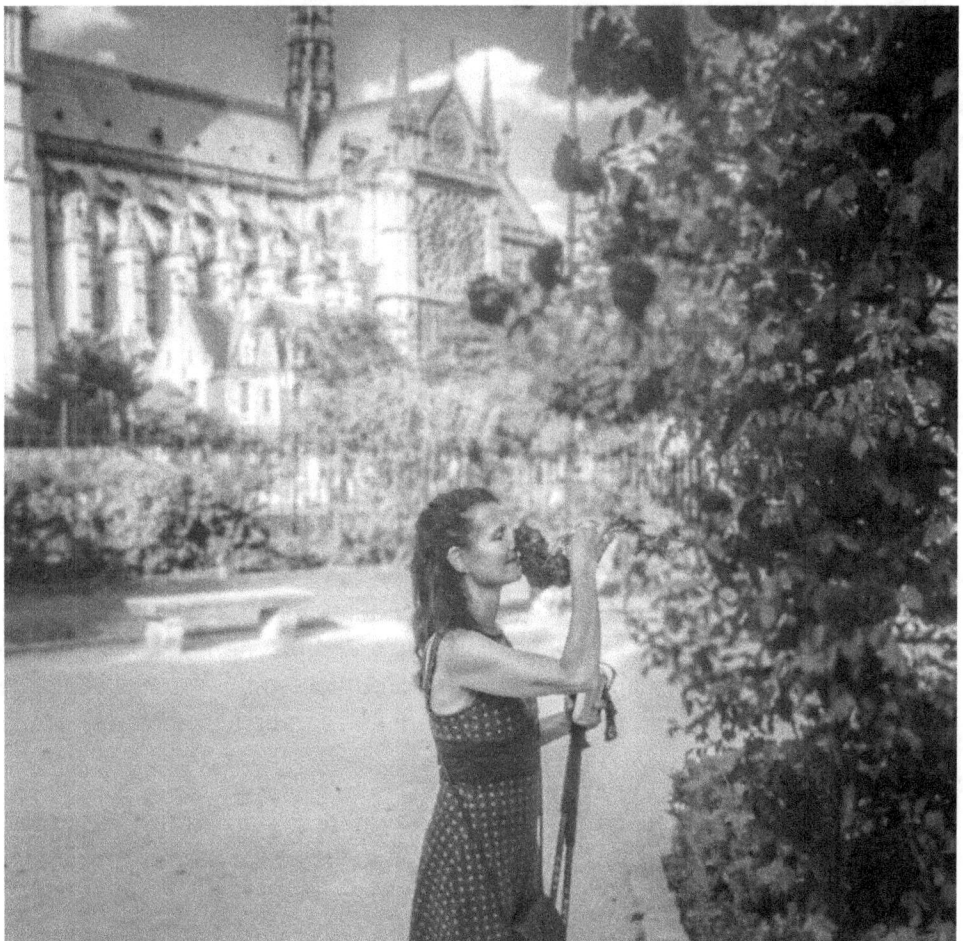

Figure 38- Karen, Paris 2012

I thank you for helping your loved one on their journey, for reading these words, and passing this love forward.

It's so difficult to write about this process, especially when it is so near the end of hours. My life goes away. How can one write about such things, the end of life? Is this the beginning of a new chapter? Where is the path? When one is dying, does one start with the end or the beginning?

Karen Morgan 1958–2013

Contributors

Caring for Karen and the creation of this work was a many-hands project. Most of these good people also stepped up to become part of Karen's core care team and were there with us through this whole journey. Here they are listed in the order their contributions first appear in the book.

Mary Kathryn LaSeur, RN, BSN, CHPN (Certified Hospice and Palliative Care Nurse)
> Mary is our neighbor, friend, and one of the true heroes of our team. Her expertise and long-earned wisdom can be found in most of the nursing and palliative care sections of this book and in Chapter 18.

Dr. Seth Fader, DO
> Seth helped author the chapters discussing pain, medications and wound care. He is board certified in Family Practice and CSWS (Certified Skin and Wound Care specialist) He practices at Swedish Medical Center. In his free time, he enjoys cooking, especially for friends and family, and triathlon training. Karen and I have been the grateful recipients of his wisdom, and his recipes.

Julia Heersche, RN, BSN
> Julia has put up with me since high school. This is no small matter. Julia has also worked in orthopedic nursing for many years. Currently she enjoys working in a progressive care unit at Flagstaff Medical Center. She also worked in caregiving through the Hozhoni Foundation and cared for each of her parents in their time. She was critical in helping Karen during some of our best and worst times and she helped immensely with consultation and writing regarding most everything to do with nursing and caregiving.

Jackie Wolfe
> Jackie works as a consultant specializing in human resources, leadership roles, and conflict resolution. Jackie's advice can be found throughout Section I. She contributed heavily to Chapter 1, Managing Conflicts in the Team. Jackie was also an important part of our caregiving team and can be found in our videos.

Marc Fendel and Jayne Simmons
> Marc is a musician, teacher, and long distance hiker. He co-wrote the section Producing and Publishing Training Videos. Jayne is the creator of Sister Sage Herbs. He and Jayne added their love, time, music, and terrific knowledge of herbal medicines to our caregiving team and wrote one of the MyLifeline posts at the end of this book. Their wisdom can be found throughout this book. Marc's music instruction videos can be found at https://www.youtube.com/watch?v=9oij0s8026w onYouTube at Music Education for All. Jayne's tinctures, balms, and other natural magic can be found at https://www.sistersageherbs.com/

Karen Conger, MS, CD, RD,
: Karen is a dietitian at Harborview Medical Center in Seattle, Washington. She focuses her training and long experience on helping people at all stages of illness to not only meet their nutritional needs, but still enjoy the pleasures of foods and eating. She contributed greatly to all sections concerning food and nutrition in Chapter 4 and 12.

Rosalind Billharz, PhD, MBA
: Rosalind assisted this project with love, and consultation. She contributed the section Infections and Compromised Immune Systems in Chapter 18 Managing Discomforts. At the time of this writing Rosalind is an instructor of microbiology, and an Assistant Professor at Pacific Lutheran University in Tacoma Washington. She has researched and authored multiple scientific manuscripts, book chapters, case studies, and scientific peer reviews.

Sue Vetter, DDS
: Sue contributed the section Oral Care in Chapter 16, Hygiene, Bathing, and Toileting. Dr. Vetter maintains a private practice in Seattle, Washington. Sue Vetter DDS http://suevetter.com/. In her spare time, she is an Affiliate Assistant Professor in the Department of Restorative Dentistry at the University of Washington School of Dentistry and is a Board Member and Faculty for OBI Foundation for Bioesthetic Dentistry. She also made the magic mouthwash that allowed Karen to enjoy food when her mouth was tender.

Gary Piscopo, ND, LAc
: Gary contributed the section Acupuncture and Acupressure in Chapter 17, Pain Management. He is a co-founding physician member of Alpine Valley Wellness Center in Wenatchee Washington, an active member of the Washington Association of Naturopathic Physicians, and the Washington Association of East Asian Medicine Association, and co-founder and CEO of Wild Brilliance Press. He and his wife Dr. Jacqueline Thomas are also long-time friends. More information about him can be found at: http://www.alpinevalleywellnesscenter.com.

Rob Winningham, PhD
: Rob contributed and assisted with Chapter 19, Dementia. Rob is even more of a brain nerd than I, and lazy too. He is a Professor of Psychology and Gerontology at Western Oregon University, and author of *Train Your Brain: How to Maximize Memory Ability in Older Adulthood* and *Cranium Crunches Workbook*. He frequently gives presentations worldwide on brain health, aging, memory, cognition, and dementia. You can learn more about Rob and memory, cognition and brain health at: http://www.robwinningham.com

Acknowledgements

No one achieves anything alone in this world. I owe so much to so many that there is no way I could ever pay it all back. I only ask that we all try to pay it forward just a little bit each day. As with most books I have a page to give thanks to some of the many good people who helped make this all possible for you, the reader. I should start with those who created the pillow of love and showed me how caregiving could be, our caregiving teams: Ann Wakeman, Anne Herrek, Amy Gest, Audrey Marshall, Chris Dunn, Chris Pope, Deon English, Elissa Ostergaard, Erik Brooks, Francis Lucerno, Ildiko Papp, Jackie Wolfe, James Negris, Janel Metcalfe, Jayne Simmons, Janet Fagan, Josh Gerak, Julia Hearsche, John Tschirhart, Karen Wang, Kaori Oto, Kim Kykendal, Marc Fendel, Mark Mendel, Mary LaSeur, Mary Lou Harris, Maureen Rigert, Mayne Tabachnick, Michelle Ness, Nancy Wilson, Paula Leffmann, Ron Hood, Seth Fader, Steve Coryelle, and Steve McFarlane,

I also thank all the wonderful people at **Mylifeline.org**. You really did save our lives and made this Framily possible.

In gathering the expertise assembled here to help you I must thank: **Kim Kobata PT BA NCS** at the **Swedish Multiple Sclerosis Center and Swedish Neuroscience Institute** for all your help with all things MS and physical therapy; **Elaine Sanchez**, author of *Letters from Madelyn, Chronicles of a Caregiver* for all your advice on caregiving and writing; **Sheila Warnock**, author of *Share the Care* and founder of Share the Caregiving organization for all the good work that you and your organization have done, and for your consultation and encouragement; **Ben Bledsoe** with Consumer Direct Care for your time and expertise. **Louise Ryan, Vickie Elting** and all the good people at the **offices of the long-term care ombudsman and National Administration on Aging** who give to people every day and gave to this project above and beyond the call of kindness or duty; **Eric Carlson** at the **National Senior Citizens Law Center** for sharing your time, your expertise and your wonderful work and books; **Edie Herman MA LMHC** for sharing your time, knowledge and the caregiving you have given; **Danielle, JP, Steve, Lisa**, and all the wonderful rehabilitation professionals at **Providence Mount St Vincent**; **Karin Hill** for your care with my Mom, and beginning to show me how to do it right; and **Mike Wattier**, Caregiver. For providing inspiration and experience.

For help with writing and editing I give thanks to: **Steve Coryelle** for your help with initial editing and your help in Karen's time; **Lu Randall** thank you for your initial editing and ideas and your work with Autism Connection of Pennsylvania; **Kris Fulsaas** for your beautiful professional editing work and the care in your caregiving; and **Judith Fielder** for your meticulous eye and excellent questions.

I also give thanks to: **Becky Kelly and her team at Kelly Productions** including **Eric Soma**, **Curtiss Marlowe**, and **Miles Lippold**, for donating your time and talent in producing the best of our videos. What an amazing time that was. I still owe you all a beer; **Derek Sparks** for your amazing work on the cover art even though we changed it several times; and **Laurel Zukerman** at **Summertime Publications**, without whom this whole project would not exist. Thank you for the spark to start and the patience to finish and all the work in between.

Detailed Contents

CAREGIVING 101:
A PRACTICAL GUIDE TO CARING FOR A LOVED ONE I
   CAREGIVING 101 II
   FOR KAREN III
   HOW TO USE THIS BOOK IV
   PROLOGUE: FACING DISEASE V
   INTRODUCTION: ADVANCED BASICS 1
   HOW DO YOU KNOW WHEN YOUR LOVED ONE NEEDS HELP 1
      Cognitive Changes 1
      Mobility Problems and Increased Risk of Falling 1
      Problems with Activities of Daily Living (ADLs) 1
    What You Can Do 1
    Dignity: Practical Considerations 2
      Respect 2
      Respect Their Choices 2
      Give Them Privacy Where You Can 3
      Acknowledge Life's Realities with Dignity, Respect, and Love 3
      Think About Their Perspective 3
      Give Them Choices at Mealtimes 4
      Exercise Your Compassion 4
    Help Your Loved One with Their Loss 4
      Anger, Sadness, and the Torrents of Emotions 5
      Things that Can Help 5
      Sources of Support 5
      Rumination 6
    A Caregiver's Loss 6
    New Ways to Do the Things They Love 7

PART I.
BEING A CAREGIVER AND TAKING CARE OF YOURSELF 9
   CHAPTER 1.
    BUILDING A CAREGIVING TEAM
    (OR, WHAT TO DO WITH ALL THE TUPPERWARE) 11
      Friends and Family: Visitors or Caregivers? 11
      Support Websites 12
    Heroes 14
      Volunteer Organizations 14
    Training Your Caregiver Team 15
    Creating a Carebook 15
      Training Your Family and Friends in Basic Nursing Skills ... 16
        Set Up Teams and Host a Training Session 17
        Gather the Group 17
        Introduce the Session 17
        Talk About the Nitty-Gritty 17
        Do Some Hands-On Training 18
        Set Parameters for Calling on Skilled Help 19
      Producing and Publishing Training Videos 19
    Managing Conflicts in the Team 21
      Who Is in Charge? 21
      Team Member Roles 21
      Clear and Respectful Communication 22
      Common Purpose 23
      Concerns that Generate Caregiver Conflicts 24
        Comfort vs. Fullness of Life 24
        Quality of Life vs. Quantity of Life 25
        How Much Care Each Person Should Give 25
        How to Do the Best Job 26
      Check Yourself If You Feel Conflict Arising 26
      Get Help from a Neutral Professional 27

   CHAPTER 2.
    CALLING IN THE PROS 29

    Finding Good Professional Caregiver Help.. 29
        Selecting the Right Professional... 30
        Going Through the Selection Process..................................... 31
    Managing Hired Help 32
        Salary and Benefits.. 32
        Payroll and Taxes 32
        Paying for In-home Caregivers... 33
    Making sure it "Feels Right"... 34

CHAPTER 3.
AVOIDING BURNOUT.. 37
    Balancing Caregiving and Work 37
    Getting Paid for Caregiving 38
    Spending Time with Friends or Connecting with Caregiver Support Groups 38
    Planning for Respite Care.. 39
        Consider Your Loved One's Needs 40
    Paying for Respite Care... 41

CHAPTER 4.
DANCING IN THE RAIN: HEALTHY HABITS FOR CAREGIVERS 43
    Embrace Stress 43
        Be Prepared... 43
        Take Breaks.. 44
        Recognize Times of Crisis 44
        Step Outside Yourself.. 45
            Calming Exercise: Four Count Breathing........................ 46
    Stay as Healthy as Can Be.. 46
        Sleep in Sleepless Times 46
        Eat Right 48
            Ask for Good Food... 48
            Plan Meals... 49
            Keep Regular Mealtimes... 49
            Eat a Balanced Diet.. 49
        Exercise for the Caregiver.. 50
        Spend Time with Friends.. 52
    Keep Your Brain Healthy 53
        Mindfulness Meditation 53
            Visual Counting Exercise.. 54
        Positive Journaling 54
        Gratefulness Journaling.. 55
        Random Acts of Kindness: Gifting.. 56

CHAPTER 5.
A BRIEF ABOUT GRIEF... 57
    Brief Acute Grieving (the Immediate Stuff)... 57
    Grief in the Longer Term (the More Subtle and Deep) 59
    Complicated Grief 60

INTERLUDE—Celebrating the Time You Have.. 63

PART 2.
LEGAL, FINANCIAL, AND INSURANCE ISSUES 65

CHAPTER 6.
THE NOTEBOOK OF IMPORTANT PAPERS... 67
    Identity Papers 67
    Medical Information 68
        Authorization to Disclose Personal Health Information 68
    Financial Information... 69
    Records of Your Wishes 69
        Advance Directives.. 69
            Medical Power of Attorney.. 70
            Living Will... 70
        POLST... 71
        Letter of Instruction and Ethical Will 71
        Will.. 72
        Durable Power of Attorney 72
    Shared Bank Accounts etc... 73
        Living Trusts.. 74
        Estate Planning (Here's Where I Punt) 74

CHAPTER 7.
    THE IMPORTANCE OF EXERCISE 75

CHAPTER 8.
    MEDICARE, MEDICAID, AND PRIVATE INSURANCE 77
        Medicare. 77
            Parts Overview 78
            Who Is Eligible for Medicare 79
            Enrollment and Premiums 79
                Getting Help 80
                Penalty for Not Signing Up Right Away 80
                Choosing a Plan or Switching to a Different Plan 81
            Getting Help Navigating the System 81
            What the Plans Cover. 82
                Med A 82
                Med B 82
                Med C (Medicare Advantage Plans) 83
                Other Medicare Plans Beyond Med C. 83
                Med D 84
                Medigap 85
            Do All Doctors and Providers Accept Medicare? 85
        Medicaid. 85
            What's Covered. 86
            Applying and Qualifying 86
                The Spend-Down. 86
                Is Your House an Asset?. 87
            Once Accepted 88
        Private Health-Care Insurance 88
            Types of Plans 89
            Knowing the Plan. 90
            Reading the Contract and Watching for Pitfalls. 90
            Having Someone Else Help You with Your Health Care 91
        Long-Term Care Insurance 91
            What Is Long-term Care Insurance? 91
            Life Insurance Policies 92
        Managing the Bills. 92
                Reconcile Provider Bills and Payer Statements 93
                Check for Mistakes 93
                Find Out Who Can Answer Billing Questions 94
                Paying the Bills 94
                Ask Someone to Help Manage the Bills 94
        Appeals. 94
                Provider Appeals 95
        Advance Beneficiary Notice (ABN) of Noncoverage 95
        Grievances and More Help. 96

    INTERLUDE—Backflips. 97

PART 3.
CAREGIVING SKILLS AND ADVICE FROM THE FIELD 99

    CHAPTER 9.
    DOCTORS. 101
        Managing Medical Appointments 101
            What to Write Down During an Appointment. 101
            Calendars to Keep Track of Appointments. 102
            Tips on Scheduling Appointments 102
            Help with Appointments. 102
        Knowing What the Letters Behind Providers'
        Names Mean. 103
            Ancillary Service Providers 104
            Other Providers 105
        Finding a Good Doctor. 105
            When and How to Fire Your Doctor 106
            What to Do If You Have Concerns 107

    CHAPTER 10.
    HOSPITALS AND OTHER MEDICAL FACILITIES 109
        Short-Term Medical Facilities (Hospitals) 109
        Helping Your Loved One During a Hospitalization 109

- Rehabilitation Facilities ... 110
  - Transitional Care Units (TCUs) ... 111
  - Subacute Care Facilities ... 111
  - Care Centers ... 111
- Comfort Care, Hospice, and Home Health Care ... 111
- Longer-Term Medical and Residential Facilities ... 112
  - Skilled Nursing Facilities (SNFs) ... 113
  - Alternatives to the Traditional Nursing Home ... 113
  - Memory-Care Facilities ... 113
  - Assisted-Living and Independent-Living Facilities ... 113
  - Adult Family Homes and Other Private In-Home Options ... 114
  - Adult Day Services ... 115
- Choosing a Long-Term or Residential Care Facility ... 116
  - Make a List of Places to Consider ... 116
  - Research Reports on the Facility ... 117
  - Call the Facility ... 117
  - Make an Arranged Visit ... 117
  - Make More than One Drop-in Visit ... 118
  - Read the Contracts ... 118
  - Other Options ... 118
  - Helping Your Loved One After They Move into a Long-Term Care Facility ... 119
  - Addressing Problems in a Long-Term Care Facility ... 119
  - Moving Out of a Long-Term Care Facility ... 120

CHAPTER 11.
MEDICATIONS ... 123
- Making a Medications List ... 123
- Giving and Storing Medications ... 125
- Keeping a Medication Log ... 127
- Using Basic Charting Techniques ... 127
  - What to Include ... 127
  - Examples ... 127
  - How the Charting Notes Help ... 128
- Paying for the Pills ... 129
- Disposing of Unused Medication the Right Way ... 130

CHAPTER 12.
FOOD AND NUTRITION ... 131
  - Weight Loss ... 131
  - Weight Gain ... 132
  - Pushing Too Hard to Get Them to Eat ... 132
- Factors that Affect Food Intake ... 132
  - Changing Food Preferences ... 132
  - Changes Involving the Tongue and Olfactory Sense ... 133
  - Early Satiation ... 134
  - Nausea ... 134
  - Sore Mouth and Throat ... 135
  - Swallowing Issues ... 136
- Techniques for Physically Helping Your Loved One Eat ... 137
  - Feeding a Person Who Has a Disability ... 137
  - Using Specialized Dishes and Silverware ... 137
- How to Use Nutrition to Keep the Gut Balanced and Moving ... 138
  - Fiber ... 138
  - Fluids ... 139
  - Movement ... 139
  - Stimulating Peristalsis ... 139
  - Balancing Intestinal Flora ... 140
  - Relaxing the Pelvic-floor Muscles ... 140
  - Finding What Works ... 140
  - Eating to Treat Mild Constipation (Two Days) ... 140
  - Eating and Diarrhea ... 141
- Approaches for Diseases and Conditions ... 141
  - Eating and Depression ... 141
    - Change in Eating Habits ... 141
    - Loss of Appetite ... 142
    - Craving for "Comfort" Foods ... 142
    - Treating the Depression ... 142

- Eating and Cancer 143
- Eating and Aging 143
  - *Living Alone* 144
- Eating and Dementia 145
  - *Early Stages* 145
  - *Middle and Late Stages* 146
- Eating and Stroke 147
- Eating and the End of Life 148
- The Brief Summary 149
  - For Weight Loss, Early Satiation, or Increased Calorie Needs 149
  - For Weight Gain 149
  - For Nausea 149
  - For Soreness in the Mouth or Throat 149
  - For Swallowing Issues 149
  - For Constipation 150
  - For Diarrhea 150
- Recipes for Shakes, Smoothies, and the Best Comfort Food Ever 150
  - Shakes and Smoothies 150
  - James's Most Wonderful Mac 'n' Cheese 151
- The Link Between Exercise, Hunger, Satiety, and Diet 152

CHAPTER 13.
EXERCISE 153
- Important Precautions 153
- Basic Guidelines 153
- Exercise Concepts (More Information Than You Want) 154
  - Endurance 154
    - *Intensity* 155
  - Strength 155
  - Repetitions (Reps) and Rep Max 156
    - *Sets* 157
    - *Volume* 157
    - *Building Strength* 157
  - Skill 158
  - Flexibility 159
    - *Classic Stretching* 159
    - *Dynamic Stretching* 159
  - Functional Exercise 159
    - *About Walking* 160
- Building a Basic Exercise Program 160
  - Day 1: Leg Strength 161
    - *Warmup and Flexibility* 161
    - *Endurance* 161
    - *Strength* 161
    - *Cool-down* 162
  - Day 2: Balance and Walking Skill 162
    - *Warmup and Flexibility* 162
    - *Endurance* 162
    - *Skill* 162
    - *Cool-down* 162
  - Day 3: Upper-body and Trunk Strength 162
    - *Warmup and Flexibility* 162
    - *Endurance* 163
    - *Strength* 163
    - *Cool-down* 163
  - Day 4: Rest Day 163
    - *Warmup and Flexibility* 163
    - *Endurance* 163
  - Day 5: Start the Cycle Over 163
- Exercise Throughout the Day 164
- Special Considerations 164
  - Exercise and Arthritis 164
  - Exercise and Orthopedic Precautions 166
  - Exercise and Heart and Vascular Conditions 166
    - *Coronary Artery Disease (CAD)* 166
    - *Congestive Heart Failure (CHF)* 167
    - *Orthostatic Hypotension* 167
    - *Claudication* 168

  Edema 168
 Exercise with COPD and other Lung Disease 168
  Use Caution with Endurance and Strength Exercises 169
  Treat Shortness of Breath Before It Occurs 169
 Exercise and Cancer 170
  Cancer-related Fatigue 170
  Metastasis 171
  Other Concerns 171
 Exercise and Infections 172
 Exercise and Multiple Sclerosis (MS) 172
 Exercise and Stroke and Hemiparesis 173
  Medical Stability 173
  Shoulder, Arm, and Hand 174
  Aphasia 175
  New Treatment Concepts 175
  Stroke-Specific Exercises 176
 Exercise and Dementia 177
  Helping a Loved One with Dementia Exercise 178
 Exercise and Parkinson's Disease 179
 Late-Stage Exercise 180

CHAPTER 14.
SLEEP 181
  The Normal Sleep Cycle 181
  Some Sleep Problems 181
 Sleep Hygiene 181
  Universal Suggestions for Better Sleep 182
  Things to Avoid 183
 Special Sleep Problems 183
  Sleep Apnea 183
  Restless Legs 184
  Sleep Jerking 184
  Nighttime Heartburn 184
  Insomnia 185
  Pain and Sleep 185
 Disease- and Condition-Specific Approaches 186
  Sleep and Depression and/or Anxiety 186
  Sleep and Aging 186
  Sleep and Lung or Breathing Problems 187
  Sleep and Cancer 187
  Sleep and Multiple Sclerosis 188
  Sleep and Parkinson's Disease 188
  Sleep and Alzheimer's Disease 189
  Sleep and Stroke 189
  Sleep and Brain Injury 190
  Sleep and Other Conditions 190
 Sleep Medications 190
  Benzodiazepines 190
  Nonbenzodiazepines 191
  Melatonin Agonists 192
  Orexin Receptor Antagonists 192
  Antidepressants 192
  Other Medications 193
  Over-the-Counter Substances 193

CHAPTER 15.
BASIC MOBILITY AND TRANSFERS 195
 Fall Recovery: How to Get Back Up 195
 Fall Prevention 196
  Fall-Risk Assessments 196
  Home Safety 197
  Medical Alert Systems 199
 Mobility Aids and Adaptive Equipment 199
  Canes 199
  Crutches 200
  Walkers 201
  Wheelchairs 202
   Features and Options 203
  Power Wheelchairs and Scooters 204
  Access Ramp 205

Slide Board	205
Lifts	205
Grab Bars and Poles	206
Bathroom Aids	207
Hospital Beds	207
Assistive Devices	208
For Grasping Things	208
For Getting Dressed	208
For Cooking and Eating	209
For Viewing and Listening	209
Obtaining and Paying for Mobility and Assistive Devices	209
Are They Medically Necessary?	210
Who Orders and Pays for Them?	210
Physically Helping Your Loved One Move	211
Standby Assist and Contact Guard Assist	212
Minimal, Moderate, and Maximal Assist	212
Practice the Techniques	213
Communicate:	214
Move Safely	215
Our Videos	215
Total Assist	216
Why They Need to Move	216
Positioning for Comfort	216
Maximum Assist Bed Mobility	217
Scooting Them Up, Down, or Sideways Using a Draw Sheet	217
Sitting Up Straight Using the Draw Sheet	218
Rolling Them onto Their Side	218
Going from Supine to Sitting at the Edge of the Bed	218
Going from Sitting at the Edge of the Bed to Transferring to a Wheelchair or Commode	219
Changing the Sheets with the Person Still in the Bed	219
Using a Mechanical Lift	219
Rolling to Prone	220

CHAPTER 16.
HYGIENE, BATHING, AND TOILETING ... 221
- Bathing ... 221
  - Adaptive Equipment ... 221
  - Setting Up and Gathering Supplies ... 221
  - The Sequence ... 222
  - A Few Tips ... 222
  - Giving a Bed Bath and Changing the Bed with the Patient in It ... 223
    - *Bed Bath and Bed Changing Supplies* ... 223
    - *The Sequence* ... 223
- Oral Care ... 225
  - Assess Their Ability for Oral Self-Care ... 225
    - *Range of Motion* ... 225
    - *Grip Strength* ... 225
  - Daily Oral Care Routine ... 225
  - Dentures or Partial Dentures ... 226
  - Oral Complications with Cancer Treatment or Other Drug Interactions ... 226
    - *Managing Oral Complications* ... 227
    - *Mouth Rinses* ... 227
    - *Treating Oral Infections* ... 227
- Toileting ... 227
  - Bedside Commode ... 228
  - Urinal ... 228
  - Bedpan ... 229
- Incontinence and Peri-care ... 229
  - Cleanup ... 229
  - Cleanup Supplies ... 230
  - The Sequence ... 230
    - *Managing Incontinence* ... 231

CHAPTER 17.
PAIN MANAGEMENT ... 233
- *How the Body Adapts to Pain* ... 233

| | *Controlling Pain* | 234 |

Measuring Pain ... 234
- A Pain Scale ... 234
- A Visual Analog Scale ... 234
- Pain Faces ... 235

Pain Medications ... 235
- Acetaminophen ... 235
- Nonsteroidal Anti-Inflammatory Drugs (NSAIDs) ... 236
- Opioids (Narcotics) ... 236
- Glucocorticoids ... 238
- Antidepressants ... 239
- Anticonvulsants ... 239
- Osteoclast Inhibitors ... 239

Nonpharmacological Ways to Help Control Pain ... 240
A Sense of Control ... 240
Exercise for Pain Relief ... 241
Transdermal Electrical Neural Stimulation (TENS) ... 242
Acupuncture and Acupressure ... 242
Counterirritants: Ben Gay, Icy Hot, and Others ... 244
Music ... 244
Joy ... 245
- *Joyfulness Meditation Exercise* ... 245
Meditation ... 245
A Sense of Purpose ... 246
Gentle Massage ... 246
Social Contact ... 247
Compassion ... 247
- *Compassion Meditation Exercise* ... 248

INTERLUDE—BUDDHA IN PAJAMAS ... 249

CHAPTER 18.
MANAGING DISCOMFORTS ... 251
Anxiety ... 251
- Signs and Symptoms of Anxiety ... 251
- Treating Anxiety ... 252
  - *Calming Exercise* ... 252
  - *Anxiety Medications* ... 253
- Managing Your Response to Their Anxiety ... 253

Fatigue ... 254
- Treating Fatigue ... 254
- Managing Their Fatigue ... 255

Shortness of Breath: Dyspnea ... 255
- Treating Acute Dyspnea ... 256
- Treating Mild to Moderate Dyspnea ... 256

Swelling and Edema ... 258
- Nonpitting Edema ... 258
- Pitting Edema ... 259
  - *Treatment Strategy 1: Returning the Fluid to the Heart* ... 259
  - *Treatment Strategy 2: Decreasing the Amount of Fluid* ... 261

Itching ... 261
Muscle Spasms and Myoclonus ... 262
- Treating Muscle Spasms ... 262
  - *Stretches* ... 263
- Preventing Muscle Spasms ... 265
- Antispasmotic and Muscle Relaxant Medication ... 266
- Myoclonus ... 267

Hiccups ... 267
Dizziness and Wooziness ... 267
- Wooziness ... 267
- Dizziness ... 268
  - *To Help Them with Their Vestibular Balance* ... 269
  - *To Help Them Better Use Their Visual Balance* ... 269
  - *To Help Maximize the Balance Sensations from the Body* ... 269

Constipation ... 270
- Preventing Constipation ... 270
- Treating Constipation ... 271
  - *Over-the-Counter Treatments* ... 271

- *Prescription Medications*..272
- *Treatment of Pelvic-Floor Muscles*..272
- **Performing an Enema**..272
  - *Gathering Supplies*..272
  - *The Sequence*..273
  - *Cleanup*...274
  - *Troubleshooting*...274
- **Diarrhea**..274
  - **Treating Diarrhea**..274
- **Wounds or Ulcers**..275
  - **Pressure Ulcers (bed sores)**..275
    - *Prevention*...276
    - *Early Detection and Stages of Ulcers*....................................277
    - *Treatment: General Ideas*..277
    - *Venous Pressure Ulcers*..278
    - *Diabetic Pressure Ulcers*..279
  - **Arterial Ulcers**..279
    - *Treatment*...280
  - **Skin Tears**...280
  - **Reopened Surgical Wounds**...280
- **Infections and Compromised Immune Systems**...................................280
  - **Hygiene Best Practices**...281
    - *The Importance of Hand Hygiene*..281
    - *Personal Hygiene Precautions*..282
    - *Visitor Guidelines*..282
    - *Food and Water Guidelines*...283
    - *Keeping Sex Safe*..284
    - *Caring for Pets and Livestock*...284
    - *Precautions When Traveling Away from Home*...............................284
  - **Signs and Symptoms of Infection**..285
- **Delirium: The Hard Road**...286
  - **Signs and Symptoms of Delirium**...286
  - **Looking for Causes**...287
  - **Medication Problems**..287
    - *Opioid Toxicity*...288
    - *Benzodiazapines—The Paradox*...289
    - *Steroid-Induced Psychosis*...289
  - **Hospital Shock**...290
  - **Managing the Hard Road**...290
    - *Help Them Keep Hold of or Regain Hold of Reality*........................290
    - *Keep Them as Comfortable as Can Be*......................................291
    - *Keep Communication Clear, Concise, and Kind*.............................291
    - *Keep Them Safe*..291
    - *A Few More Thoughts on Delirium*...292

CHAPTER 19.
DEMENTIA 293
- **Diagnosing Dementia**...293
  - **Types of Diseases Causing Dementia**.......................................294
    - *Protein-based Dementia*..294
    - *Vascular Dementia and Vascular Cognitive Impairment (VCI)*...............294
    - *Mixed Dementia*..294
    - *Alcohol-Related Brain Disorder (ARBD)*...................................294
  - **The Most Common Diseases Causing Dementia**...............................295
    - *Alzheimer's Disease*...295
    - *Vascular Dementia*...295
    - *Parkinson's Disease and Parkinson's Associated Dementia*.................295
    - *Lewy Body Dementia*..296
    - *Frontotemporal Dementia*...296
- **Treating and Managing Dementia in the Early Stages**..........................296
  - **Medications**..297
  - **Brain Preservation**...297
    - *Healthy Habits for Brain Health*...297
    - *Prehab*..298
- **Managing Dementia in the Middle and Late Stages**.............................299
  - **Understanding How Memory Works**...299
    - *Putting These Concepts to Practical Use*.................................300

	Training the Memory in Late-Stage Dementia	300
	Helping Them Orient	301
	Communicating Strategically	301
	Managing Unwanted Behaviors	302
	Using Monitors and Alarms	303
	Taking Care of Yourself	304

CHAPTER 20.
NEAR THE END 305
    Physical Changes 305
    Metaphysical Changes 305
    As the Body Shuts Down 306
    Leave Nothing Unsaid 306
  Our Vigil 307
  Time with Karen, My Lifeline Post May 29, 2013 307
    Dear Friends, My Lifeline Post written late May,
    posted June 4, 2013 308
    My Lifeline Post May 30, 2013 309
    Morning, My Lifeline Post June 3, 2013 309
    Vigil, My Lifeline Post June 5, 2013 309
    From Mary Lou, My Lifeline Post June 5, 2013 310
    1:42 a.m., My Lifeline Post June 6, 2013 310

EPILOGUE 311

CONTRIBUTORS 312

ACKNOWLEDGEMENTS 314

www.ingramcontent.com/pod-product-compliance
Lightning Source LLC
Chambersburg PA
CBHW081333080526
44588CB00017B/2603